The Courage to Fail

The Courage to Fail

A Social View of Organ Transplants and Dialysis

Second Edition, Revised

Renée C. Fox and Judith P. Swazey

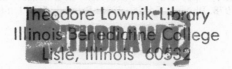
The University of Chicago Press
Chicago and London

Renée C. Fox is a professor in the departments of Sociology, Psychiatry, and Medicine at the University of Pennsylvania, where she is also the first Annenberg Professor of the Social Sciences.

Judith P. Swazey is a professor in the Socio-Medical Sciences Department at Boston University School of Medicine and in the Department of History at Boston University and is a member of the Special Scientific Staff (Pediatrics) at Boston City Hospital.

Portions of chapter 4 were published in the December 1973 issue of the *Hastings Center Report,* © 1973 by the University of Chicago

The University of Chicago Press, Chicago 60637
The University of Chicago Press, Ltd., London

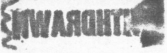

Library of Congress Cataloging in Publication Data

Fox, Renée C.
   The courage to fail.

   Bibliography: p.
   Includes index.
   1. Medical innovations—Social aspects. 2. Transplantation of organs, tissues, etc.—Social aspects.
3. Hemodialysis—Social aspects. I. Swazey, Judith P.,
joint author. II. Title.
RA418.5.M4F68   1978   362.1'9'795   78-56332
ISBN 0-226-25943-9
ISBN 0-226-25944-7 pbk.

Contents

Preface to the Second Edition

Since the publication of the first edition of *The Courage to Fail,* we have continued to follow the course of organ transplantation and dialysis, and in 1976–77 we carried out new firsthand research in preparation for this revised edition. Transplantation and dialysis still exemplify the range of medical and social phenomena and issues that motivated us to do our original study in 1968. During the past decade, the field has been altered both by the medical developments that have and have not occurred in human organ transplantation and by the passage in 1972 of Public Law 92-603, providing Medicare funding for the treatment of end-stage renal failure.

In response to these developments, we have written two new chapters (10 and 11) and recast our final chapter. We have dispensed with the brief epilogue that dealt with developments between 1970 and 1974. We also have omitted our chapter on "a sociological portrait of the transplant surgeon," because it was misinterpreted by many readers as a eulogy. It was perceived this way, in part, because we did not state that we drew the "portrait" from the language and ideology of the transplanters themselves or tell why we intentionally did so.

In preparing this new edition, we have become more aware of the extent to which we have systematically tried to discern and analyze key attitudes, values, and beliefs of transplant and dialysis physicians through their distinctive professional language. We are increasingly impressed with the degree to which the feelings and the outlook of such physicians are coded into their technical language. Many of the insights in the new chapter on transplantation in the 1970s come from our attention to the meaning conveyed by their use of phrases like the "terrible" graft versus host disease associated with bone-marrow transplantation and the "climbing Mount Everest phase" of liver transplantation.

The purpose of this new edition is not only to update the transplantation-dialysis picture, but also to present new conceptual insights about the process of therapeutic innovation and to consider the medical, ethical, and social implications of the "democratization of dialysis."

Preface to the First Edition

The Courage to Fail grew out of the meeting of a sociologist (Fox) and a biologist and historian of science (Swazey) at the Harvard University Program on Technology and Society in the fall of 1968. Although trained and working in different disciplines, we discovered a common professional involvement in medicine. Both of us had been consistently interested in how a social scientific perspective could provide insights into the content and evolution of biomedical research, and into its societal and cultural ramifications.

Our collaboration began when Dr. Emmanuel G. Mesthene, director of the Technology and Society Program, asked us to examine the long-range implications for American society of new and nascent biomedical developments. Independently, each of us concluded that the most fruitful type of investigation would be one that focused on an area of biomedical innovation sufficiently advanced to permit detailed empirical study. We felt that concentrating on subjects such as genetic engineering and behavior control, which in 1968 were only beginning to yield up knowledge and clinically applicable techniques, would launch us on an inquiry that, for us, was too futuristic and speculative.

This was the reasoning behind our decision to make an in-depth study of organ transplantation and chronic hemodialysis. The choice of these two therapeutic innovations was prefigured in several ways. From 1951 to 1954, one of us (Fox) had been a participant observer on the metabolic research ward (F-Second) of Boston's Peter Bent Brigham Hospital. During that period Ward F-Second's clinical investigators conducted pioneering work on the artificial kidney and performed the world's first human kidney transplant (Fox 1959). The other (Swazey) had spent 1966–68 with a research group established by the Technology and Society Program to explore a range of current and prospective biomedical technologies and their societal consequences. Among the topics this group examined, she found the biological and medical as well as social aspects of transplantation and dialysis particularly engrossing (Mendelsohn, Swazey, and Taviss 1971).

The form this book finally took was shaped by certain research decisions we made at the beginning of our study. As we reflect five years later on the "natural history" of our work, we are intrigued that a number of the basic methodological decisions we made in the first stage of our inquiry were formulated without fully discussing the conceptual approach to transplantation and dialysis that underlay them. From the outset, for example, we agreed that we would not confine our fieldwork to participant observation in a single transplantation or dialysis unit. Although we did not articulate it at the time, this implied that we were seeking a broader perspective on these therapeutic innovations than a microcosmic study could provide.

A threefold approach to transplantation and dialysis, albeit at first implicit, guided our research. To begin with, we were interested in studying these biomedical innovations primarily from the viewpoint of the research physicians engaged in them. As the reader will find, this does not mean that we excluded the experiences of transplant and dialysis patients. But even when we write about patients, we do so with emphasis on the insights their stories give us into the social and cultural dynamics of medical research with human subjects. In part, our concentration upon clinical investigators expresses our interest in the history and sociology of medical science. Beyond this, it reflects our desire to contribute to a sparsely documented aspect of modern medicine. In this connection, we have observed that research physicians are more receptive to having social scientists like ourselves portray their world than to undertaking this task themselves. The norms that regulate their community are as stoical as they are scientific, constraining them from communicating to others about the nonmedical and especially the stressful aspects of their vocation.

Second, as our focus on the research physician implies, we thought of transplantation and dialysis as constituting a paradigmatic case that exemplifies the attributes and process of therapeutic innovation. For us, transplantation and dialysis present virtually the whole range of medical and social phenomena that characteristically accompany biomedical research and its clinical application. In addition, they have generated some new phenomena that can be expected to accompany future medical developments. Most important among these are what we term the "gift-exchange" dimensions of both transplantation and dialysis.

Finally, we saw transplantation and dialysis in a broader societal perspective. We shared the intuition that the ramifications of these developments were significantly related not only to changes in contemporary medicine, but also to more general changes in our society's "common conscience." The issues that were being highlighted both in the professional literature and in the mass media in 1968–69 alerted us to these metamedical considerations. Heart transplantation was at its peak. The symbolic significance of the human heart and the definition and meaning of death were being discussed intensely. A great deal of concern was expressed about the problems of allocation of scarce resources that the availability and distribution of human organs and artificial kidney machines posed. And there was a growing preoccupation with the quality of life that these bold interventions in the human condition afforded the recipients of transplants and dialysis.

With the foregoing perspective on transplantation and dialysis, we began our work with a thorough review of past and current medical literature, to familiarize ourselves with the scientific and clinical state of the art and with the sorts of psychological, ethical, and social problems that physicians and patients involved with these procedures were encountering. In addition to studying the professional literature, we undertook a systematic content analysis of the copious treatment of transplantation and dialysis by the mass media. To ensure a comprehensive survey of newspaper coverage, we subscribed to a national press clipping service for two periods of five months each in 1969 and 1970. We maintained an up-to-date knowledge of the professional and popular literature throughout the four years of researching and writing this book.

A particular kind of fieldwork constituted the core of our research methodology. We traveled throughout the United States, spending from several days to a week at most of the country's major transplantation and dialysis centers. At each center we conducted detailed interviews with patients and their families and with members of transplant and dialysis teams, including internists, surgeons, immunologists, psychiatrists, nurses, social workers, laboratory technicians, and bioengineers. Subsequent to our visits, we maintained a regular correspondence with many of our informants. Our trips to these centers also included attendance at medical team conferences, rounds, and out-patient clinics, analysis of patient charts, observation of transplant surgery and of in-hospital and home dialysis, and visits to research laboratories. There were two transplant centers that we studied more continuously, making regular visits to each unit over a twelve-month period.

The two major themes around which our research evolved were gift exchange and uncertainty. It cannot be said that we discovered the gift dimension in transplantation and dialysis. At the time we began our study both the popular and the professional literature were filled with references to organ donations as gifts of life. The Uniform Anatomical Gift Act had been drafted and was being adopted by state legislatures. And articles on home hemodialysis emphasized the extraordinary life-giving service that was performed by family members who were responsible for running a relative's artificial kidney machine.

However, although the label "gift" was being applied to transplantation and dialysis, the notion of the gift had not been conceptualized in a way that yielded insights into its broader medical and social significance. Medical articles that alluded to these gift phenomena, for example, were written largely from a psychiatric perspective, emphasizing the relationship between the independence–dependency needs of the patient, the live organ donor or the dialyzer and their respective capacities to withstand the stresses that these treatments entailed. Whereas the medical literature highlighted the psychic strains and characteristic defense mechanisms that dialysis and transplantation evoked in patients and their relatives, the mass media were more inclined to underscore the heroic, sacrificial, and scarce nature of the gifts being proffered and received through these treatments.

By winter 1968 we not only were steeped in the literature but had conducted a series of interviews and begun participant observation in a renal transplant unit. Our field experiences persuaded us that no matter what the individual personality characteristics and motives of donors and recipients in organ transplantation might be, all "givers" and "receivers" in this transaction underwent a common set of experiences. It suddenly occurred to us that what we were observing was gift exchange as it was classically introduced into social science literature a generation ago by Marcel Mauss (Mauss 1954).[1] Mauss pointed out that however spontaneous and expressive gift exchange may be, it nevertheless entails three "symmetrical and reciprocal" obligations: receiving and repaying as well as giving. The further our work advanced, the more we were impressed with how various phenomena that we recurrently observed resulted from these obligations. We noted that donor and recipient could become bound to one another in either a transcendent or a tyrannical way. And we also were impressed with the problem of receiving a gift of such magnitude that it cannot truly be reciprocated. These observations now took on larger meaning for us. As we gained knowledge of the social dynamics of hemodialysis, we realized that here too the norms of gift exchange applied, though not in the same literal sense as with organ donation. In turn, this new outlook on dialysis and transplantation led us to identify the gatekeeping role that the medical team plays as an integral part of the gift-exchange process. Through their screening activities, the physicians ultimately establish who is to give and who is to receive these potentially lifesaving treatments.

The second major theme that structured our research comprised the problems of uncertainty that are inherent to medicine in general and that are encountered with particular frequency and acuteness in clinical research. Therapeutic innovations like transplantation and dialysis involve research physicians and their patient-subjects in explorations of the medical unknown that are as perilous as they are promising. In this shared situation, physicians and patients are cast in social roles that make them specialists in uncertainty. Our formulation of the problems of uncertainty that transplantation and dialysis entail progressively came to include phenomena as diverse as the biological mysteries of the rejection reaction, the ambiguities of the relationship between clinical experimentation and therapy, the problematic aspects of the clinical moratorium, and the dilemmas involved in allocating various kinds of scarce resources.

The twin themes of gift exchange and uncertainty expanded and took on new dimensions as we continued to collect case materials. Each field trip we made was designed to further investigate specific aspects of the data and concepts we had thus far developed. In addition to what we expected to gain, these trips provided new empirical materials and generalizations that carried us beyond our original starting points.

For example, we went to Montreal in February 1970 explicitly to discover why the Montreal Heart Institute had publicly announced a moratorium on cardiac transplantation. In the course of our interviews with cardiac surgeons there, we became aware of the subculture to which they seemed to belong. They had received specialized training at the same centers as surgeons conducting heart transplants elsewhere. Very strong affect—in some cases positive, in others negative—linked them to the larger but still restricted circle of men engaged in cardiac surgery. Furthermore, their attitudes toward the human heart, death, work, commitment, and achievement struck us as being distinctive. These insights gained in Montreal influenced our subsequent interviews with transplant surgeons in other cities. What might almost be called the world view that they expressed in their conversations with us, as well as through their daily rounds which we also observed, led us to construct an ideal typical picture of the transplant surgeon which we call a "sociological portrait."

In a comparable fashion, a trip to Houston to interview Dr. Michael DeBakey and Dr. Denton Cooley about their experiences with cardiac transplantation amplified the concepts already guiding our research and opened up new lines of inquiry. In this setting, the "courage to fail" ethos of such surgeons was dramatically exemplified for us. We also began to see its applicability to all the participants—patients and their families as well as other medical professionals—in the entire transplantation and dialysis endeavor.

Our trip to Houston took place after Dr. Cooley had performed the first clinical implant of a complete mechanical substitute for the heart in a patient named Haskell Karp. This surgical "first" had attracted worldwide publicity. It had been accompanied by a priority dispute about the artificial heart's development. It had raised ethical questions concerning the quality of informed, voluntary consent obtained from Mr. Karp, and about the adequacy of the social control mechanisms that are supposed to govern such innovative medical acts. Finally, when the decision was made to remove the artificial heart and implant a human organ, a controversy had arisen over the propriety of flying a dying patient from Massachusetts to serve as Mr. Karp's heart donor.

The more we reflected on it, the more it seemed to us that in "the case of the artificial heart" problems of uncertainty and gift exchange converged with the ethos of transplant surgeons in ways that threw into sharp relief complex issues fundamental to the ethics of medical experimentation. Because this case synthesized many of our essential concerns, we asked and were granted permission to return to Houston and study it in detail. Like "the heart transplant moratorium," "the case of the artificial heart" became a major chapter in our book.

A final illustration of how our perspective on transplantation and dialysis, our guiding themes, and the results of our fieldwork mutually interacted is provided by our experiences in Seattle. We journeyed there initially to talk with Dr. Belding Scribner, whose development of a cannula-shunt apparatus had made chronic hemodialysis possible and had led to Seattle's becoming the mecca of dialysis centers. Discussions with Dr. Scribner and his associates not only enriched our data on dialysis, but also expanded what we meant by the allocation of scarce, life-maintaining resources. The Seattle group had dared to experiment both with community involvement in the establishment and support of a dialysis treatment center and with the processes and criteria of patient selection for treatment. Their involvement of laymen on the admission committee for the treatment program and their early attempts to use measures of "social worth" in the decision-making about who should receive dialysis and who not had focused national attention on them. To a certain degree this was deliberate on their part, for Dr. Scribner and his colleagues were intent on raising the consciousness of both the medical profession and the public about the seriousness and complexity of the selection issue, and about those aspects of it that would be irreducible even in a more just and equitable allocation system. The Seattle physicians were also grappling in a more outright way than most medical groups with the "quality of life" and "the right to die" concerns that had been generated by the capacity to keep terminally ill persons alive indefinitely.

In the course of our first interviews in Seattle, we heard many allusions made to the "case of Ernie Crowfeather." For this medical team, Ernie had come to personify the whole spectrum of painful problems that dialysis and transplantation can entail. When Dr. Scribner urged us to devote a chapter of our book to Ernie's story, we concurred. For as we learned more about Ernie's history we too came to see his case as "the epitome of all the problems."

The foregoing reflections on how and why our research evolved as it did provides a clearer picture of this book's structure and content than would a more conventional summary of the flow of chapters. For our book is organized not only around the analytic themes and issues that we have highlighted, but also around the series of individual and institutional case studies from which they grew. Thus the underlying logic of the book resides in the fact that each chapter adds new empirical materials and new generalizations to the original starting points, drawn from the progression of medical and social settings in which we worked.

The title of our book, *The Courage to Fail*, expresses our sense of the deepest and broadest implications of transplantation and dialysis. It epitomizes the bold, uncertain, and often dangerous adventure in which medical professionals and their patients are engaged. All have a high vested interest in the success of their endeavor. In their shared value system, a primary measure of success is the sheer survival of patients undergoing transplantation or dialysis. Beyond survival, it is hoped that these procedures may give patients an improved state of health that will enhance the quality of their lives. Success also means progress in medical knowledge and technique that may come from their collaborative research. For some of these physicians, and for some of their patients as well, professional and public recognition for their pioneering roles is another integral part of success.

Not only courage in the face of great uncertainty is required of physicians and patients in the transplantation and dialysis situation, but also the courage to give and receive what is asked of them. With the possible exception of giving birth, transplantation entails the most literal gift of life that a person can offer or accept. And chronic dialysis similarly involves its participants in a continual process of exchanging life for death. Because of the meaning and magnitude of what is being transmitted, both dialysis and transplantation demand courage in the face of the gift.

The probability of failure in transplantation and dialysis is high. These therapeutic innovations are in a stage of development characterized by fundamental scientific and medical uncertainties, and they are applied only to patients who are terminally ill with diseases not amenable to more conventional forms of treatment. In this context, the death of the patient is the archetype and pinnacle of failure for all concerned. Confronting this situation with courage is an ultimate value shared by physicians and patients. As they themselves recognize, the supreme form of courage that participation in transplantation and dialysis asks of them is "the courage to fail."

We have chosen our title with full consciousness that it evokes religious associations. (Its relationship to the title of Paul Tillich's renowned theological work *The Courage to Be* is apparent.) For we believe that the largest and perhaps most enduring significance of organ transplantation and dialysis lies in the ethical and existential questions they raise. Problems of uncertainty, meaning, life and death, scarcity, justice, equity, solidarity, and intervention in the human condition are all evoked by these therapeutic innovations. Transplantation and dialysis have played an important role in making such moral and metaphysical concerns more visible and legitimate in present-day medicine.

But involvement with these matters does not seem to be confined to medicine. Rather, we have the impression that in many different domains of our society there is increasing preoccupation with the same questions of values, beliefs, and meaning. These questions, and the concern with them, are as religious as they are ethical. They are rooted in the Judeo-Christian tradition of our culture and in this sense represent a reaffirmation of our "common faith." At the same time, however, the growth of interest in these problems that is now observable in our society, and especially the degree to which they are manifesting themselves in medicine, suggests that reformulations of quite fundamental aspects of our societal value system may be under way. A rapprochement seems to be occurring between scientific and religiomoral orientations toward health and illness, life and death. In this regard, *The Courage to Fail* is a case study not only of therapeutic innovation in modern society, but of more general processes of social and cultural change.

Acknowledgments

Throughout the course of preparing this volume we have received invaluable help from many sources. The study was made possible by the continuing support of the Harvard University Program on Technology and Society and by the initiative and sponsorship of its director, Dr. Emmanuel G. Mesthene.

We extend our deepest thanks to the medical professionals and their patient colleagues who so freely and generously shared their knowledge and experiences with us. We are further indebted to the several physicians who critically reviewed those portions of the manuscript based upon our visits to their institutions.

Four persons, Dr. George Baker and Dr. Paul Russell of Massachusetts General Hospital, Professor Talcott Parsons of Harvard University, and Professor Charles E. Rosenberg of the University of Pennsylvania, reviewed the entire manuscript for us. We are grateful to them for undertaking this task. Professor Willy De Craemer of York University in Toronto, Canada, provided valuable sociological insights and encouragement at many points in our research. For this, and for his reading of various portions of the text, we extend our appreciation. To Dr. Lawrence K. Altman, our sincere thanks for sharing with us his materials on the case of Ernie Crowfeather.

We are indebted to Mr. Alex Capron, Esquire, of the University of Pennsylvania School of Law and to the Honorable A. Leon Higginbotham, Jr., U. S. district judge for the Eastern District of Pennsylvania, for their assistance in obtaining legal documents associated with the *Karp* v. *Cooley* lawsuit, and for their guidance in analyzing them. Judge Higginbotham's penetrating commentary on the case was not only indispensable to our intellectual understanding of its nuances, it also encouraged us to attempt a criticism of the legal process involved.

For their aid in preparing various stages of the manuscript, our thanks go to Judith Burbank, Jane Draper, Nancy Friedman, Susan Goldman, Michelle Rappaport, Margaret Collins, and Debby Snyder. Finally, it is not an exaggeration to say that this book could not have been written without the understanding of Peter W. Swazey and his active belief in our work. To him, and to Beth and Woody, a very special thank you.

Quotations from Paul A. Freund, ed., *Experimentation with Human Subjects* (New York: George Braziller, 1970); L. K. Christopherson and D. T. Lunde, "Heart Transplant Donors and Their Families," *Seminars in Psychiatry* 3 (February 1971): 26–35; and David Sanders and Jesse Dukeminier, "Medical Advances and Legal Lag: Hemodialysis and Kidney Transplantation," *UCLA Law Review* 15 (1968):377–80 are used by permission of the publishers.

The Courage to Fail

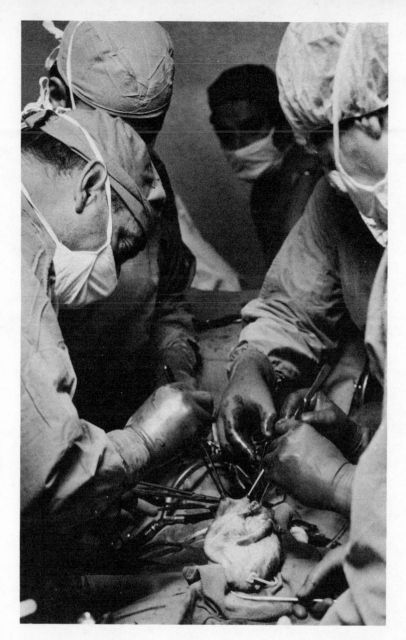

From Genest 1969, p. 32

1

Patterns in Therapeutic Innovation: Transplantation

1

Gift Exchange and Gatekeeping

The donor who offers a part of his body for transplantation is making an inestimably precious gift. The acutely ill patient who receives the organ accepts a priceless gift. The giving and receiving of a gift of enormous value, we believe, is the most significant meaning of human organ transplantation. This extraordinary gift exchange, moreover, is not a private transaction between the donor and the recipient. Rather, it takes place within a complex network of personal relationships that extends to the families, the physicians, and all the members of the medical team who are involved in the operation. Within the network of these relations, a complex exchange occurs through which considerably more than the organ itself is transferred.

The development of transplantation has created options that did not previously exist for warding off death, saving life, demonstrating an ultimate kind of concern for another person, and expressing transcendent meaning. At the same time, organ transplantation takes place under circumstances that impose constraints upon the persons involved, and within an interactive framework that structures the situation for them in ways that limit and bind as well as open and free. The freedom to give or to receive an organ is neither absolute nor random. These freedoms are mediated and governed by the norms of gift exchange, on the one hand, and by an at once biological, psychological, and sociological screening process that we refer to as "gatekeeping" on the other.

In his classic anthropological work *The Gift*, Marcel Mauss pointed out that although gift exchange is an expressive set of acts through which something symbolic and interpersonal as well

5

as material is transmitted, it is not totally spontaneous. Rather, it is structured by a triple set of norms: the obligations to give, to receive, and to repay, which Mauss defined as "symmetrical and reciprocal" (Mauss 1954). By this he meant that under certain socioculturally defined circumstances, an individual or a group is supposed to offer a gift to a particular person. In turn, the person (or persons) to whom the gift is proffered is expected to accept it. The recipient is then under social and moral pressure eventually to balance out the exchange by giving the donor something of equivalent worth. Failure to live up to any of these entwined expectations produces disequilibrium and social strain that affects the donor, the recipient, and those closely associated with them.

Looked at in a certain way, the donation of an organ is one of the most dramatic and supreme forms of gift giving extant in contemporary society. It has not yet reached the point of institutionalization where it is obligatory, or even considered to be an ordinary act. Nonetheless, organ donation is impelled as well as regulated by the norms of gift exchange of which Mauss wrote.

The obligations to give and receive that animate and structure organ transplantation are not inexorable or automatic. They are usually triggered when the physician first suggests to a patient and his family that a transplant might be considered. Self-screening and medical-team screening processes are then set into motion. In kidney transplantation, for example, the patient must first reach at least a tentative decision about whether he wishes to receive an organ. At the same time, his relatives are passing through the first phases of a parallel process, appraising themselves and each other as possible candidates for the live donation presumed to offer the patient his best chance of life.[1] Concurrently, the medical team is beginning to exercise their gatekeeping functions. They launch a series of procedures designed to test not only tissue compatibility but also the physical and psychological eligibility of donor and recipient to undergo and withstand organ exchange.

If, from these multiple points of view, no suitable live donor is found, the medical team may suggest a cadaver transplant. Screening for cadaver donations (which occurs in all organ transplants except those of live-donor kidneys) involves tissue typing, the consent of the donor or his next of kin, determination of the occurrence and cause of the donor's death, and the acquiescence of the recipient.

We have called these screening processes "gatekeeping" because they allow only certain individuals to give or receive an organ. Their goal is to optimize the patient's chances for survival and to offer him as enduring, active, and meaningful a posttransplant life as possible without undue physical, psychic, or social harm to himself, the donor, or their families. The transplant team recognizes that being willing and able to give an organ has important emotional, social, and spiritual meaning for many individuals and family groups. And so an implicit secondary goal of these screening processes is not unduly to deprive such persons of the opportunity to act as donors and to protect them (as well as the recipient in cases where a live-donor transplant is being considered) against psychic injuries if the medical team decides they are not eligible to give an organ.

At the same time, because physicians realize that close relatives of the patient are subject to a great deal of social and psychological pressure to offer a kidney, they feel themselves to be under a "great moral obligation . . . not to persuade . . . , or . . . over-persuade" a family member to do so (United Nations Economic and Social Council 1970). Physicians have used the term "moral blackmail" to conceptualize a subtle but very powerful form of organ extortion that can inadvertently result from their zealousness. This appreciation of the extraordinary pressures upon family members to donate an organ, and physicians' emphasis on their responsibility not to reinforce or exploit these pressures, is analogous to what Francis Moore has described as the ideal "posture of 'informed consent' in therapeutic innovation." It is "not a matter of trying safely and sanely to explain to a volunteer what is going to be done," he has written, "but rather the much more difficult task of explaining alternatives to a worried patient who wishes, above all else, to have the experiment carried out on him" (F. Moore 1970, p. 366).

C. H. Fellner and S. H. Schwartz have contended that "the medical profession looks upon the motivation of the living organ donor with distrust and suspicion," partly because they are skeptical of the "altruism" of the potential donor's motivation and hold it in "disrepute." Transplant teams, Fellner and Schwartz argue, are unduly concerned about the psychopathology that may impel certain individuals to volunteer, especially those unrelated to the recipient. Physicians' misgivings about the true motivation of the live donor may, in fact, be largely a projection of their own guilty reluctance to "inflict irreversible damage on a healthy person" (Fellner and Schwartz 1971). Although this point of view is psychologically suggestive, we feel that it underestimates the role that the clinical insights and ethical sensitivity of transplant team members play in what Fellner and Schwartz would consider their overly cautious and suspicious attitudes toward live volunteer donors.

Some of the fundamental sources of the medical profession's disquietude about the "true" motives that account for live organ donation and the "real" meaning of such an act have been most clearly expressed in the form of arguments for and against the use of living donors who are unrelated to the recipient. Such a gift raises what Abram has called the "psychological dilemma": "Is donating such an organ a 'gift' . . . to save another's life based on completely unselfish motivation, or is it based on masochism and unresolved guilt?" (Abram 1972, p. 54). Even more fundamentally, the question involves physicians' collective "view of human nature" (Sadler and Davidson 1971, p. 99). Do they individually and as a professional group have "faith in the altruistic principle," and in the more than occasional capacity of "ordinary people" to act with "healthy altruism derived from genuine moral concern" (Bevan 1971)? Or have they thrown "altruism into disrepute" (Fellner and Schwartz 1971) through their failure to believe that many people are capable of giving of themselves to suffering others, even to the point of offering one of their organs to a "stranger"?[2]

When an organ transplantation seems appropriate, then, a number of persons in different statuses and roles participate in deciding whether a transplant will be carried out, what type it will be, who the donor will be, and so on. Because so many people share in this decision, no individual is totally free to give or receive an organ. But it is also true that a dying patient is not absolutely free to refuse a transplant now that this alternative exists. He is perhaps especially constrained to accept one when a member of his own family offers such a gift. Correlatively, as the act of organ donation becomes more institutionalized, we are all increasingly subject to social pressures to make this kind of gift. In those cases where one is faced with a dying relative whose life could possibly be saved by a live organ donation from a family member, the Maussian "obligation to give" is maximized. The final gatekeeper in organ exchange is the physician. Acting on behalf of the transplant team, the patient, and possible donors and their relatives, as well as for himself, he makes the ultimate judgment. The physician's role here is as sociological and moral as it is medical. He acts as mediator and interpreter in the complex social system called into play by the transplantation situation. In this capacity, he weaves his way back and forth among the patient, candidate donors, their families, and the wide range of specialists who constitute the transplantation team. His role here is like that of the superior of a religious order who, in the name of higher ethical and spiritual values, controls what gifts can be offered and received by the members of the community he represents.[3] The physician is not free to abnegate his responsibility, nor may he exercise it arbitrarily or coercively. He must base his decision on biomedical, psychological, and sociological criteria that are acceptable within his profession.

In certain respects, the physician is under pressure to decide in favor of an organ transplantation. He is propelled toward it by his own professional and personal motivation to do everything possible to save the life of his dying patient, as well as by the strong desire of the patient's family. He is also pushed in this direction by his role as a clinical investigator with the responsibility to advance medical knowledge and technique as well as to care for patients. And the desire of some research physicians to "pioneer" and to be recognized for their trailblazing contributions may act as an inducement to perform transplantations.

Counterbalancing these factors that "push" a physician toward the transplant option are a number of "pull" factors that tend to deter him from it. The "pull" factors may include his medical opinion that the patient's condition is not serious enough to warrant transplantation, or that the risks attending the procedure outweigh its possible benefits; failure to obtain the necessary quality of consent from either the prospective recipient or donor; the medical and moral conviction that he should not prolong the patient's suffering through the use of these heroic means; and his reluctance to be judged irresponsible or flamboyant by his peers.

In sum, the option of organ transplantation is set down in a matrix of interacting persons—the prospective recipient, candidate donors, the members of their families, the physician and his professional colleagues—who together constitute a small but intricate social system that facilitates organ transplantation in some ways and impedes it in others.

The Gift and Its Implications: Five Cases

The following cases were gathered in the course of our participant observation with two groups engaged in kidney transplantation. They will be focal to our analysis of the gift-exchange and gatekeeping aspects of transplantation.

Mrs. Amico

When we first heard the renal transplant team discuss Mrs. Amico,[4] they seemed to feel that her psychological problems, particularly her extreme depression, ruled her out as a kidney recipient. The medical team was trying to "straighten her out physiologically" to see what kind of psychological improvements might be effected. Dr. Emerson, an internist, pointed out to the team that "it is hard to evaluate Mrs. Amico's depressed state in terms of eligibility for a transplant, because disease, debility, and the fear of death can tip someone over into a state of psychological disturbance." In addition to her being "a tough emotional problem—almost suicidally depressed," Dr. Emerson was afraid that Mrs. Amico's cardiac problems would preclude her being a kidney recipient. Dr. Richards, the surgeon who headed the transplant team, described Mrs. Amico as a "domineering person" who had married late in life after a successful career. Since no potential family donor was known, Dr. Richards told the group, Mrs. Amico would have to go on chronic dialysis to stay alive until a cadaver donor might be found; and once this was done "we would be stuck with her—for we could not tell her 'we're sorry, but this Thursday we don't think you can keep your dialysis appointment.'"

Eventually, Dr. Emerson got Mrs. Amico to admit that a related donor did exist—her father. But Mrs. Amico did not want her father to give her a kidney. She could not bear to be indebted to him for such a gift. When the father came to the hospital for donor-compatibility tests, he was described by Dr. Richards as a "sixty-seven-year-old fossil, in training to be a donor by dieting, and so forth." The psychiatrist working with the transplant team told the group that he hoped nothing would preclude the father's serving as a donor, for the act would be "the high point of his life," the first time he and his daughter had ever been close. When Mrs. Amico learned how much her father really cared for her, she was deeply moved. This reconciliation between Mrs. Amico and her father, who turned out to be a "reasonably good tissue match," provided the solution for the transplant team. Mrs. Amico was finally placed on the transplant "ready list." Dr. Richards noted in group rounds that "Mrs. Amico was the closest the group had come to turning a patient down for emotional reasons; but now I'm glad we accepted her, because she seems to be accepting the rigors of treatment so well." After her transplant, Mrs. Amico had a series of continuing medical complications, including being "on the thin edge" in terms of her cardiac condition. She died several months after receiving her father's kidney.

Billy Watson

Billy was introduced to the renal transplant team as "a ten-year-old boy, 42 inches tall and weighing 48 pounds." Billy has nine siblings, ages four to fourteen years. When his parents were first approached about the possibility of a transplant for Billy, "they reacted in an irrational way, but since then have come to realize that he is failing rapidly. He has had three hospitalizations for heart failure, has had to withdraw from school, and is suffering from advanced renal insufficiency." The presenting physician noted that Billy was felt to be too young and small for chronic dialysis, given its retarding effects on growth and development. The medical problems in his case were described as "very interesting," presenting the transplant group with the question of whether they could achieve a "successful" transplant with such a small child.

Billy was evaluated for more than two months by the transplant team, and during this time members of the team, singly and in group meetings, expressed their anguish over how to resolve the case. Billy's mother proved to be the best donor in terms of tissue compatibility. She wanted passionately to save Billy's life by giving him one of her kidneys, but the medical team felt reluctant to encourage or even permit a mother with responsibility for nine other children to subject herself to the immediate and long-term risks of a live organ donation. Dr. Richards once said that Mrs. Watson's zealous desire to help Billy, irrespective of the consequences for herself and her family, was analogous to the biblical parable of the one stray sheep. Mrs. Watson told the team that the other children were aware of Billy's critical illness, and that in many ways he was the family favorite. The transplant team's social worker was worried about the strength of Mr. and Mrs. Watson's marriage, and about how much support the parents could give each other and Billy throughout the transplant experience. Mrs. Watson seemed to be using the kidney donation as a tool to manipulate her relationship with her husband, for she implied to the social worker that she would get a divorce if she did not prove to be a suitable donor and Mr. Watson would not volunteer. Dr. Emerson stated, with respect to this problem, that "if we think for nonmedical reasons that she won't be a good donor, we will tell her the tests are no good. Billy is so sick we don't have time to procrastinate much longer. I'm afraid we'll be damned if we do and damned if we don't in this case."

After Billy's case had been discussed for over a month, we asked Dr. Emerson whether transplantation had closed off a physician's option: that of deciding not to treat a young child like Billy, but rather letting him die in a relatively short time from the fatal course of his disease. Dr. Emerson replied, "We've kind of created a monster we don't know how to handle. The mother has pushed us into doing a transplant on Billy. It's our responsibility to handle this [to accept or not accept such a case]. The physician is beginning to see laymen who ask, 'Why are you keeping my eighty-nine-year-old mother alive?' but this is a very different thing from asking, 'Why are you keeping my little Billy alive?'" In a group meeting, Dr. Emerson stated, "I honestly don't know if Mrs. Watson will be used if the group is not in some sort of moral accord on having her serve as donor. And yet it's a question of letting Billy go if we don't use his mother."

When we talked with Dr. Richards after Billy's case had been discussed for over two months, he said: "I have that little boy on my mind all the time. It's terrible. I don't know what to do. The mother wants to help so much. Do I have the right to prevent her? She knows it could succeed; it's not wild stuff, like Krebiozen. Mrs. Watson feels that it's the same thing as running into a burning building to save her son. I suppose I haven't made up my own mind about doing a transplant on Billy, although the whole group is moving in that direction." Our notes after talking with Dr. Richards included the following entry: "The constellation of excruciating issues raised by Billy's case include: Is this a 'normal' family, psychologically? Is Mrs. Watson's motivation for wishing to donate 'acceptable' or 'pathological'? Irrespective of her motivation, should Mrs. Watson be granted the right to donate a kidney to one child when she has nine others to care for? Might it not be more rational and more merciful to let this small boy die, rather than to keep him alive for what will probably be only a short time, given the advanced state of his disease and his youth?"

Shortly after our talk with Dr. Richards, Billy received a kidney from his mother. Billy's physicians acknowledged that they reached the decision to do the transplant because, in the end, they could not simply stand by and let him die. Seven months later, Dr. Emerson reported to us that Billy was "back in school and doing just fine."

Margaret Ryan

Margaret Ryan, age twenty-four, had three sisters and a brother "all anxious to donate" a kidney. The best donor, in terms of tissue compatibility, proved to be her younger sister Kathleen, but Kathleen had an anatomically abnormal double collecting system in her left kidney. Although she had no apparent kidney problems and was in good health, the transplant team was concerned about the possible medical consequences of taking the normal kidney for Margaret and leaving Kathleen with the structurally abnormal one. An older sister had two normal kidneys, but she was not as good a tissue match. The transplant team went through a torturous decision-making process about using Kathleen as a donor. Part of the difficulty in making the decision stemmed from a lack of basic data on the future likelihood of renal complications for Kathleen were she left with one anatomically atypical kidney. The greatest risk, one doctor commented, might occur if Kathleen became pregnant, because pregnancy places an added burden on kidney function. In this case, the group decided that Kathleen was unlikely to marry. She was a pious Catholic girl whose history of broken marriage plans suggested she might have religious and emotional conflicts over marrying.

The decision about using Kathleen as a donor was most visibly upsetting to Dr. Richards, who showed a strong affection for both her and Margaret. The morning after Margaret's transplant, Dr. Richards was extremely depressed at the transplant team's meeting. During surgery he had discovered that Kathleen, the donor, had a double renal vein as well as a double collecting system. "It was a dandy situation," he commented wryly. He breathed an audible sigh of relief when an attending doctor reported that he had just seen Kathleen and she was "doing OK."

Two weeks after the transplant, Margaret was getting over a rejection episode and generally doing well. Said Dr. Richards at rounds: "She really feels wonderful. It's a great reward just to talk to her, she is so grateful. I sure like keeping her around, because she is such a jewel."

Susan Thompson

Susan is a twenty-six-year-old unmarried woman who works for an airline. She was admitted to the hospital for the fifth time with chronic renal failure of unknown etiology. For the past year she had been maintained on "borderline compensation" with a special diet, but her condition was deteriorating. She had begun to experience growing fatigue, nausea, and vomiting, with dehydration and increasing azotemia (excessive amounts of nitrogenous materials in the blood). She entered the hospital for rehydration, and transplant plans were set into motion.

Susan explicitly stated that she wanted to have a live-donor transplant rather than to go on dialysis. She likes to travel and has occasion to do so as an airline employee. She felt that dialysis would keep her at home. Each of her parents was considered as a donor (she is an only child). Her father was eventually disqualified, primarily for physical reasons. Susan's mother expressed her willingness to be a donor, but the medical team had reason to believe that on an unconscious level she did not really want to give Susan a kidney. The team noted, for example, that while Mrs. Thompson was being worked up she developed gastrointestinal problems and heart palpitations. As soon as she was told that she would not be the donor for her daughter, "she changed for the better." Mrs. Thompson does not know, nor does her daughter, that she was turned down for psychological reasons. There is no entry in Susan's chart, or in that of either of her parents, that states why neither live-donor candidate proved acceptable. Mrs. Thompson was told that she could not be a donor because she was "not a good tissue match."

Susan had strong objections to a cadaver transplant, because she had heard that the outcome with this type of transplant was not as good as with a live-donor one. The medical team thus was left with only two recourses: to put Susan on dialysis or to let her die from the natural course of her disease. They chose to put her on dialysis. The nursing notes describing Susan's first day on the machine read: "Patient anxious. Does not want 'dumb machine.' " The second day's notes included the observation that, "today, when Susan roused herself and began to vomit and shiver with a chill, she exclaimed over 'what a mess' it was to be on the machine." We asked the dialysis nurse whether the team had to have the consent of the patient for beginning dialysis, for it was clear that Susan was not happy with this option. The nurse said, "Right now Susan is very sick, and somewhat unbalanced mentally as well as physically" as a result. She was not considered in a fit condition to give or withhold consent, and so it was her parents who were authorized to give it. Once the patient was in better condition, the medical team reasoned, it was her right to decide whether she wanted to stay on dialysis. They assumed that she would be more "rational" and thus more inclined to assent to dialysis after the procedure had alleviated some of the toxic metabolic effects of chronic renal failure that could cause either depression or hyperexcitability in the central nervous system.

Marvin Ziegenfuss

Marvin Ziegenfuss, a seventeen-year-old boy, was transferred to the University Hospital's renal unit from his hometown hospital with a tentative diagnosis of Goodpasture's syndrome. The clinical picture of this relatively rare disease, which occurs predominantly in young adult males, is characterized by hemoptysis (bleeding from the lungs), anemia, proteinuria (protein in the urine), rapidly advancing renal failure, and imminent death. Neither the cause of the disease nor any definitive therapy has been established (Benoit et al. 1964).

When Marvin entered University Hospital, he was in early renal failure and had been bleeding extensively from his right kidney since a renal biopsy had been performed on it. His past history included a year of petit mal seizures, characterized by loss of awareness and by confusion. Soon after admission to University Hospital, Marvin had a number of grand mal seizures. One of his admission notes provides a good summary of the diagnostic and therapeutic uncertainties confronting the renal team:

Impression: 12 months of hemoptysis and newly discovered hematuria with renal biopsy apparently consistent with acute glomerulonephritis or Goodpasture's syndrome makes diagnosis of Goodpasture's syndrome tempting. No description on biopsy however of arteries—and polyenteritis nodosa could also fit this picture. The seizure disorder could be explained by central nervous system involvement (?temporal lobe) with similar process but this must be examined with EEG, skull films, brain scan and possible lumbar puncture. Acute episode of increased renal failure appears to be secondary to renal biopsy—we may have lost the right kidney. Steroids have been started and may ameliorate the pulmonary problem, but there is no evidence that the progression of renal disease in Goodpasture's syndrome is affected. Bilateral nephrectomy with renal transplantation should be considered if review of pathology specimens confirms diagnosis.

Within a week of Marvin's admission, the renal team agreed to do a right nephrectomy because of the continuing hemorrhage from that kidney. A renal team note read: "The question has been raised of bilateral nephrectomy but we feel this should not be done at this time since the left kidney may respond to future treatment with antilymphocyte globulin [ALG], and the diagnosis is not completely established." Thus, the renal team adopted a policy of "watchful waiting" until a diagnosis of Goodpasture's syndrome could be substantiated.

Even after pathologic study of Marvin's right kidney had strengthened the probability that he had Goodpasture's syndrome, the problem of selecting a therapy continued to be acute.

I have seen the slide of his kidney and he has severe proliferative changes compatible with a diagnosis of Goodpasture's. We could not reasonably recommend removal of the remaining kidney because (1) his function may stabilize and be able to maintain him; (2) we have no room for him in our chronic dialysis program; (3) we have not even discussed transplant possibility with the parents yet. This leaves us with only an attempt to arrest his disease process. This could be tried with (1) ALG, (2) Imuran and/or (3) steroids. We cannot get ALG at present. Therefore we suggest that he be placed on Imuran and steroids in order to try for a remission. We will follow closely and may have to dialyze intermittently as we go.

Following removal of his right kidney, Marvin's blood-urea-nitrogen level [BUN] remained high, necessitating intermittent peritoneal dialysis. He was also experiencing intractable pain in his right flank and seemed to need regular doses of narcotics to tolerate the discomfort. The renal team felt that his pain was partly psychogenic, and they were also concerned about his becoming addicted to the pain-killing drugs. They thus asked Dr. Holmes, a psychiatrist, to see him.

Dr. Holmes found Marvin to be a pale, withdrawn young man who spoke only in monosyllables and appeared to be depressed, although he denied any such feelings. He expressed worry about the kind of life he would have if he was put on the artificial kidney machine. His concern focused on the dietary restrictions that hemodialysis necessitates. He said he could not stand these restrictions; he was sure that his parents understood this and therefore would concur with the idea of a transplantation. Marvin seemed to have been encouraged by a kidney recipient on his ward to look forward to the kind of life a transplant could offer him.

Dr. Holmes learned that Marvin is the third oldest of six children, whose parents are devout Mennonites from a rural area. The church had given the Ziegenfuss family a great deal of support, both financial and emotional, since Marvin's illness.

Marvin's father is forty years old and, Dr. Holmes felt, is a relatively passive and accepting kind of person, defensive about expressing his feelings. His mother, thirty-eight, wears the traditional garb of Mennonite women: a long, unadorned dress of somber color, hair drawn back and bound in a net, and a small cap on her head. She and her husband frequently stated their fundamentalist belief that "everything is in God's hands." Although stoical in nature, Mrs. Ziegenfuss was considered by the psychiatrist to be more openly expressive about her feelings than her husband. Partly because of their fundamentalist religious conceptions, both parents were initially convinced that Marvin's symptoms were due to the immoral, unhealthy practices—drinking (beer) and smoking—in which he had begun to indulge.

During the short stay at his local hospital, Marvin denied his illness to such an extent that he threatened to discharge himself and return home. Marvin's doctor had to ask Mr. Ziegenfuss to explain the gravity of Marvin's illness to him, and make him realize his life was in danger unless he cooperated. According to Mr. and Mrs. Ziegenfuss, Marvin did not speak to them at all for the first two weeks after his transfer to the University Hospital. Mr. Ziegenfuss felt that Marvin was angry at him because "I told him that if he didn't take care of himself he would die." However, Marvin's mother felt that Dr. Holmes's visits with her son had "begun to open [him] up and [help him] talk a little bit more."

When Dr. Holmes first broached the subject of a live-donor kidney transplant, Mr. Ziegenfuss stated his conviction that if Marvin wanted a kidney, he would have to ask them for it. Mr. Ziegenfuss went on to say that parents today are inclined to give too much to their children without reflection and that the children, in turn, take all they receive for granted. He seemed to feel that Marvin was indifferent to the sacrifice his parents might be making if one of them acted as a donor. At this point, Dr. Holmes was "concerned that [Mr. Ziegenfuss's] ambivalence about giving an unrepayable gift of a kidney to his son might be a source of serious difficulty in the future." In contrast to her husband, Mrs. Ziegenfuss seemed unequivocally willing to make a donation from the outset. Subsequently, however, Mrs. Ziegenfuss expressed some hesitancy over whether she and her husband had done the right thing in offering to serve as donors. Further questioning revealed that in addition to her reluctance to counter her husband's reasoning, she was worried that they might have held out a prospect to their son that he would not have thought of or wanted on his own initiative. Both parents seemed lucidly aware, as Mr. Ziegenfuss said one day, that "Marvin is dying fast." But they did not expect to be completely at ease about the religious justification for giving a kidney to their son. Their religious beliefs did not rule out all forms of medical intervention, but they did wonder whether they might be going against God's intentions by doing something so extraordinary as allowing a live organ to be removed from one of their bodies and transplanted into their son.

When Dr. Holmes discussed Marvin's case with a group of psychiatric residents, the residents questioned whether a transplant was indicated for a patient who might be ill with an autoimmune disease like Goodpasture's syndrome, which would strongly compound the problems of rejection and infection, and one, moreover, whose prognosis was known to be "uniformly terrible." And even if a kidney transplant seemed to be indicated, the residents speculated, should Marvin's parents be asked to sacrifice a kidney in the face of the probability that Marvin would still die within the next few years? At this same case conference, Dr. Holmes said he sensed that the renal team was also anxious and uncertain about what they ought to do in this case. Although they had concluded that Marvin's personality characteristics did not make him a good chronic dialysis candidate, the pros and cons of a transplant, live or cadaver, seemed less clear-cut to them. In turn, the physicians' indecision was picked up by Marvin and his parents and reinforced their own doubts.

When Marvin was asked his feelings about accepting a kidney transplant from his parents, he said: "They can offer if they want to. After all, they're parents. Of course, if they want me to die, they can do that too."

On the basis of the interviews with Marvin and his parents, Dr. Holmes concluded that neither of the parents should be permitted to give an organ to their son, even if they proved to be compatible donors, but should be told that they were disqualified on grounds of histoincompatibility. He thought that Marvin should be maintained on chronic hemodialysis for a period of time and then, if the renal team thought it appropriate, he should be placed on the list for a cadaver transplant.

In the days following these psychiatric interviews, according to Dr. Holmes, Marvin "somehow picked up his father's desire to be asked for the organ and did so. . . . Family communications appeared to increase, with more and more sharing of feelings about operations, and so on, among them." These developments, along with the assurance that the costs of a transplant would be covered by the hospital, changed Mr. Ziegenfuss's outlook. He began to "appear increasingly comfortable" to the physicians. The psychiatrist, as well as the renal team members, now agreed that Mr. Ziegenfuss's willingness to donate a kidney was sufficiently informed, voluntary, and conflict-free to make him a suitable donor. Subsequently, the final results of the tests showed that from the standpoint of histocompatibility Marvin's father was an acceptable donor, and his mother was not.

Once some of the conflicts with his parents had been resolved, Dr. Holmes reported that Marvin began to "look different (better)." He even expressed a different attitude toward dialysis, maintaining now that if a transplant was not successful, he was sure he would be able to live out the rest of his life by means of the artificial kidney.

Shortly after the renal team had agreed to accept Marvin for a live kidney transplant from his father, his remaining kidney was removed. Some two months after his initial admission to University Hospital he was discharged and became an out-patient who returned to the hospital twice a week for hemodialysis. In the weeks that he has been awaiting a transplant, Marvin's only new medical problem has been a fractured left ankle, a complication that the renal team feared might be due to the effects of dialysis. Marvin, however, finally admitted that he had broken the ankle at a fund-raising party given for him by his hometown friends. A neighbor had complained to the police about the party's noisiness. When the police arrived in a patrol wagon, the teen-agers, in a panic, ran out onto a balcony, and the balcony collapsed, causing the guest of honor's injury!

Gift-Exchange Aspects of Live-Donor Transplantation

Whenever a live-donor kidney transplantation is being contemplated by a medical team, the close relatives of the candidate-recipient are subject to pressure to offer themselves as donors. Beyond the biomedical reasons that favor a live organ donation, its symbolic meaning virtually compels every family member at least to consider making such a gift. For the gift of an organ signifies the transcendent personal willingness of the donor to give unsparingly of himself to prevent the death of his child, sibling, parent, or spouse; and it is a powerful way of bearing witness to the integrity and solidarity of the family as a social system.

Both these meanings of donation were present in the case of Billy Watson, and both contributed to its psychological and ethical complexity. His mother's ferocious desire to save his life by giving her kidney to him whatever the risk to herself and the welfare of her nine other children, and his father's apparent reluctance to do so in spite of the threat to his marriage and paternity that not volunteering would pose, jeopardized the Watson family in different ways.

The characteristic structure and dynamics of the family system in a given society influence not only the degree to which various relatives are expected and motivated to donate an organ, but also the amount and type of strain to which they will be exposed if they either offer or refuse to do so. On the basis of the ideal-typical characteristics of the modern urban American family, for example, we would predict that the parents of a child or a young, unmarried adult who was a candidate-recipient would be more predisposed to give an organ to their son or daughter, and less ambivalent about doing so, than other kin. For before full adulthood and marriage, an individual's closest and strongest family bond is considered to be his relationship to his parents. Furthermore, the ideal of uncontingent parental love and of the willingness of parents to "make sacrifices" for their children as an expression of this love is firmly institutionalized in many sectors of our society. This is associated with the mother's role even more than with the father's.[5]

However, the case of Marvin Ziegenfuss is rather particular in this regard. On one level of consideration, his mother seemed willing to donate a kidney to her son. At the same time, on fundamentalist religious grounds she shared her husband's initial inclination to feel that the tendency of many parents to give unstintingly to their children constituted poor moral training, precisely because it led to the kind of attitude their own son had expressed: "They're parents, and so they ought to do it." Here we have an instance of a mother trying to discipline her inclination to give to her child, out of deference to religiomoral convictions and what she believes to be the authoritative opinions of her husband. Further complicating this case were the strains in the father-son relationship that ensued from the turbulent, defiantly antipuritanical stage of adolescence through which Marvin was passing.

Another facet of gift exchange is revealed by this case. Mr. Ziegenfuss's belief that Marvin should "ask to receive" raises the question whether it is normatively appropriate in any gift transaction for a potential recipient to request that the gift be made. In the purest kind of gift exchange, either the donor knows that he is socially required to make a particular gift or he spontaneously wants to do so. As we have already implied, what complicates organ donation in this regard is that this is an exceptional act of giving and receiving that is still not fully institutionalized. Thus what one ought or ought not to do in this context is ambiguous.

In our type of family system, sons and daughters are not ordinarily supposed to give of themselves to their parents, defer to them, and care for them to the same extent that parents are expected to do for them. Quite the contrary, sociologically as well as psychologically, an individual's ability to set up and autonomously maintain his "own life" and "own family" is taken to be an important measure of his adequacy and maturity. These seem to us to be some of the reasons why live organ donations from offspring to parents might be more stressful, as well as less frequent, than organs given by parents to children.[6]

From a certain sociocultural point of view, the most appropriate live organ donor would be an adult patient's spouse. The husband-wife bond has primacy in American kinship. The love of husband and wife does more than unify them as marital partners. It "makes genitor and genetrix out of husband and wife . . . creates the blood relationship of parent and child," and symbolizes the "enduring diffuse solidarity" that ideally ought to exist between all members of the nuclear family (Schneider 1968, pp. 38, 50). But though the spouse thus may be the family member most appropriate and most willing to donate his or her organ, husbands and wives are usually excluded from doing so because they are related by marriage rather than by "blood." This means that there are no biogenetic reasons why they are likely to exhibit a high degree of blood- or tissue-type compatibility. This discrepancy between motivation and eligibility is a potential source of strain in a family, not only for the husband and wife but also for the whole kinship unit that they have created and are supposed to unify through their mutual love.

The spouse of a potential organ recipient has a strong emotional interest in the willingness of a sibling or parent to make such a gift to the patient. But the spouse is also susceptible to a great deal of apprehension about the implications of his or her mate's accepting the organ. For the spouse is likely to be aware that the bond forged between a parent or sibling donor and the recipient might lead to the kind of identification and debtor-creditor relationship that could undermine the transplantee's solidarity with his conjugal family. Therefore, a recipient's spouse may experience conflict between an overweening desire to have the patient's life "saved" by a live-donor organ transplant and anxiety over the sociopsychological consequences of accepting such a gift from a transplantee's parent or sibling.

Similar counterpressures may occur when one's spouse is a prospective donor for a sibling or parent. The spouse's desire to donate could be interpreted as illegitimately putting loyalty to a brother or sister or parent before love and responsibility to husband or wife and children, as the following case illustrates.

Several hours after Mr. Jorgenson was accepted by the transplant team as a prospective kidney recipient, his older brother Edward called the team's renologist (Dr. Cohen) to ask, "Anything I can do, Doc?" Dr. Cohen told Edward he could come to the hospital for blood typing, which he subsequently did. When he returned for tissue typing, Edward informed Dr. Cohen that his wife "categorically opposed" his acting as donor to his brother. Dr. Cohen suggested that Edward and his wife talk the situation over with their family doctor. The family physician later called Dr. Cohen and said that this was "an extremely difficult situation." In his opinion, Edward did want to donate his kidney, but his wife vehemently disapproved. "Her psyche is delicate," the family doctor stated, "and she is clearly the dominant person in the marriage." He thought it was possible that in addition to brotherly devotion, Edward was motivated to offer his kidney by a wish to break out of his submissive relation to his wife. In light of the family doctor's report, and his own appraisal of the family dynamics involved, Dr. Cohen decided to tell Edward he was not an acceptable donor because he was not a compatible tissue match with his brother.

Another sociopsychological consequence of such an organ exchange can be that of emotionally tying a married donor and a sibling recipient so closely to one another that it threatens the relationship of donor and recipient to their spouses, children, and other kin. The most extreme instance of this sort we know is the case of a thirty-five-year-old married man who received a kidney from one of his four siblings, an unmarried older sister. After the donation, in the words of the attending transplant physician, the sister "felt absolute control over her brother, as if she had castrated him." When the patient was discharged from the hospital he went to his sister's home to convalesce, rather than returning to his wife and children. He ultimately rejoined his own family, and soon after died of pneumonia.

This potential conflict is heightened because siblings generally constitute the best donors from a genetic point of view. Unmarried siblings, of course, are not subject to the constraints against donating that may be implicitly or explicitly imposed by marriage partners. But in a case like Margaret Ryan's a sibling might hesitate to act as donor on the grounds that she ought not to jeopardize her eligibility for the future responsibilities of marriage and parenthood. This kind of reasoning inhibited the transplant team from immediately accepting Margaret's sister as a donor. In a sense, medical professionals here played the role that one might expect parents to exercise in some cases. That is, a mother or father might well try to dissuade a son or daughter from donating an organ to a sibling on the premise that although the risk involved might be appropriate for parents to undertake, it surpassed brotherly or sisterly obligations or prerogatives. In families where relations between parents and offspring are particularly vexed, one might expect siblings to be especially insistent on acting in loco parentis by offering a kidney to their afflicted brother or sister.

These conjectures, based on our field materials and on sociological reasoning about the nature of the American family system, are borne out by Roberta G. Simmons's review of seventy-nine cases considered for kidney transplantation by the University of Minnesota Hospital over the period 1 February 1968 to 15 January 1970 (R. G. Simmons et al. 1970). In her data, as in ours, it becomes clear that the prospect of a live organ donation creates a situation that lays bare the microdynamics of entire families. The life-or-death circumstances that surround it and the extraordinary gift it entails bring to the surface the structural strengths and weaknesses of a family and the collective life history in which they have been played out.

One family pattern that seems to occur repeatedly in the live organ transplant setting is the "black-sheep donor" syndrome.

Case B.U. — Twenty-eight-year-old woman: The patient had four siblings. Her sister was ineligible medically. The parents approached two of her brothers, both of whom were willing. The third brother was a so-called black sheep. He had left home when young, had been in jail for bad debts, was divorced, and did not visit the family. However, the patient had remained close to this brother and she wished him to be the donor. She wrote him to this effect, and to the surprise of the family he did donate. [Simmons, Fulton, and Fulton 1970, p. 11; see also Eisendrath 1969]

This is perhaps the most literally sacrificial act of all. A member of the family who is considered to be particularly deviant offers himself as a donor, or is offered by his relatives. Collective punishment, self-immolation, an attempt at expiation and redemption are mixed in this at once vindictive, guilt-ridden, altruistic, and quasi-religious behavior. It points up the great complexity and essentially symbolic nature of what is being given and taken in organ exchange.

Transplantation teams recognize the implications of giving an organ and as a consequence know how devastating it might be to a prospective family donor, the candidate recipient, and the kinship unit to which they both belong, to reveal that the donor was unsuited for psychological reasons. Thus, although Susan Thompson's doctors believed that her mother was too ambivalent to be permitted to donate a kidney to her daughter, they told Mrs. Thompson that she was ineligible because of tissue-type incompatibility. Furthermore, nowhere in her chart, or her husband's or Susan's, was an official note made recording the real reason for her elimination. In an unplanned, consensual way, these protective mechanisms have been independently instituted by several of the kidney transplant groups with which we are acquainted. That physicians are willing to violate at least two important norms of medical ethics by telling a deliberate untruth and by withholding a chart entry indicates how grave they consider the consequences of revealing "psychological incompatibility."

As in Mauss's gift-exchange paradigm, once a live organ donation is offered to a potential recipient, he is under some obligation to accept it. In principle, he can refuse it. However, to do so not only would reduce his chances of life, but would also imply his rejection of the donor: his motivation, qualities, and the family bonds he epitomizes. What Mrs. Amico would have been refusing had she not accepted her father's kidney was the full measure of his love for her expressed in the form of a living part of himself. In addition, she would have deprived him of a transcendent, religious kind of experience. As Dr. Richards and the team psychiatrist both pointed out, for Mrs. Amico's father the act of donation was a "high point" of readiness, fitness, selflessness, and commitment that constituted the "supreme moment" of his life.

C. H. Fellner and J. R. Marshall, among others, have examined the significance of organ exchange to the donor.

We were much more impressed by reports from all our donors that the act had turned out to be the most meaningful experience of their lives, of substantial impact in that it had brought about changes within themselves that they felt were beneficial. There appeared to be two overlapping phases to this experience. The first began just prior to and continued through the immediate postoperative period, usually a month or two. During this phase they received a good deal of attention from their families and friends and also from strangers who had heard about their sacrifice either by word of mouth or by reading about it in the local newspapers. . . . They said that this attention made them feel "good," "noble," "bigger," "happier," and generally increased their self-esteem. They all added, some with disappointment, that this attention rapidly diminished and they ceased to be celebrities.
It was at this point, later, that they noted what we called the second phase: namely, certain changes in their attitudes or ideas about themselves, which they considered more lasting. These changes were mostly expressed in phrases like these: "I feel !ike I am a better person. . . . The whole of my life is different, I've done something with my life. . . . I feel . . . kind of noble, I am up a notch in life. . . . I have done a lot of growing up. . . . I am much more responsible . . . now I can do anything." [Fellner and Marshall 1970, p. 1249]

In turn, receiving an organ from a relative obliges the patient to try to return to the donor something comparable to what he has been given: in effect, to discharge the "debt" he has incurred. Mauss has indicated that this state of owing, with its accompanying constraint to repay, is inherent in all forms of gift receipt. But in the case of organ transplantation the magnitude and meaning of what has been exchanged are so great that finding a mode of repayment adequate to release the donor and recipient from a continuing creditor-debtor relationship may become difficult.

In coping with this deep feeling of obligation, recipients tend to exhibit what psychiatrists have termed "ambivalent dependency" in the following form: "It's a debt that can't be repaid.

We've got to be a lot closer by virtue of what he [the donor] has done. . . . Even when he does things that annoy me, I won't complain, because, yes . . . I am indebted" (Crammond 1967, p. 1225). The donor may feel that this kind of gratitude is excessive. One donor reported that he felt disturbed that the recipient treated him as a "small god," was "overenthusiastic" and "will do anything I say" (Crammond et al. 1967, p. 1218). But, either unconsciously or consciously, many live donors not only feel that the recipient is extraordinarily obligated to them, but also that he ought to be identified with and bound to them in special ways. A more common pattern is a tendency for the donor to exhibit a greater degree of "proprietary interest" in the state of health, activities, and personal life of the recipient than he did before transplantation. "He's being unfair to himself and to me [by going back to work so soon] . . . . After all, it's my kidney. . . . That's me in there" (Crammond 1967, p. 1226). It has also been noted that when the recipient's body rejects a transplanted kidney, the donor may experience anger and chagrin, as if a part of himself had been repudiated, wasted or lost, proved inadequate, or allowed to fail.

> A 43-year-old married teacher received the transplant of a kidney donated by her sister; the organ was rejected after one month. While awaiting a second transplant she developed hepatitis and died six months after her initial surgery. Following the rejection of the transplanted kidney, the donor wrote to the patient, venting her anger at the failure of the kidney to function. [Eisendrath 1969, p. 382]

These were some of the eventualities in the mind of the psychiatrist-consultant for the case of Marvin Ziegenfuss when he expressed his initial "concern" regarding the "serious difficulty in the future" that could be caused by the "ambivalence" of Marvin's father over "giving an unrepayable gift."

Cadaver Organ Transplantation and Gift Exchange

Cadaver organ transplantation does not usually involve the same sorts of family-based obligatory demands on the prospective donor as does a live-donor organ exchange. But all of us are nonetheless subject to a number of normative pressures toward participating in the act of organ exchange after death. Because of the amount of information and publicity accorded organ transplantation in recent years by the mass media and by voluntary health agencies, people are increasingly aware that they can arrange to make parts of their bodies available for transplantation after death. The advent of cardiac transplantation, in particular, has stimulated the creation of a number of new institutional arrangements to facilitate donation, such as the Uniform Anatomical Gift Act, and national, regional, and local programs to register prospective donors, like the Living Bank in Houston, Texas, the Medic Alert Registry, and the Uniform Donor cards distributed by the National Kidney Foundation. (The donor card arrangement permits a person to will his organs for transplantation simply by signing a wallet-sized card in the presence of two witnesses.)

One preliminary study of responses in Minnesota to a 1970 campaign to publicize the need for organ donation and to interest persons in obtaining donor cards suggests that certain kinds of social and cultural factors are important in determining whether individuals will seriously consider such an action. R. G. Simmons, J. Fulton, and R. Fulton drew a random sample of eighty-two donor-card volunteers from the thousands of persons who requested a card to sign and compared them with a group of their neighbors of the same sex who had also been exposed to the campaign but had not asked for a card. The donor card volunteers were found to be "more highly educated, less conservative and less committed religiously, more favorable to science, more active in charity work, more willing to attempt new things, and more likely to hold unconventional and secular attitudes toward death and death rites, than . . . those in the comparison group (Simmons, Fulton, and Fulton 1970, p. 25).

When individuals express a desire to bequeath one or more organs for transplantation, they often phrase it in the following way: "If anything should happen to me, I'd like someone to be able to use my kidneys or heart." A variety of motives and beliefs seem to underlie the desire to offer such a gift. To be of use in a way that helps others is an expression of our at once pragmatic and humanitarian Judeo-Christian tradition. Cadaver organ donation provides this opportunity in a new form. Many prospective donors imply that their death will be endowed with "more meaning" because they will pass on a life-giving heritage to another. That they often regard this act as a way of "living on" in and through someone else suggests a latent drive for immortality.

Another sentiment commonly voiced by those contemplating a cadaver donation is the desire to "help others through medical science," a value that is widely held in American society.

When the dying patient or, often, his family is asked to consider permitting an organ to be taken for transplantation immediately after death is pronounced, they are subject in a more immediate and magnified form to the same pressures that act upon the healthy person to serve as a donor after death. Partly for this reason, the convention has developed that the doctor attending the dying prospective donor, or pronouncing him dead, shall not be a member of the transplant team. This arrangement helps to protect the donor-candidate and his relatives against the eventuality of a transplant physician's undue eagerness to obtain an organ for his patient. And it comparably shields the transplant team from being accused of predatory behavior by emotionally distraught relatives of a cadaver donor.

Families of cadaver donors have frequently stated that they felt impelled to assent to donation for essentially religious motives. This is particularly true in the case of the heart, which even in our scientifically oriented society has magicoreligious meaning. The development of cardiac transplantation has revealed that the heart is still widely viewed as the seat of the soul or spirit, the source and repository of love, courage, and the highest, most human emotions. For example, the father of a young woman donor said that the gift of her heart endowed her "otherwise meaningless death with a measure of dignity and worth," and the mother of a young child donor affirmed, "We think God had a purpose in taking Mike, if we know it's going to help someone else." For the wife of another donor, "It's a wonderful feeling. I suppose this is one of the compensations of being the wife of a heart donor . . . the feeling someone who was very dear to me is still taking part in life." A situational reason that the gift of a heart takes on this significance for the next of kin is that a high percentage of cadaver donors are young people who die prematurely, often in vehicular accidents or by suicide. Families have also expressed the hope that the donation may be a redemptive act for the deceased, making up for his sins of omission or commission.

Because of the significance that the gift of a cadaver organ may have for the donor's family, it is not surprising that they may experience a "double grief reaction" should the recipient die: for the "final demise" of their relative as well as for the passing of the person in whom a part of him resided. As the brother of a heart donor put it when the recipient died, "Strangely, we feel a double loss, one over a person very close to us and one for a person we never knew." In turn, the recipient who does not retain an organ has been known to experience guilt because he feels that he has willfully rejected both the organ and its donor. These phenomena suggest that the gift of an organ may be unconsciously perceived by donor and recipient as an exchange through which something of the donor's self or personhood is transmitted along with his organ.[7]

There is some evidence that this double grief reaction may occur because the donors' families have not fully resolved the feelings of loss, anguish, anger, and guilt that normally accompany bereavement and mourning (Lindemann 1944). At least one transplant group has found that by offering heart donors' kin help in dealing with death and grief they have been able to prevent them from grieving a second time after the recipient dies. This is not only because these donors' families seem to have more completely accepted the death of their relative than they would otherwise have done, but also because they exhibit less of a tendency to think of the recipient as a substitute family member (Christopherson and Lunde 1971a).

In discussing the norms that structure the gift-exchange aspects of live-donor transplantation, we cited some of the obligations of candidate-recipients to accept an organ. The "sick-role obligations" to cooperate with the medical team in an attempt to get well and resume normal responsibilities constituted one set (Parsons 1952, pp. 436–39); the obligation not to blatantly reject the volunteer donor's gift or his person was among the others. These normative pressures to receive apply equally to patients being considered for receipt of a cadaver transplant.

One of the major factors impelling a patient to reach out for and accept a kidney transplant, whether live or cadaver, is the physical and psychic suffering he may experience on hemodialysis. In the words of Abram, Moore, and Westervelt (1971):

One has to work with dialysis patients to fully appreciate the investment which they make in the new kidney. To them it is a salvation, a way to escape the dependency and illness of hemodialysis. For many, the experience of hemodialysis is only

måde tolerable by the expectation of renewed life after they
get their kidney transplant.

Susan Thompson expressed something of the despair Abram
describes when she found herself on the kidney machine. Marvin
Ziegenfuss was also emotionally propelled toward a transplant
by his strong feelings that the dietary and other restrictions to
which he would be subjected on hemodialysis would be intolerable. For some patients, "seeing my blood outside my body,"
running through coils of synthetic tubing, is deeply distressing.
Many regard the machine in an anthropomorphic way, as a
"miraculous . . . powerful monster . . . with an almost frightening
hold on my life," a "rigged roulette wheel," reducing me to a
"half-robot, half-man." "I don't want to be buddy-buddy with
the machine," exclaimed one patient, expressing some of the
resentment, anger, and fear of dehumanization that drive many
end-stage kidney patients toward transplantation (Abram 1968;
Borgenicht, Youngner, and Zinn 1969).[8]

The gift of an organ from a dead donor, like that from a live
one, sets up feelings of identification, indebtedness, and special
kinds of responsibility in the recipient. These feelings are vividly
illustrated by the poem and quotation that follow.

Organ Transplant

I drank,
my arteries filled with fat;
the ventricle went lax
and a clot stopped my heart.

Now I sit
in St. Petersburg sunshine.
No whiskey;
wearing a girl's heart.

My blood has adopted a child
who shuffles through my chest
carrying a doll. [Reed 1970]

I had a few bad dreams two or three nights in a row. I thought
that maybe my new kidney wouldn't function. I had a strong
feeling that I had a part of another man's body; a man that I
didn't even know. One day I lay in bed, and I tried to visualize

the kind of a person whose kidney I had. First I felt a little guilty because I was taking it from him. Then I realized it was a gift from his family. But every once in a while I think of it as a foreign body, and if I treat it all right, it will probably stay with me and do all right. My attitude changed from a kind of despair to one of new hope. It's just like starting a new life. [A change of attitude 1969]

Recipients of a cadaver transplant and their families frequently want to say thank you in some way to the deceased donor's relatives. However, many transplant centers have established the convention of keeping the donor, the recipient, and their respective families anonymous. Through this social control mechanism the medical team tries to minimize the extent to which the recipient and his family feel beholden to the donor and his kin. They also seek to reduce the tendency of the donor's family to identify with the recipient, to think of him as a substitute relative, or to make claims upon him. Furthermore, this insulates the recipient and his family from being influenced by their knowledge of the donor's person, character, social background, or life history. The degree to which this protection may be needed is suggested by the following remark, made by the father of a boy heart donor to the father of the young girl who had received it from him: "We've always wanted a little girl, so now we're going to have her and share her with you."

The Physician's Gatekeeping Role

Although the selection of recipients for organ transplantation is exacerbated by the shortage of suitable donors, the elimination of a supply-demand problem would only ease, not resolve, the decision-making process that the medical team must go through with each candidate recipient. The case of Billy Watson dramatically exemplifies some of the state of the art and ethical problems that compound the gatekeeper's selection function, raising as it does the question whether a ten-year-old boy with terminal kidney disease should undergo a transplant, or whether extraordinary measures of any kind ought to be taken to save his life. Another range of issues is represented by the case of Susan Thompson, involving her refusal to accept a cadaver transplant, her resistance to dialysis, and her desire for a live transplant for which, in the end, no family member proved eligible. Marvin Ziegenfuss's case posed still other perplexities: Would it be appropriate and justifiable to do a kidney transplant on him, when this is such a highly experimental form of therapy for the rare, imperfectly understood Goodpasture's syndrome with which he is afflicted? Should his father's fundamentalist "you must ask to receive" attitude psychologically disqualify him as a suitable live donor?

As these cases indicate, there is as yet no clear-cut, uniformly applicable set of criteria that enable the medical team to select a patient for kidney transplantation. To begin with, unambiguous evidence has not yet been established to "indicate whether a given patient at a given time is better off with a graft or with maintenance dialysis" (Scribner and Blagg 1968). If transplantation is favored, the medical criteria for a kidney recipient are "relatively simple" to list, although not always easy to decide upon in a particular patient.

The patient should have irreversible renal disease from which life expectancy is limited to a few weeks or a few months. He must not have a major element of infection. . . . A normal lower urinary tract must be present. Other serious disease processes must be ruled out. Vascular, cardiac, or neurologic changes which are secondary to the renal failure should be judged reversible. [Starzl 1964, p. 11]

The chief of one of the renal transplant teams we observed pointed out that in addition to these medical criteria, in order to be considered "appropriate for a transplant" a patient must

have sufficient emotional stability to understand the procedure, to face it, to bear the uncertainty, the possibility of crises, the eventuality of multiple transplants and dialysis, and prolonged separation from the family postoperatively.

The age of the candidate-recipient, with its sociological as well as biomedical implications, and his family status and responsibilities also may be evaluated.

Given the uncertainties and complexities that still surround the selection of renal transplant patients after nearly two decades of clinical experience, it is little wonder that the criteria of recipient eligibility for newer procedures, such as heart and liver transplants, are even less well defined. For example, it is difficult for physicians to predict the course of a patient with seemingly irreversible, terminal coronary artery disease. One cardiologist working with a heart transplant team told us dejectedly that "most of the criteria used to decide how many weeks or months the patient has to live are baloney. The type of patient who is a suitable candidate for cardiac transplantation, if it is to be carried out at all, is a patient who is going downhill in the hospital in spite of receiving top care."

Transplant teams have developed a number of criteria for screening and selecting organ donors that structure and guide this aspect of their gatekeeping functions. Like the standards that define recipient eligibility, however, these criteria are by no means unequivocal.

The major biomedical criterion for both live and cadaver transplants is the availability of a nondiseased donor organ that is reasonably compatible with the recipient's tissue type. Various medical uncertainties complicate this precondition. For one thing, there is some uncertainty over whether the presence of any disease process in the donor renders the organ to be transplanted "unhealthy" in ways that may not be revealed by the tests routinely administered to evaluate its function. For another, there is considerable debate among physicians concerning the importance of a close tissue match, especially for cardiac transplants, in forestalling rejection of the transplant.

Nor is the question of when the donor is actually dead a settled one. With the development of new techniques of resuscitation and the advent of cardiac transplantation has come an effort to institutionalize a redefinition of death as the absence of brain function rather than the cessation of breathing and heartbeat. Although these brain-death criteria seem to have been generally accepted and put into use at transplant centers, they are not uncontroversial, particularly with respect to issues such as how long a flat brain wave must last before death is pronounced.

Live-donor kidney transplants confront the physician and his colleagues with the problem of deciding whether giving one of a pair of organs will subject the donor to excessive risk. Some of the medical uncertainties and moral ambiguities involved are exemplified by the issues the transplant team had to weigh in considering Mrs. Watson as a donor for her son Billy, on the one hand, and Kathleen Ryan as a donor for her sister Margaret on the other. In the Ryan case, the decision was made to allow Kathleen to donate in spite of a structural abnormality in the kidney she would have left. On the operating table, as the transplant was taking place, another anomaly was discovered that had not shown up in the screening tests. Thus, as a consequence of limitations in the current state of medical knowledge and technique the team inadvertently exposed the donor to more hazard than they had either predicted or intended.

In assessing the eligibility of a live donor to make a gift of one of his organs, the physician must also consider a number of psychosocial factors. Most of these are associated with the gift-exchange dimensions of transplantation that we have already discussed. In the cases of Mrs. Amico's father and Billy Watson's mother, for example, the nature of their motivation and the consequences of the donation had to be evaluated: the degree of voluntariness and spontaneity; the "normality" and ambivalence; the meaning both to the donor and recipient; the implications for the personality integration and functioning of each of them; the extent to which the transplant might "bind" them one to the other or fuse their identities; the impact on other close relatives and on their families, viewed as social systems. Even with the consultant help of psychiatrists, psychologists, and social workers, many of the judgments made here are highly intuitive.

The role that the psychiatric consultant for Marvin Ziegenfuss inadvertently played through his interaction with the boy and his parents is interesting to consider. One of the unanticipated consequences of his interviews is that they opened up channels of verbal and emotional communication within the family, so that relations were generally improved, and father and son were brought to the point where an organ exchange between them was possible. Thus, in a sense the psychological help the family received encouraged them to go through with the live-transplant option. This raises some question about whether the psychiatrist's therapeutic impact might have constituted a form of persuasion, incompatible with the spontaneous, voluntary consent that ideally should have been obtained from Marvin and his father.

Finally, no matter how scrupulous and subtle a medical team may be in their screening, they are left with the uncertainties that ensue from the marginal and still not clearly defined medical and social status of the live donor. He is neither sick nor a patient in the conventional sense of these categories, but a well person to whom the physician permits deliberate injury in order to help a dying individual who *is* his patient. Sociologically as well as medically, neither the rights nor the obligations of the live donor have yet been clearly delineated. "We haven't lost a donor yet" is a quip one hears members of a transplant team make from time to time. What they are saying, obliquely, is that they know the day will come when a live kidney donor will lose function in his remaining kidney, through disease or injury. In effect, they are bracing themselves for the painful and still unknown ethical and medical ramifications of this eventuality.[9]

The gatekeeping role, as we have indicated, is full of uncertainty and strain for the transplant physician. That these physicians work as part of a team complicates it even further. The transplant team is made up of members of different specialties (internists, surgeons, immunologists, psychiatrists, nurses, social workers, etc.). This division of labor and sharing of responsibility provides a certain amount of mutual support, but it also means that divergent points of view, not always easy to reconcile, will have to be taken into account. For instance Dr. Emerson, an internist, felt more strongly than Dr. Richards, a surgeon, that Mrs. Amico should be disqualified as a kidney recipient because of her cardiac disorder. There was some disagreement between internists, as well as between internists and surgeons, over whether Kathleen Ryan should be permitted to serve as donor to her sister. Miss Romano, the social worker on the same transplant team, challenged physicians' decisions when it seemed to her that they had erred in their consideration of the "financial component" of transplant screening. Sometimes she pointed out that the cost of the transplantation and attendant care would impose a serious strain on the recipient and his family. In other instances she voiced concern over what she regarded as a tendency to choose as recipients patients who could bear the expenses of a kidney transplant ("Are you going to choose on a financial basis?").

The social worker's comments call attention to one dimension of the much larger problem of allocation of scarce resources that complicates the selection of recipients. The number of patients admitted to transplantation is limited not only by restricted funds, but also by the availability of suitable organs, medications such as the newer immunosuppressive drugs, hospital beds, facilities such as artificial kidneys, heart-lung machines, and intensive care units, and specially trained medical professionals. For example, in contemplating the treatment of Marvin Ziegenfuss, the renal team found itself without a supply of ALG, temporarily without a vacant place on their chronic hemodialysis program, faced with the possibility that, for psychosocial reasons, the family would not be able to provide a live donor, and also confronted with the likelihood that if they undertook surgery of any kind (nephrec-tomy or transplantation or both), Marvin's kidney, lung, and neurological complications would necessitate recurrent admissions to the intensive care unit. It is within this framework of a multi-faceted scarcity of resources, then, that the physician makes his intricate decision as to which terminally ill patients shall be offered the extraordinary option of a transplantation, and which shall not.

Such decisions are rendered all the more difficult because an especially close relationship, at once personal and collegial, often grows up between patients and the medical team in the transplant situation. This relationship is the product of many factors, includ-ing the grave, long-term illness of the patients, the imminent possibility of their deaths, their continuing, intensive contact with the team, and the specialized care they receive, with its attendant experimental risks. In the face of these conditions, patients and the medical professionals caring for them tend to become mutually identified in what amounts to a positively sanctioned transference-countertransference relationship (see Fox 1959, pp. 86–109). This was visible, for example, in Dr. Richard's feelings about Margaret Ryan. It quickened his motivation to provide her with a kidney transplantation, increased his depression when surgery did not go as well as he had hoped, and heightened his pleasure in her promising posttransplant course.

A strong emotional identification with their patients disposes physicians to do everything they can to prolong their lives, how-ever drastic the means or however reluctant the patient is to undergo the potentially life-saving procedure. The following en-tries made by Dr. Davis in Mr. Lyon's chart illustrate the degree of involvement he felt in trying to bring his dying patient to accept a transplant—to the point where he came close to violat-ing the norms of voluntary consent.

I spoke to Mr. L tonight about the question of renal transplanta-tion. It is obvious that he practices a great deal of denial. States that he does not think or know his kidneys are bad enough to warrant operation. Also he is very afraid of operative risk in general. Is reluctant to ask his sister to donate. Also states family has left everything up to him. Because of the potentiality of an unusually good donor, who is most likely perfectly emotionally motivated, I think the matter should be pursued. We enforce need for operation by clear statement of renal condition. Have a few of our healthy, successful patients talk to him and allay his fear.

. . . Have talked repeatedly to patient about transplant, but he remains petrified and denies illness. . . . Disease getting ready to plunge downhill. . . . Patient close to accepting surgery. Contact transplant group about hemodialysis. . . . Peritoneal dialysis instituted. Sister typed.

The case of Mr. Lyon throws into bas-relief what one might term the existential significance of the role of gatekeeper: those aspects that some physicians half ruefully say force them to "play God." The screening responsibilities of the transplant physician endow him with the awesome prerogatives of permitting some persons to donate or to receive a so-called gift of life and of closing off this option to others. In a dramatic form, the acts of choosing certain individuals to participate in a transplantation and of not choosing others bring the physician face to face with age-old moral and religious questions. When is it justifiable to prolong human life? And when should the physician allow life to end?

The cases around which this chapter turns demonstrate how difficult and how erroneous it would be to take a simple stand on the kinds of questions raised by organ transplantation in its present stage of development, or to make absolutist policy recommendations. Should live organ transplantation between close relatives be prohibited or tabooed, on the grounds that the psychic and interpersonal stress it entails for most donors, recipients, and kin is too great and far-reaching? Or are these stresses sufficiently counterbalanced to warrant continuing this type of transplantation, given the symbolic meaning of live transplantations as well as the fact that it offers a better prognosis for survival from end-stage kidney disease than any other medical therapy currently available? Is the postoperative existence of different categories of transplantees (patients who have received kidney, heart, liver, or lung transplants) sufficiently long, active, and meaningful, and free enough of anxiety and pain, that their lives are worth fighting for and holding onto? Or is the "quality of life" that certain kinds of transplantations afford more dubious than this? Are the essentially "situation ethics" guidelines that transplant physicians are using in their function as gatekeepers appropriate and adequate? Or is there a need for the medical profession purposively and collaboratively to develop more general ethical rules? Would such codified principles help to provide greater distributive justice and mercy for patients and their families as well as greater emotional economy for physicians and their transplant teams?

One might ask whether many of the sociopsychological phenomena and problems now associated with organ transplantation are temporary, largely by-products of its lack of convention or routine. Other observers of the transplantation scene have suggested to us that as the act of donating bodily organs becomes more institutionalized, it will also become more "ordinary." They contend that the current "mystique" that surrounds it will gradually be dispelled, along with the nonrational meanings that organ transplantation now holds for donors, recipients, and their families.

We would not deny that organ transplantation can be expected to undergo a process of comparative rationalization and demystification. But, we would argue that some of the core attributes of the gift-exchange and gatekeeping aspects of organ transplantation we have singled out cannot be reduced beyond a certain point. They are not merely epiphenomena of the present early "state of the medical art." Nor, for that matter, are they purely consequences of certain personality characteristics of individual donors and recipients (e.g., "passive dependency," "domineering" traits, or "appropriative" tendencies) or of the dynamics of particular kinship units. In our view, so long as organ transplantation is regarded and defined as a gift or a donation, it will be subject to norms of giving, receiving, and repaying, with their attendant social, cultural, and psychological functions and strains. As long as organ transplantation continues to be indicated, it would be utopian to imagine that the problems of scarcity associated with it will ever be so perfectly resolved that physicians, patients, and families will no longer have to make choices about who may give and receive an organ, and under what circumstances. The day may come when medical science better understands and controls the body's immunological defenses, so that organ transplantation will no longer be performed only when patients are terminally ill. But until that time it will be linked with the kinds of life-and-death matters that are conducive to magical reactions and religious responses.

2

Specialists in Uncertainty:
The Problem of Rejection

"Wouldn't it be nice to know why he is doing so well?" This ironic statement was made by an immunologist as newspapers heralded the fact that it had been seven months since Dr. Philip Blaiberg had received his still viable transplanted heart. With characteristic medical humor, the immunologist was commenting on the many unknown factors and unsolved problems that beset the field of organ transplantation.

Problems of uncertainty[1] are inherent in all areas of medical practice, and thus to some degree all medicine can be said to be experimental. Some of these uncertainties come from limitations in current medical knowledge and techniques; others stem from the physician's own incomplete mastery of a rapidly expanding body of concepts, information, and skills; still other uncertainties grow out of difficulties in distinguishing between personal ignorance or ineptitude and the open-ended, imperfect state of medical science, technology, and art.

Physicians working in innovational fields like transplantation and dialysis, however, have a special professional relationship to uncertainty, investigation, and experimentation. They deliberately work in the realm of the uncertain and unknown, focusing on those questions that medicine still has not answered and seeking to make some headway with their solution. At once clinicians and investigators, these research physicians have a dual role. They care for patients whose diseases are not well understood and can be only imperfectly treated by present-day medicine. They also conduct studies of these maladies, using some of their patients as research subjects. The research physician's ultimate goal is to advance medical knowledge and technique to the point where such diseases can be prevented. Until he reaches that goal, he seeks a treatment that "will become steadily more reliable, more effective in humanely extending useful life, and . . . less costly" (Russell 1969*b*, p. 665). The information gained through particular clinical research projects may or may not prove immediately relevant and helpful to the disorders of the patient-subjects who have consented to be involved, and the studies inevitably expose them to some degree of discomfort, risk, or potential harm.

Because of the uncertainty inherent in their work, research physicians, as well as their patient-subjects, are constantly confronted with difficult clinical problems. Above all, they face more numerous and grave problems of therapeutic limitation than most other physicians. They can seldom cure their patients; more often they can only ameliorate their condition, and frequently they can do little more than postpone their death. They must work with patients whose condition is already precarious. Here, for example, is the way one transplant surgeon describes the patients he considers suitable candidates for a heart implant:

> I think that we must face the fact that in the beginning stages of a procedure as radically different as cardiac replacement, one is going to have to take patients who are far from ideal candidates, most of whom have not only irretrievable heart disease but also hepatic [liver], renal [kidney] and pulmonary [lung] disease, because that is part of the entire picture of irreversible, end-stage cardiac failure. Obviously these are going to add to the risks in the initial phases of this operation, but I think we have to accept them. . . .
> To sum up, I think there are really no contra-indications for cardiac transplantation at this early stage except that patients might be too well to need it. [C. W. Lillihei, in Shapiro 1969, p. 17]

The uncertainties that pervade transplantation and dialysis at this stage in their development are fundamental and various. Their clinical implications are serious. Physicians and patients involved in these areas must have special capacities to meet the unknown and the "failures" that accompany it. This chapter is a case study of one set of problems of uncertainty critical to organ transplantation. These problems are all related to the phenomenon of rejection: "the innate and unrelenting intolerance of individuals to grafts of other people's tissues and organs" (Billingham

1969, p. 1020).[2] Although the rejection phenomenon had been encountered in kidney transplant experiments with animals, the magnitude of the problems it would pose for human recipients could not be fully perceived until the start of clinical trials. In June 1950 in a Chicago hospital, Mrs. Ruth Tucker underwent the first recorded human kidney transplantation, from a cadaver donor. Eight months later her surgeon, Dr. Richard Lawler, again operated on Mrs. Tucker, seeking to discover why the new kidney's excretion of urine had begun to steadily diminish.

> now they would be able to see the implanted kidney again and determine whether it had changed. Possibly they were all inwardly prepared for an unpleasant surprise. Nevertheless, it was a shock when the bed of the left kidney lay exposed before them.
> The kidney they transplanted seemed to have vanished. Only after looking carefully did they find a shrunken remnant which was no longer functioning, obviously no longer producing urine. Ruth Tucker's organism . . . had fought a secret defensive battle against the foreign tissue. . . . The host body had obviously attacked the transplanted kidney and destroyed it. [Thorwald 1971, p. 99]

More than two decades after Mrs. Tucker's case, virtually all commentators on transplantation agree that an insufficient understanding of the mechanisms underlying the rejection of a transplanted organ continues to be the "central obstacle . . . to the wider applicability of transplantation as a remedy for disease" (Russell and Winn 1970, p. 786). Or, in the more colorful prose of a newspaper account, reviewing the first year of cardiac transplantation:

> 97 times, surgeons said, "Yes, we are ready," and 97 times relatives of dead or dying persons said, "Yes, you may take his heart." But in "Year Two" of human heart transplants, Nature is still saying, "No." For it is Nature's law that a human body should reject "foreign" tissue, whether it be a virus or a borrowed heart. [Heart transplant surgeons find rejection big obstacle 1969]

As this quotation implies, the fact that rejection is the central problem of uncertainty in transplantation is a medical and scientific irony. The implantation of an organ is itself a complex surgical act which can now be performed with great proficiency. Yet again and again a technically perfect operation turns out to be a prelude to an immunologically destructive process that cannot be controlled by surgical means.

This chapter will focus on three sets of uncertainty problems associated with the phenomenon of rejection and attempts to control it in the transplant recipient. The first of these concerns the still indeterminate role that donor-recipient tissue typing plays in decreasing the likelihood and the magnitude of a rejection reaction. A second group of uncertainties centers on the many unresolved questions about the properties and value of the various medical regimens that have been tried to forestall or control such a reaction. In turn, these uncertainties generate a third cluster of problems: those of the often unanticipated and intractable side effects of immunosuppressive therapy.

Rejection: An Immune Response

The phenomenon of rejection began to be defined in 1943, when Gibson and Medawar made a systematic comparison of the outcome of skin autografts (grafts in which the same person is both donor and recipient) and homografts (in which donor and recipient are different persons). This study was followed by Medawar's now classic work on skin homografts on rabbits, through which he established the basic pathophysiology of the homograft reaction and its immunologic nature. He defined rejection as an immune response and assigned a central role in rejection to the white blood cells, or leukocytes, which contain the antigens that sensitize the body to foreign proteins—whether they are disease-causing bacteria or grafted skin. In 1952, through their studies of renal homografts in the dog, Dempster and Simonsen demonstrated that these conclusions were applicable to tissues other than skin.

As is so frequently true in the evolution of science, a number of entrenched beliefs about transplantation and rejection had to be questioned before such fundamental progress could be made. These false trails included the failure to distinguish between the properties of autografts, which have a high probability of permanent success, and those of homografts, which do not; the assumption that the tendency to reject a graft of tumor tissue was due to its malignant nature rather than to its more general status as foreign tissue; the supposition that all immunological processes and responses were mediated by antibodies, present in the serum of the blood; and the belief that rejection was a powerful and inexorable reaction.

Once researchers understood that rejection was an immune reaction to a foreign protein, an attack on the problem became possible. There were two strategies that could be pursued. Researchers could try to choose transplanted tissue that was less "foreign," looking for a method of tissue typing analogous to the typing of red blood cells that made blood transfusion possible. If other tissues beside blood could be typed, and a match made between donor and recipient, the rejection reaction could be circumvented. Alternatively, physicians could take on the immune reaction itself and try to suppress it through a variety of means. It is typical of scientific research that both strategies were pursued simultaneously.

Tissue Typing

Human tissue typing was made possible by the discovery of the first human leukocyte group, reported in 1958 by Jean Dausset. On the basis of this finding Dausset proposed that white blood cells, like red blood cells, might be classified into various groups (Rapaport and Dausset 1968a, p. 52). The importance of tissue typing in transplantation was recognized at once, and programs for matching human organ donors and recipients were soon being worked out. Dr. Thomas Starzl recounts the origins of the first such program, in 1964. At the time of his first series of kidney transplants at the University of Colorado, from November 1962 to March 1964,

there were no practical means of assessing in advance the biologic suitability of donor-recipient combinations. The only immunologic screening that was systematically applied preoperatively was designed to avoid red blood cell incompatibilities. Consequently, the transplantation itself served as a test system in which the recipients of histoincompatible kidneys were presumably weeded out either by death or by loss of their homografts at varying times after the transplantations. Realizing this to be the situation, a six-month moratorium on new cases was declared at the University of Colorado from March to October, 1964. During this time a program was planned, in collaboration with Dr. Paul Terasaki of Los Angeles, which for the first time would attempt donor selection by prospective histocompatibility matching with serologic methods. [Starzl 1969, p. 246][3]

Three principal lines of work have been pursued in the development of tissue-typing methods for transplantation: a more complete and accurate identification of leukocyte groups; confirmation of the now generally accepted view that leukocyte groups are in fact the locus of the active transplantation antigens; retrospective studies of organ donors and recipients (chiefly kidney) to analyze the success or failure of transplants between compatible and incompatible donors and recipients.

Tissue typing is still in its early stages and is surrounded by medical uncertainties. Dr. Paul Terasaki (developer of the Terasaki typing scale) points out that

genetically determined transplantation antigens have been shown to be of importance with every . . . organ and in every species thus far studied. The principal question to be answered is to what *degree* histocompatibility antigens will be of importance when their influence is modified by currently available means of immunosuppression.

A precise answer to this question cannot now be formulated because of deficiencies of the tissue typing methodology currently being used to identify donor-recipient incompatibilities. [Terasaki, in Starzl 1969, p. 22][4]

In view of these limitations in knowledge, the question has been raised about the wisdom of using histocompatibility typing as an important criterion for donor selection. To Terasaki, as to others in the field of transplantation immunology:

The justification for this continued practice comes from the fact that recipients of HL-A compatible kidneys[5] have generally fared better clinically than those who have not had this advantage. Not only has their survival been at a higher rate, but they have also had less histopathologic damage to the homografts as well as better renal function. The most striking benefits of compatibility have seemed to accrue at a considerable time after transplantation. Thus, the risk from early homograft repudiation was often not closely correlated with the degree of incompatibility. However, with the passage of time, a divergence of results became more clear between the matched and mismatched cases. [Terasaki, in Starzl 1969, p. 26]

The most recent period of discussion regarding the role of tissue typing in preventing rejection, insuring survival, and deciding whether a particular transplant should be performed in the first place came with the initial surge of heart transplants. Transplant surgeons had hoped that the heart might be less antigenic than the kidney, thus lessening the need for a good match between donor and recipient. An eminent cardiac transplant surgeon, Dr. Norman Shumway, recalls three bases, cultural as well as biological, for such a hope:

[the heart] is a far less complex tissue than either skin or kidney and perhaps therefore less antigenic. Also, the heart is a large dose of antigen and conceivably might force an antigen-antibody stalemate. Finally, teleologically, perhaps the animal would be reluctant to shed such a vital foreign tissue! [Shumway, Angell, and Wuerflein 1968, p. 172]

The value of tissue typing, particularly if the heart proved to be less prone to rejection than other organs, was heatedly debated at the first "summit meeting" on heart transplantation, held at Cape Town in July 1968. The discussion revealed the degree of uncertainty and discord that prevailed seven months after Dr. Christiaan Barnard's first heart implant. It also dramatized the emotional significance for the convening surgeons of making cardiac transplantation depend on securing a good match:

Dr. J. Mowbray: Well, firstly, about typing. We are now trying to extrapolate, as happens so much of the time, from kidney or liver experience to the heart. If we were to take the kidney experience and ask what is the use of typing, the answer is that the groups with the best matches appear to have stable renal function; the groups with the worst matches do not have stable function and within a 4–5 year period are likely to have to lose their kidney because it does not function. To extrapolate this to the heart presumably means to lose their life at the end of 4–5 years. . . . One of the important things to notice is that the only way that you can tell that a kidney is not doing well at a year (or even 2 years) or before that time, is to biopsy it. A kidney shows much worse damage on biopsy than anybody believed could be true with an organ that functions so well. . . . We should be selecting by typing to get the best match because it may prevent the troubles that may appear in 3 or 4 years' time if some of these patients are alive then.
Professor Barnard: Would you go so far as to say that you would select your recipient, if you have more than one recipient, on tissue typing?
Dr. Mowbray: Oh, undoubtedly. If you have a limited number of donors and have to do a limited number of transplants, and if you have to select a few recipients. . . .

Dr. Cooley: . . . Sometimes one overlooks the fact that the clinical urgency may overrule the other factors. . . . Suppose the surgeon has one man who is dying before his eyes with heart disease, and a donor who is ABO compatible with even a reasonable tissue cross match. To my thinking, one should not deny that recipient the possibility of even a 6-month life. . . . I would not want my immunologists to stay my hand simply because we did not have an adequate tissue match.

Professor Barnard: Did you use tissue typing then just as a sort of research study?

Dr. Cooley: In our first 3 cases we did not have facilities for tissue typing in our hospital. We had to send our tissue typing off to Terasaki. The results of the typing were available after the transplantation had been performed.

Professor Barnard: Let me pose the problem of a patient who, you think, can still last for 6 days; he is not dying today. You have a donor with ABO compatibility and the immunologists tell you after tissue typing that he is not a good match.

Dr. Cooley: This, of course, would be an important feature. You must realize also that the donor will die within 12 to 24 hours. If the transplant is purely elective and the recipient may live for 1–2 weeks, then I think that one may hesitate to do the transplant. But none of our cases had better than a C rating on tissue typing. I think the decision will always be difficult. . . . We should not be too strict with indications for cardiac transplantation at this early stage because even immunologists will agree that an occasional grossly mismatched patient under good immunosuppressive therapy can achieve a good functional result from a transplanted kidney, and apparently the latitude with a transplanted heart is even wider than with the transplanted kidney. So I don't want to have too strenuous or stringent restrictions placed upon us in selection of donor and recipient.

Professor Barnard: So I think it is agreed that today we would wait only for ABO compatibility.

Dr. Ross: By that you mean that you wouldn't wait for tissue typing before you performed the transplant?

Professor Barnard: Well, we would perform tissue typing.

Dr. Ross: And only use it retrospectively?

Professor Barnard: Yes, retrospectively.

Speaker: Is everyone in agreement with that?

Professor Barnard: This is a statement I am making. I am asking you whether you agree with that.

Speaker: We haven't agreed with that.

Dr. Stinson: I say I can't agree with that.

Dr. Botha: I won't. . . .

Dr. Kantrowitz: I think it might be worthwhile to take a poll of the members of this Panel, to see how important each of you considers the tissue typing to be. I think ABO groups are, of course, mandatory, and additional tissue typing is desirable but not essential.

Dr. Ross: I think there is one other relevant point, and that is how long it takes to get the tissue typing through. If you have to fly to Los Angeles, we will say that is one factor. . . . on the whole, we . . . have to wait 2–3 weeks for a donor. In that case, most of our heart transplant cases become acute cases, because we have to take the first donor that comes along. Now, if this is the case with everybody here, and if you can get your tissue typing back in 2 hours, would you ever turn down a donor?

Dr. Kantrowitz: Well, we did.

Professor Barnard: Do you think that was correct?

Dr. Kantrowitz: I don't know.

Professor Barnard: The point is this, you used a worse donor then?

Dr. Kantrowitz: No. We did not operate on this patient. This is a patient 2 weeks ago. We got a donor and we waited for the tissue typing. The immunologist said that this was the worst possible match.

Professor Barnard: And the patient died?

Dr. Kantrowitz: We did not do the operation and the recipient went on to die about 2–3 days later.

Professor Barnard: Well, that is what Dr. Cooley has been saying. You do not have the recipient's interest at heart, when you do a thing like that.

Speaker: On the contrary, he has the recipient's interest at heart.

Professor Barnard: He couldn't have it at heart, because the recipient died. He couldn't have done worse.

Speaker: Well, it depends. . . .

Professor Barnard: This is a suitable time to conclude, as we have agreed on all the points. [Shapiro 1969, pp. 21–23, 60–63]

By spring 1969, assessment of the first 140 heart transplants had established that the heart was not, after all, a "privileged" organ with respect to rejection. At a meeting of the American College of Cardiology, stimulated by a report of the first 17 transplants by Cooley's team, DeBakey and other transplanters were widely quoted in the press as now holding that "tissue typing before surgery in an attempt to get a good match appears to be a prerequisite if we are to achieve long-term success" (see Nora et al. 1969). DeBakey stated he would now try for a C+ or B match whenever possible, as experience had shown that D matches stand almost no chance of a six-month survival. And Dr. Eliot Corday, a past president of the College of Cardiology, declared that the importance of prospectively typing the donor and recipient and of obtaining a good match were the two major new concepts resulting from the first year's experience with cardiac transplantation in man.

The value of tissue typing, however, at least by present methods, remained equivocal. The most experienced and successful of the heart transplant surgeons, Norman Shumway, was in less than full accord with the move toward more stringent requirements for donor-recipient histocompatibility that followed analysis of the first year's results with heart transplants. "At this moment," he stated in the fall of 1969, "we are in no position at all to make a categorical statement about the acceptance of donors on the basis of histocompatibility alone" (Stanford heart transplant team plans few changes in program 1969).

The pressure of timing makes it particularly difficult for cardiac transplants to rely on the still uncertain techniques of tissue typing. But in the more established field of kidney transplantation, the significance of matching donors and recipients also is uncertain. Questions have been raised by Starzl and his associates on the basis of an exhaustive analysis of short- and long-term survival in 189 kidney recipients at Colorado Medical Center. In the Denver series, histocompatibility matching by the Terasaki scale (A-D antigen match classification) correlated "partially" with the outcome only in sibling-to-sibling transplants: "the designation of an A match endowed a slight advantage in terms of survival and quality of homograft function as well as a highly significant advantage in terms of the histopathologic appearance of the kidneys at various times postoperatively." In contrast, in the cases of parent-to-child or nonrelated donor transplants, "the A-D grades failed to conform to any identifiable spectrum of outcome" (Starzl et al. 1970, p. 462).

During a personal interview, Starzl reflected on the poor correlations between typing grades and survival, function, or histopathology in his transplant series. "Tissue matching is important, but as it's been done until now it really hasn't helped very much. It's probably time to look at matching from a different point of view. The concept of tissue typing is a good one, but the expression of data has been insufficient. We probably haven't been measuring what we should have been measuring."

Immunosuppressive Therapies

At the same time that these attempts at tissue typing and matching were being pursued, researchers explored the strategy of trying to suppress the immune reaction. During the first years of kidney transplants, massive doses of whole body irradiation, sometimes accompanied by bone marrow infusions, were used in an attempt to check rejection. At the Peter Bent Brigham Hospital in Boston, for example, six kidney recipients were treated with irradiation between May 1958 and April 1960. "In all of these patients," Moore states, "the pressure of clinical necessity in a desperate situation forced the decision to go ahead." But in Boston, as at other centers,

the many failures with whole body irradiation, the difficulties in achieving a balance of survival after the sledgehammer blow of damaging x-rays, made it clear to all concerned that a better method . . . must be found for breaching the immunosuppressive barrier and making it possible to transplant tissues without rejection. [F. Moore 1965, pp. 104, 112]

A major step in breaching the rejection barrier was taken in 1959, when Drs. Robert Schwartz and William Damashek reported their classic experiment on "drug-induced immunological tolerance." They showed that a state of tolerance to an antigen could be induced in rabbits by daily injections with 6-mercaptopurine, an antimetabolite then in use in the treatment of cancer.[6] Within a few months, transplant researchers such as Dr. Roy Calne in England were applying Schwartz and Damashek's work to kidney transplantation, attempting first to control rejection in dogs. These studies, plus retransplantation experiments in which the kidney was returned to the original donor dog several days after transplant, undermined what now began to be viewed as the too "mystical" and unduly pessimistic belief that rejection is an unremitting, irreversible process.

By April 1960, as a result of extensive studies with the dog model developed by Dr. Joseph Murray, a kidney transplant patient at the Brigham had been treated with 6-mercaptopurine. During this same period, Dr. George Hitchings of the Burroughs Wellcome Research Laboratories synthesized azathioprine (Imuran), a drug closely related to but less toxic than 6-mercaptopurine. To Dr. Murray, "the current state of kidney transplantation may be said to have started in [March] 1961 with the use of azathioprine in a patient who survived for 36 days [before dying of a drug-induced toxicity]" (Murray 1966a, p. 57). His colleague, Francis Moore, vividly recalls the spirit that animated this period of transition "from the laboratory to the hospital."

During the next three years (after the first patient in the spring of 1960) 13 others were operated upon at the Brigham Hospital, with drugs as immuno-suppression for kidney transplantation. Then, starting in the spring of 1963 at this hospital, and at several others in this country and abroad (particularly in Richmond, Denver, Paris, London, and Edinburgh) the experience with kidney transplantation was expanded very rapidly indeed. Exploration was commenced on a much larger clinical scale. The doctors in all of these hospitals were seeking to establish a new routine that would be safe, practical, and effective. All of these experiences were based on the assumption that it would be possible to obtain long-term survival in a patient, maintaining him in good health, with both his own diseased kidneys removed, a homotransplanted kidney in place, and achieving immuno-suppression by means of a drug. This assumption of clinical success was based wholly on the animal work in the laboratory, and its reality—which stimulated so many other workers—was first achieved in the case of Mr. M. D. He was operated upon April 5, 1962, and for the first time gave substance to the growing conviction that drug immuno-suppression would make homo-transplantation possible. [Moore 1965, p. 134]

A crucial innovation during the phase of early clinical trials with drug immunosuppression was the use of double drug therapy, consisting of azathioprine and a steroid, prednisone. Cortisone had been discovered in adrenal secretions in 1936, and in the early 1950s it was shown that hormones of the steroid family could affect a wide range of immunosuppressive responses. But, as Starzl observes, the value of steroids in treating rejection was not appreciated until their clinical use was begun—showing once again the uncertainties involved in extrapolating from the animal model to man.

There were essentially no preceding laboratory data to indicate that the benefit with this now universally accepted combination of agents would be as great as proved to be the case. Indeed, the first publication on experiments in animals was a belated confirmation of the far more convincing observations already made in humans. It is difficult even in retrospect to ascribe priority for standardization of azathioprine-steroid therapy to any single authority or transplantation group. What is clear is that by late 1962 the two drugs were being used together in one way or other and with varying degrees of conviction about their synergism for the prevention or reversal of renal homograft rejection in at least one British and three American centers. Since then, comparable regimens have been adopted throughout the world. . . . With the combined use of azathioprine and prednisone the previous air of hopelessness about the prospects of successful clinical renal homotransplantation was dispelled almost overnight, and with good reason. It became apparent that many patients dying of terminal renal disease could be restored to relatively good health and that the benefit was apt to be long lasting, especially if a kidney was transplanted from a blood relative (Starzl 1969, pp. 242–44; see also Starzl 1964, chap. 14).

But the wave of hopefulness that greeted the innovative use of azathioprine and prednisone did not last. Prolonged experience with this drug combination proved disappointing. A tenaciously high posttransplantation mortality rate belied investigators' early conviction that these two drugs alone could restore "many patients dying of terminal renal disease . . . to relatively good . . . long lasting . . . health" through a kidney transplantation (Starzl 1969, p. 244). At the same time that it clinically disheartened research physicians, and to some degree disenchanted them with the synergistic capacity of this pair of drugs to prevent or reverse rejection, it also provided them with a powerful incentive to seek better pharmacological means for doing so. The trials of ALG therapy were the result.

Interest in today's third major immunosuppressive agent, anti-lymphocyte serum (ALS) dates from the experiments of Metchnikoff in 1899. (ALS is an antiserum produced by injecting lymphocytes from a donor of one species into a recipient of another species.) Although ALS has been "under episodic investigation" since the turn of the century, it was not until 1961 that B. H. Waksman and his colleagues showed that it is an effective therapy against homograft rejection. Several other research groups working with ALS soon confirmed this. The discovery that ALS can impair the homograft reaction triggered a decade of intensive study of its properties and potentialities for controlling rejection, and also those of its globulin derivatives (ALG).

One of the first clinical trials of ALG therapy was undertaken in 1966 by Starzl and his associates. Drawing on experience gained from animal experiments, they used ALG in a triple drug combination, with azathioprine and prednisone. Because of the high risk of a reaction from injecting a foreign protein such as

ALG, it was administered only during the first four months after transplant surgery. In a report on the first fifty-eight renal transplant patients to receive ALG, Starzl detailed the reasons for launching the trials:

A trial of ALG therapy was begun at the University of Colorado in June 1966 because of dissatisfaction with the results obtained using azathioprine and prednisone together in the preceding 4 years. During that time, the mortality during the first 12 postoperative months after intrafamilial renal homotransplantation had remained almost fixed at about 30% despite the acquisition of extensive experience, adjustments in the way in which azathioprine and prednisone were administered, the use of ancillary measures such as local homograft irradiation, and even the application of histocompatibility matching. [Starzl et al. 1969, pp. 448–49]

During these first years of its clinical assessment, ALG was widely acclaimed as a highly effective new weapon in the battle against rejection. It was reported, for example, that in the early Denver trials of ALG, "the one year survival after consanguineous renal homotransplantation was in excess of 90 percent, the ultimate kidney function was superior to that in comparable past cases, the quantities of azathioprine and prednisone necessary to achieve these results were decreased, and lethal septic complications were virtually eliminated" (Starzl 1969, p. 255). Although triple drug therapy is generally acknowledged to have reduced mortality and improved homograft function, however, Starzl and his team have found that ALG causes no improvement in a third measure of immunosuppressive effectiveness. In a study of 189 recipients, "the grafts under treatment with triple drug therapy were in no better condition [regarding tissue injury] than kidneys sampled at comparable times in the double agent era" (Starzl et al. 1970, p. 464). Moreover, as we shall see, some serious negative side effects of ALG have been discovered by researchers, who are now more somberly considering their implications.

In sum, then, since the rejection barrier first began to be breached in the early 1960s by 6-mercaptopurine, "chemical immunosuppression has been in no small measure responsible for the level of success presently enjoyed by clinical transplantation" (Russell and Winn 1970, p. 851). At the same time, the continuing pervasiveness of the rejection problem is suggested by the estimate that, in kidney transplants, "about 75 percent of related living donor transplants and 95 percent of cadaver donor transplants have one or more episodes of threatened rejection" (Hume 1968, p. 125). Transplanters continue to regard the uncertainties and limitations that still cloud the treatment of rejection as the major obstacle to further significant increases in the "success" rate of human organ transplantation. A look at some of these problems enhances one's appreciation both of the gains that have been made and of the distance yet to be traversed.

To begin with, immunological researchers have only a limited understanding of *how* the various classes of immunosuppressive compounds act against rejection. Coupled with this is the puzzle of how to explain cases of relatively long survival in animals who have received various organs with no immunosuppressive therapy, and in some human kidney recipients before the advent of azathioprine and prednisone. The mild rejection and consequent long-term survival of many pigs receiving liver transplants with no immunosuppressive therapy has evoked particular interest and has given rise to the same hope once expressed for the heart: that in terms of antigenic response, the liver may be one of the "easier" organs to transplant (see Starzl 1969, chap. 11).

The most basic clinical problem with the immunosuppressive agents now in use—antimetabolites, steroids, and ALS/ALG— is that "they do not suppress immunologic processes selectively, but interfere with synthetic processes and cell replication widely throughout the body" (Russell and Winn 1970, p. 851). Starzl admits that "nonspecific" immunosuppressive treatment is tanta- mount to "using a bludgeon where a therapeutic scalpel would be preferable" (Starzl 1969, p. 227). The clinician using these drugs is faced with a dilemma: the interruption of lymphocyte activity and other cellular processes throughout the body that is necessary to check rejection simultaneously increases the patient's susceptibility to severe, massive, and often mysterious kinds of infection. As Dr. Anthony Walsh bluntly declared, "What we must avoid is a successful graft in a dead patient" (Walsh 1969, p. 178). His warning is substantiated by Dr. Paul Russell's statement regarding the loss of kidney graftees:

Infection is the major threat. Our estimate is that some 85 per cent of patients who die following transplantation do so with obvious clinical infection which contributes more or less to their deaths. Pulmonary infection is particularly common and it is well known that bizarre organisms occur in an unexpectedly militant state in the tissues of such patients rendered passive by constant immunosuppression. [Russell 1969*b*, p. 660]

The problem of infection also confronts heart transplant physicians and patients. For example, the Stanford Medical Center transplantation team reported that infection killed five of twelve patients who died after a heart implant, that the twelve patients had a total of forty-one separate infections, and that 25 percent of a series of twenty transplant recipients had pneumonia caused by aspergillus, a fungus "which rarely causes disease in the general population."

The development of clinically usable, selective methods of combating rejection remains a prime goal of transplant immunology. One approach being studied in animal models is the induction of tolerance in the transplant recipient, a process in which his "immunologically competent cells (small lymphocytes) become unable to initiate the synthesis of a restricted range of antibodies."

In animals, the barrier that the homograft response imposes has frequently been overcome by treating the recipient with donor antigens, thereby inducing a state of tolerance or paralysis. If human recipients could be made to tolerate a graft, the clinical dependence on immunosuppressive drugs would be greatly reduced. The way in which antigens paralyze lymphocytes is still a mystery, although it seems that direct interaction of antigens with lymphocytes is involved. [Transplantation immunology 1968, p. 834; see also Schwartz 1968]

In addition to the problem of infection, the immunosuppressives themselves can cause grave side effects, some of which were unanticipated before clinical trials. A particularly difficult problem is posed by child kidney recipients, in whom immunosuppressive therapy causes distinct retardation of growth and maturation, with attendant psychosocial problems. In both adults and children the cortisone group of drugs "is particularly well known for severe side effects ranging from peptic ulceration, often with acute complications, to pancreatitis, severe dissolution of bone, retardation of healing, and psychoses" (Russell 1969b, p. 660). Less life-threatening but of considerable psychological impact for the recipient are the cosmetic effects of high-dosage steroid therapy—notably the florid, bloated "moon face" it induces. The jolly and healthy appearance of the transplant recipient pictured in the mass media may be partly a side effect of his steroid therapy.

An example of the potentially damaging effects of azathioprine was uncovered in laboratory trials of liver transplants when ex-

perimenters found that the drug was toxic to the dog's liver—
the very organ it was being administered to protect. It remains
uncertain whether azathioprine is similarly toxic to the human
liver, although a high incidence of liver damage has been seen
with 6-mercaptopurine in cancer chemotherapy.

Various undesirable side effects of ALG have also come to
light through animal and clinical trials. In the first clinical cases,
it became evident that ALG may cause pain and swelling at the
injection site, fever, hives, generalized rashes, and, most seriously,
anaphylactic (shock) reactions to the foreign protein. Other
problems have caused even more serious doubts about both its
efficacy and its safety. For example, analysis of the first 18 heart
transplants performed in Houston indicated that after one to two
weeks the effectiveness of ALG in man is significantly reduced
because the serum stimulates antibody formation against itself
(Heart transplant safeguard falters 1969, p. 784); the ALG then
may be inactivated or may form antigen-antibody complexes
that can settle in the kidneys and produce toxic nephrosis. Another serious limitation of ALG therapy has been the inability
of its manufacturers to standardize the dose. Without standardization, each new batch must be administered on a trial-and-error
basis, increasing the likelihood of negative side effects.

Perhaps the gravest concern about ALG therapy has been the
discovery of a probable link with cancer. In 1968, the *Journal
of the American Medical Association* reported that a significant
number of kidney recipients (15 of 400) had developed "spontaneous" cancers of the lymphatic system. "At the moment," one
of the discoverers of the first four cases of malignancy stated, "it
appears that the incidence will be low enough so that the clinical
use of these [transplantation] procedures will not be vitiated"
(Neoplasms: A complication of organ transplantation? 1968,
p. 246). As of fall 1970, there were forty known cases of
de novo malignant neoplasms in kidney recipients, eleven of
which had been reported by Starzl's unit at Denver (Starzl, Penn,
and Halgrimson 1970).

Given the problems and ambiguities that surround ALS/ALG,
one of its chief clinical developers, Thomas Starzl, recognizes
that although its immunosuppressive effect is clear,

other avenues of inquiry remain open including whether the
benefit of ALG is outweighed by its side effects, if there is really
a need to add globulin therapy to that with the standard drugs

or if this practice will lead to increased survival, how the globulin might be refined and made less toxic, and what improved schedules of administration could be evolved for clinical use. [Starzl et al. 1969, p. 448]

In spite of all these problems and uncertainties, medical investigators continue to express what they consider to be rational optimism about the imminent possibility of understanding and controlling rejection.

The limitations of non-specific immunosuppression including ALS seem altogether too great to me for this form of treatment to endure. We must move to specific alteration. This will come first for the recipient, I believe, but we should not exclude the possibility of some form of directed alteration of donor specificity. As these advances are made, transplantation treatment will become steadily more reliable, more effective in humanely extending useful life, and even less costly. [Russell 1969*b*, p. 665]

what we most look forward to hearing at the next transplantation congress [in 1971] is new discoveries of fact or principle which will come as a complete surprise to us, discoveries of a kind which we are quite unable to foresee. Such is the vitality of transplantation research that we need not doubt that several such discoveries will, in fact, be made. [Medawar 1969, pp. 668–69]

In reviewing the history of research on the rejection phenomenon and immunosuppressive theory, we have been struck by the patterned phases through which this investigation has passed. These successive periods are characteristic of the process of clinical research. They follow from the attitudes and value commitments of investigators as well as from the cognitive and technical properties of the medical-scientific pursuit of knowledge.

Initially, clinical investigators respond to new discoveries with enthusiasm and hope. It is not only their intellectual excitement over solving a scientific problem that accounts for their buoyant reaction, but also their expectation that the advances made will allow them to care for patients more effectively. But with every such breakthrough new uncertainties, therapeutic limitations, and negative aspects are gradually discovered. That unwanted side effects are frequently not predicted is not only the result of chance elements in the way that knowledge unfolds. It also results from the tendency of clinical investigators to deal with uncertainty by focusing on the positive, forward-going aspects of their search. Gradually, investigators recognize and acknowledge the new problems they have uncovered. In their publications, they typically write first of "encouraging results" and later of "discouraging results."

Once the difficulties have been acknowledged, research physicians often deal with them by finding that they have favorable "spin-off" implications. Transplantation researchers, for example, now recognize "a significant risk of neoplasia" (de novo malignancy) owing to immunosuppressive therapy and assert that this risk is simply "part of the price for success after renal transplantation" (Starzl et al. 1970, p. 455). But many of them also argue that the cancerogenic effects of immunosuppression may provide the kind of critical insights into the development of malignancies that could lead to their prevention or cure.

the value of transplantation studies cannot be measured simply by the number of transplants that succeed. In addition to the planned studies, the gain to other, apparently unrelated, fields is sure to be of major importance. For example, the observation that patients on chronic immunosuppressive therapy after renal transplant have a significantly higher incidence of lymphomas and other neoplasms suggests that the cellular rejection process, which is a nuisance in transplantation, may provide a vital defense against the proliferation of abnormal cancer cells. This exciting lead is now being pursued in laboratories directed to the study of neoplasms. The cancer workers undoubtedly are seeking to enhance what the transplanters are trying to suppress.

A better understanding of the immunological processes involved in rejection will clarify the pathology of an assortment of diseases, such as rheumatic diseases, nephritis, and multiple sclerosis, that seem to involve "auto-immune" processes. The immunological studies might even provide a new approach to the problem of arteriosclerosis, which is the major cause of damage to the hearts that have been replaced by transplantation. [Dole 1969, p. 1036]

To some degree and for a certain time, this "spin-off" effect may encourage researchers to pursue a particular line of investigation that has proved as intellectually and clinically troublesome as promising. But how long research physicians maintain such scientific optimism in the face of uncertainties and their consequences for patient-subjects, or go on feeling that there is justification to continue what they are doing, depends on where on the spectrum from experiment to therapy they believe a particular clinical innovation falls. As we shall see in the next chapter, the discussion that has gone on for two decades about the status of kidney transplantation, and more recently about cardiac transplantation, is not primarily a surgical argument. The debate is largely concerned with the problems of rejection that we have considered. Thus the uncertainties associated with tissue rejection are central to what we call the experiment-therapy dilemma as it manifests itself in organ transplantation.

3

The Experiment-Therapy Dilemma

"Dilemma: a situation that requires one to choose between two equally balanced alternatives; a predicament that seemingly defies a satisfactory solution."

American Heritage Dictionary

Being a clinical investigator has its problems. A lot of the research you do is of no benefit to patients, and there's a real possibility that you can do them harm. So, in order to do research you've got to close your eyes to some extent, or at least, take calculated risks with the patients on whom you run the experiments. . . . Still, you almost never attain the ideal research. . . . You rarely get to the basis of the problem you're investigating, because it's touch and go all along the way with these patients. Their care and welfare have to be taken into consideration. . . . So, you usually end up by compromising your research goals and standards. [Fox 1959, pp. 55–56]

In this statement, a young research physician expresses the strain he experiences in trying to reconcile the roles of clinician and investigator. Under optimal conditions, the clinical investigator's dual responsibilities are complementary. His investigative work bears directly on the diagnosis and treatment of his patients' conditions, which in some sense it benefits, and conversely, his clinical activities on behalf of his patients also advance his research.

The difficulty is that patient-care and research responsibilities are not always in perfect accord; sometimes they may openly conflict. Some of the tests and procedures the research physician conducts with patients may not be directly relevant to their illness or potentially beneficial to them. Their primary purpose is to obtain scientific information. Characteristically, when research physicians discuss this type of medical experimentation, they are likely to preface it with the remark that "it would be interesting to try" X procedure. In those instances where clinical trials *are* predominantly therapeutic in intent, innovative therapy may expose the patient to discomfort and risk. Given the high degree of uncertainty with which the clinical investigator works, possible adverse effects of the treatment being tried cannot necessarily be predicted. Further, what he does to aid or protect his patient-subjects may either preclude or undermine an experiment he would have liked to bring to its logical conclusion.

The research physician's attitude toward the two facets of his professional role might aptly be described as one of structural ambivalence.[1] His ambivalence originates in the social structural properties of his professional role rather than in his personality attributes. On the one hand, he is inclined to insist on recognition of the degree to which he is clinically and therapeutically oriented. We recall, for example, the experimental surgeon who bellowed at us that he performs innovative operations for only several hours a day and spends the rest of his day "seeing patients like any other physician." In their writings about their work, many investigators underscore its clinical or therapeutic nature, in distinction to "pure experimentation."

> we are concerned with a few of the ethical questions of therapeutic innovation raised by the application of new treatments to sick people. These are initial trials, carried out in human patients, of drugs or operations that may benefit the subject. This is the largest single category of medical experimentation— if that is a suitable term for therapeutic innovation—currently practiced at the clinical level. [Moore 1970, p. 359]

> I do object slightly to the idea that cardiac transplantation is human experimentation. From our point of view as physicians, it should be considered clinical investigation. [And from the recipient's perspective] these are patients who are desperate, who are staring death in the face, and for whom there is at the moment no other possible treatment. [Shumway, in Stinson, Dong, Iben, and Shumway 1969, p. 187]

Some investigators express their clinical commitment in a dramatically urgent way, stressing their responsibility to the dying patient, particularly their "moral duty" to do everything they can to "save him."

> A point I think we mustn't stress so much [in discussing candidates for heart transplants] is . . . that the patients must have a will to live. I think many a man in the terminal stages of heart failure . . . who is really sick and has a poor blood supply to the brain from poor cardiac output, would say: "Oh please

leave me alone, I want to die." But I don't think that the patient can decide whether he wants to die or not. I think that as doctors our duty is to give the patient all the therapy and all the treatment that is available to us. [Barnard, in Shapiro 1969, pp. 266–67]

It is objectively true, to use Starzl's phrase, that the clinical investigator is greatly "preoccupied with the therapy" necessary to the complex care of his patients (Starzl 1969, p. 144). At the same time, there is often a note of hypersensitivity and defensiveness in the investigators' assertions about how clinically oriented they are, which may be a response to several factors. Present-day researchers are still concerned that their work in no way be identified with the types of medical experiments conducted in Nazi Germany. "It would be difficult to overstate the impetus this uniquely tragic European experience gave to studies of the ethics of human experimentation. Out of a concern with the violence done to human beings came an interest in defining precisely the conditions under which human experimentation might take place" (Graubard, in Freund 1970, p. vii). Research physicians are also reacting to the considerable emotional stress of caring for patients under such conditions of uncertainty and such therapeutic limitations. As we shall see, the strain they feel is intensified by their typically close and continuous relations with the patients who are also their subjects. A telling sign of the tension physicians experience in this connection is their tendency toward counterphobic gallows-humor jokes about how impotent they often are in dealing with patients' illnesses and impending death.

Dr. Pierce: Dr. Cooley not only has the most survivors, but he has also tied for having the most autopsies.
Dr. Cooley: I am the recipient of a dubious honor. [Shapiro 1969, p. 202]

Dr. G: How is Mr. X's condition? [a patient suffering from infection and other complications after a kidney transplant]
Dr. H: Well, his kidney is better, but the rest of him sure isn't so good.

The other side of the research physician's ambivalence makes him emphasize that his research with human subjects is important for the advancement of scientific understanding as much as for its potential therapeutic implications. For example, a clinical investigator describes the ideal work situation as one in which "potentially significant discoveries in the animal laboratories can be tested in the wards with a minimum delay; conversely, observations on patients will influence the direction of basic research" (Starzl and Marchioro 1965, p. 372). In another context, he also expresses something close to nostalgia because now that immunosuppressive drugs exist it is no longer possible (justifiable) to study the effects of an untreated rejection reaction in patients. "The brilliant studies of Hume and his colleagues . . . assume a special significance since it is unlikely that opportunities will ever again be available to study the fate of untreated homografts in humans. . . . The importance of [these] studies in understanding the pathologic physiology of rejection can hardly be overestimated" (Starzl 1964, pp. 142–43).

As the foregoing implies, the research physician is concerned with striking what he terms a proper, equitable, or justifiable balance between the investigative and the clinical aspects of his role. In his equation, this balance is partly contingent on two complex phenomena: the quality of the "informed, voluntary consent" he has obtained from his patient-subjects and the "quality of life" the proposed treatment may offer. To leave aside for now the difficult problem of evaluating how informed and voluntary consent has been, or whether a patient's life has been improved, physicians reason about the relationship between these variables and the balancing of their roles in the following fashion. "My patient has given me permission to do this experiment in the expectation that it may benefit him physically, psychically, and/or spiritually. Therefore, I am acting in a legitimate 'physicianly' way. I am not acting just as an impersonal experimenter."

The research physician's attempt to equilibrate his clinical and investigative responsibilities is related to a basic problem: determining how experimental and/or therapeutic a new operation, drug, or other procedure is at a given time in its development and for a given class of sick persons. This classificatory aspect of the experiment-therapy dilemma is an issue whose import goes far beyond semantic preciousness or academic hairsplitting. It affects research physicians and their patient-subjects in fundamental ways. The evaluation of a particular medical or surgical procedure's status is a primary criterion for deciding on whom and in what circumstances it may justifiably be used.

The stage of development of a treatment like hemodialysis or transplantation is frequently conceptualized and discussed in a way that is too dichotomous and static—either as "experiment" or "therapy." Therapeutic innovation is more accurately viewed as a process or a continuum that moves from animal experiments to clinical trials with terminally ill patients beyond the help of conventional therapies, then to the use of the treatment on less and less critically ill patients.

This evolution is not necessarily unbroken and in one direction. At one end of the spectrum, investigators frequently are conducting parallel or interrelated programs of animal and human study. They may work back and forth between the laboratory and clinic, testing data obtained from animal work on patients and patient findings on animals. As a clinical program develops, they may encounter unanticipated problems that constitute setbacks to physicians and patients. Most notable are grave side effects of a new treatment, such as the suspected link between ALG and neoplasms mentioned earlier. As we will detail in chapter 6, in this phase of a therapeutic innovation's development there often is a clinical moratorium: the clinical use of the new treatment is suspended.

The decision to slow down a clinical program may also be prompted by a "crisis of success." Thus, once "relatively protracted" kidney homograft function was obtained in "considerably more than half the cases," it became

essential to systematically obtain data which [would] help those institutions to plan maintenance care and to establish a long-term prognosis for chronic survivors before a new series of homografting procedures [was] begun. For this reason, a six-month delay on new cases was decided upon at the University of Colorado, beginning in March, 1964, during which time additional information could be obtained about the adequacy of late homograft function; the frequency, severity, diagnosis, and treatment of delayed rejection and the incidence of indolent urologic and other complications. [Starzl 1964, pp. 189–90]

But whatever its stage of development, clinical investigation entails an interplay between research and therapy, and the balance shifts as the new treatment evolves.

Physicians do not have standardized and unevocative terms to designate the stages of development of a new therapy clearly and objectively. Quite to the contrary, we have been struck by the elaborate, equivocal, or emotional quality of some of the language used. For example, a research physician describes the early efforts to apply renal transplantation to the treatment of terminal kidney disease as a "pioneer era doomed to failure" in which the "risk imposed" and the death rate were both "exorbitant" (Starzl and Marchioro 1965, p. 369). And he characterizes a later phase in kidney transplantation—the period when immunosuppressive therapy consisted of a double-dose regimen of azathioprine and prednisone—as one in which this procedure had become "an effective but incompletely characterized form of palliative therapy" (Starzl and Marchioro 1965, p. 372).

An even more striking example of the difficulty physicians have in verbalizing "what is experimental" and "what is therapeutic" is provided in the following exchange between six prominent specialists working on transplantation problems.

Kilbrandon: I thought we had been talking about therapeutic surgery. What is experimental surgery?
Reemtsma: This is a qualitative distinction. . . . In dialysis or transplantation when we use the term experimental we mean that we are uncertain of the outcome, but we are attempting to help those patients. This is unlike experimental work in which cancer cells are injected in volunteers to see what happens and which does not claim to help the patient. Yet removal of the stomach for an ulcer is an experiment and so is taking an aspirin for a headache, in the sense that they may or may not work. Perhaps we have over-sold the experimental nature to ourselves and to others in our determination to convince people that we are doing procedures with an uncertain outcome. We should be aware that these procedures are undertaken with therapeutic purposes in mind.
Kilbrandon: But is a kidney transplant regarded as experimental surgery?
Woodruff: We are in danger of equating experimental procedures with procedures which have a relatively low success rate. I think this is a mistake, but even on this basis I would not regard kidney transplantation as experimental. In my own unit over the last twelve months, six patients have received renal transplants and all of them are still alive. In another condition for which four people were treated over the same period, all the patients are dead, yet the operation in those cases was a perfectly legitimate and orthodox one.
Schreiner: There is no alternative treatment to surgery for some conditions at present, but there is an alternative to renal transplantation.
van Rood: Is not the distinction between experimental and normal surgery simply that in experimental surgery you want to get information while in the other kinds of surgery you are

trying to treat the patient? The fact that by carrying out surgery on a doomed patient you can get information doesn't make it experimental.
Kilbrandon: A transplant involves two operations: is one experimental and the other therapeutic?
Reemtsma: I object strongly to this distinction. [Wolstenholme and O'Connor 1966, pp. 164–66]

Physicians' difficulties in ascertaining the overall experimental-therapeutic status of a procedure, and thus when and on whom it may rightfully be tried, have several sources. To begin with, they are partly related to ambiguities in the criteria physicians use and in their characteristic way of reasoning about the problem. What Joseph Fletcher has called "mathematicated decisions" based on "a statistical morality" are generally invoked to try to resolve this issue (Fletcher 1969, p. 236). Physicians use probabilities and percentages to estimate factors such as the differential diagnosis of a disease and its course under varying circumstances—especially its prognosis in response to alternative treatments. (This mode of reasoning, of course, is not peculiar to the clinical investigator; it is inherent in all medical practice.) Here, for instance, is how one cardiac transplant surgeon told us he reasoned about eligibility for a heart transplant and about an acceptable or nonacceptable mortality rate.

One weighs the mortality of the disease against the mortality of the operation. In the case of coronary artery disease the majority of patients die in a very short time, but not all of them do. The survival rate from heart transplants has to be definitely better to be justified, because the patients go through a great deal and the surgical team does also. We don't know yet if the mortality rate has or has not been acceptable in cardiac transplantation. A one percent mortality is not justifiable in elective preventive surgery, such as a gallbladder operation. But in curative surgery an acceptable mortality varies with the seriousness of the condition involved. A 50 percent mortality is not bad if you are sure that the patient would die without surgery. In fact, under the circumstances where you're 100 percent sure the patient is going to die [of his disease] any operative mortality rate is acceptable. It's the in-between cases that are hard, the ones where you can't say for sure that the patient is going to die. One criterion we used for heart transplant eligibility was that the patient must be hospital dependent; but then we realized that the heart recipient was hospital dependent too.

Similar questions must be faced by the renal transplanter. What chance of survival would the terminally ill kidney patient have without a transplant? What other potentially effective forms of therapy are available? What are their assets and liabilities, compared with a transplant? In this context physicians invoke the concepts of relative "success" and "failure," categories of central importance in evaluating the "experimentalness" of a treatment and its consequent suitability for patients with different grades of illness. The major criterion for "success" or "failure" is the statistically expressed death rate of patients treated in this way: both their immediate posttreatment mortality and survival rates and the ultimate life expectancy of what one research physician terms "chronic survivors." How "high" or "low" a death-survival rate is considered to be is determined by comparing it with the "results" of other treatments in varying steps of development, as well as by estimating what patients' prognoses would have been had they not undergone the procedure. For example, in 1969 Dr. John Merrill expressed why he regarded kidney transplantation as no longer so experimental:

Transplantation of the kidney, at least between related donor-recipient pairs, is now a clinically feasible procedure. A recent analysis of more than 2000 human renal allografts reported to the Transplantation Registry indicated that the two-year survival rate for sibling donor-recipient pairs is approximately 80 per cent. The results of recent transplantations of cadaver kidneys shows a success rate comparable to that of open heart surgery for acquired valvular disease. [Merrill 1969, p. 1030]

In addition, physicians also appraise success and failure in qualitative terms, trying to judge the meaningfulness and utility of the clinical improvement during patients' period of survival, however short or long it may be. According to this calculus, a procedure that is in clinical use but is "still very experimental" would be one in which the problems of uncertainty are numerous or of basic importance; the death rate is "high"; and the survivors generally "do not do very well", so that the only "suitable human candidates" are patients so totally incapacitated that their death is imminent.

Although research physicians have worked out an informal method for assessing the experiment-therapy status of a drug, operation, or other treatment, this does not provide detailed, clear-cut indicators for making at least three critical decisions: (1) How can the physician tell that his work with laboratory animals has solved the conceptual, empirical, and technical problems presented by a therapeutic innovation sufficiently to warrant trying it on human subjects? (2) How can he determine whether the survival and success rates of his clinical trials "justify" his continuing to apply this procedure to patient-subjects? (3) What sorts of results definitely indicate that on both scientific and ethical grounds the new treatment can be administered to patients who are less than terminally ill?

But the ambiguity of the criteria used to locate a therapeutic innovation on the experiment-therapy continuum is not the only source of the difficulty. The problems are augmented by research physicians' emotional involvement in both the investigative and therapeutic aspects of their dual role. Characteristically, they are caught up in the intellectual challenge of discovering, testing, and developing a new therapy. Their zeal to make such a treatment "more than an experiment" is not just a consequence of their scientific absorption. It is also associated with their sense of "clinical urgency": their pressing desire to keep their dying patients alive and, beyond that, to be able to palliate, if not cure, their desperate and complex illnesses. This clinical fervor may lead a research physician to overestimate how far a treatment has progressed toward the therapy end of the experiment-therapy spectrum. Or it may impel him to be too aware of its uncertainties, limitations, and dangers and thus to be excessively cautious. Research physicians are also professionally motivated to qualify in the eyes of their colleagues as "authentic and acknowledged pioneers" in their fields (Cournand 1969, p. 1018). Their desire to be recognized as the first to discover or try something of clinical import may incline them to overestimate its therapeutic status; yet their desire to be viewed as rigorous investigators may dispose them to emphasize how experimental a procedure or drug still is.

Many of the core issues involved in assessing the experimental/ therapeutic status of a treatment are epitomized in the development of kidney and heart transplants. Kidney transplantation is the earliest, best-developed type of organ graft. It has passed through a number of phases in the experiment-therapy spectrum. Cardiac transplantation has a shorter history and falls closer to the experimental end. A comparison of their status throws light on some of the subtler aspects of the experiment-therapy dilemma. As we have noted, the process of therapeutic innovation typically involves overlapping steps. In the earliest stage of developing a procedure or a drug, where uncertainty and risk are at a maximum, investigators work with animal subjects. Thus the dramatic impact of the first human-to-human heart transplant in 1967 was lessened for those familiar with the more than sixty-year history of cardiac transplantation, dating from the dog-heart experiments done by Alexis Carrel in 1905 and including the 1964 attempt by Dr. James Hardy and his colleagues at the University of Mississippi to transplant a chimpanzee heart into a sixty-eight-year-old man. Similarly, the techniques of kidney transplantation had their beginnings in the 1902 reports of animal studies by the Viennese surgeon Dr. Emerich Ullmann and, more importantly, in the work of Carrel a few years later.

Laboratory study, as Moore points out, "puts the stamp of human and ethical acceptability on therapeutic innovation more than does any other characteristic. Preliminary laboratory trial is the only way to provide information, however incomplete or inadequate, that might lead to an acceptable informed consent" (F. Moore 1970, p. 511). The importance of animal trials is not lessened by their limitations. Chief among these is the difficulty of developing an animal model in which one can reproduce a condition found in a sick person or test a treatment. Between 1951 and 1953, for example, Dr. Joseph Murray, at Boston's Peter Bent Brigham Hospital, perfected the now standard animal model for kidney transplantation, drawing upon techniques pioneered by Ullmann, Carrel, and other earlier workers. This model —a bilaterally nephrectomized (both kidneys removed) dog with a homotransplanted kidney—in turn became the prototype for the experimental and clinical transplantation of other organs, such as the heart, liver, and lungs.

An extensive period of animal work, however, can seldom answer all the questions that will be posed by the human patient. There are limitations in extrapolating from the best of animal models to the critically ill human being, and in many cases it has not been possible to truly reproduce the human disease condition. For example, years of painstaking work have not enabled transplant researchers to produce in the dog either the type of chronic renal failure that has been the major indication for human kidney transplants or the type of congenital heart disease that now signals the need for a human heart implant. Nor, as we have seen, have the immunological problems that still dominate transplantation been solved through years of animal experimentation, though enormous strides have been made and will probably continue.

The personal background of the individual clinician—his acquaintance with the disease and his general sophistication in the field—and the capabilities of his institution to carry out the many aspects of a complicated procedure such as a heart transplant are also important prerequisites for therapeutic innovation. But in most clinical research, however readily one may list preconditions such as animal experimentation and personal and institutional expertise, there are no neat guideposts signaling to physician-investigators that the time has indubitably come to move from animal to human trials. Rather, this transition is a phase in clinical research, irrespective of the nature of the procedure, that is inherently "premature" and for that reason is often judged to be controversial and sometimes "immoral." This inherent prematurity, as we shall see in detail, was a root cause of the turbulent reception of human heart transplantation, both by medical professionals and by laymen.

The difficulties of predicting the outcome of the first clinical trials or of clearly defining their goals compound the difficult decision to launch human trials. Francis Moore has recalled the mix of uncertainties and hopes in the decision to attempt kidney transplants from unrelated donors at the Peter Bent Brigham Hospital:

By 1951, Dr. Thorn and Dr. Merrill had accumulated a large experience in treatments done on the artificial kidney. Increasingly, they saw patients for whom the artificial kidney offered little hope. Kidney transplantation was needed, and it was time for a renewed trial.

. . . The contemporary work of Simonsen and Dempster had not yet been published. The few other recorded human transplants in the literature carried very little information. Dr. Gordon Murray and his colleagues in Toronto had evidently completed four kidney transplantations with only short-term survival in three. In the fourth, the transplanted kidney was thought to be alive and making urine for 15 months. Unfortunately, there were no reported studies of renal function or biopsies to show the microscopic appearance. Therefore, it was impossible to state whether the kidney was alive and functioning well.

Using the artificial kidney to tide the patient over preoperative and postoperative intervals, kidney transplantation was now to be given a trial in patients in whom there was no outlook for long-term survival except by repeated dialysis treatments on the artificial kidney.

. . . Just as in any new scientific undertaking, the final result here was not clearly seen at the outset. It was hoped that the transplanted kidneys might function longer than was previously reported in animals, or that the general advances in surgery, medicine, and biology would permit some unexpected success in transplantation. There was every reason to expect something new when all the techniques of modern medicine and surgery were applied. This expectation alone justified the undertaking, and the first patient was operated upon by Dr. Hume on April 23, 1951. [F. Moore 1965, pp. 69–71]

As is vividly documented by the mortality figures from the beginnings of human kidney and heart transplantation, the initiation of the clinical phase of a new therapy is a stressful and discouraging period for a research group. Given the combined result of the many unknown and uncontrolled factors at this level of experimentation and of the drastic illnesses of the patients, "successful" outcomes are rare and ephemeral. Failure and death rates are high. By 1963, when the era of immunosuppressive drug therapy was just beginning, 194 kidney transplants had been reported in the literature. Of the 103 nontwin transplants in this total, fewer than 10 percent survived for more than three months (Goodwin and Martin 1963). Figures from cardiac transplantation are comparable: of the 162 transplants reported through 30 May 1970, 104 recipients had died within three months of surgery.

Figures like these take on substance in Moore's description of the "black years" of kidney transplantation at the Peter Bent Brigham.

In the early days of transplantation, between 1952 and 1962, this was an era during which the infant field was most readily subject to criticism. . . . Several of the patients operated on for kidney transplantation at Peter Bent Brigham Hospital during the "black years" between the introduction of whole body radiation and the discovery of immunosuppressive chemotherapy were admitted with no kidneys whatsoever. Each had had a single kidney removed because of injury or mistaken identity, and there was no alternative. Repeated dialysis was then in an infant stage, and any concept of maintaining a person for weeks, months, or even years under dialysis alone was simply out of the question. . . . In all of these the outlook without operation was nil, and the standards for acceptability of operation were therefore lowered to give the patient at least some chance for recovery. In many of these early desperate attempts, experiences were gained which later made it possible to raise the standards of acceptability for other patients with less urgent situations. [F. Moore 1968, pp. 384–86]

As kidney transplantation began to emerge from these "black years" there was still "a dismal picture of repeated failures and only an occasional success" (Starzl 1964, p. xi). But to those in the field, a new stage was reached when, in 1959, Murray performed the first successful transplant between a nonidentical donor and recipient. Looking back on this event, in 1964 Starzl expressed the conviction that, "An operation which can in the individual case provide five years of relatively healthful existence, as has been the case in Murray's . . . transplant . . . cannot be said to be without significant worth at least in the isolated case" (Starzl 1964, p. xi). By 1964, enough transplants had been carried out for Starzl's textbook *Experience in Renal Transplantation* to be published. He stated frankly, however, that "the place, if any, of renal hetero- or homotransplantation in the treatment of terminal renal disease is not yet clear. To say that the problem of homograft rejection has been satisfactorily solved is folly. The converse view that this means of therapy has no real value would, however, appear to be an equally limited attitude" (Starzl 1964, p. xi).

In 1963, when Starzl was preparing his text, the Human Kidney Transplant Registry was inaugurated. This is a formal centralized method of collecting from renal transplanters around the world data on variables such as the age and sex of donors and recipients, the number of live and cadaver donors, the relationship of live donor to recipient, the recipient's disease, pre- and intraoperative treatment of the recipient, types of immunosuppression used, onset of kidney function, renal and nonrenal complications, transplant and patient survival figures, and the final cause of the recipient's death. The registry has become a major tool in physicians' attempts to evaluate the status of renal transplantation. It is premised on the kind of mathematicated probability reasoning characteristic of physicians that we discussed earlier. For example, the eighth registry report, which analyzed data gathered through 1 January 1970, summarized the cumulative results of human kidney transplantation as follows:

The collected experience of 3645 kidney transplantations, of which 40% were performed in 1968 and 1969, provides data for the following calculations of transplant survivals. Kidneys from consanguinous living donors have a 78% one year survival and a 75% two year survival; kidneys from cadaveric donors have a 52% one year survival, and a 41% two year survival. The only survival group showing statistically significant improvement over the Seventh Report is in the one year survival from cadaveric donors. None of the other groups individually had significantly improved survival rates but when all are analyzed collectively the slight improvement of each group represents a significant trend. Two thirds of patients with a functioning kidney at one year are rated "completely normal" in their activities. [Murray, Barnes, and Atkinson, Eighth report of the Human Kidney Transplant Registry 1971]

Despite the wealth of data available in the Kidney Registry, and although human renal transplants have been carried out for nearly two decades, there is no easy agreement in the field on the overall experimental-therapeutic status of the procedure. In 1970 there was general agreement that the survival rate had become more "decent," making kidney transplantation a "generally practical aspect of human biology" (F. Moore 1968, p. 385). But this statement is subject to a wide latitude of interpretation. Numerous investigators have contended that renal homotransplantation is "increasingly accepted as a regular clinical service," that a "majority of cases are clinically successful," and that it is "now the therapy of choice for selected patients with end-stage kidney disease." In making such evaluations, research physicians do not mean that kidney transplantation has proved to be a "curative procedure" or a "definitive treatment" of "routine therapeutic usefulness" in the "ordinary practice of medicine." They acknowledge that renal grafting still provides a "fertile area for clinical investigation." This is a euphemistic way of expressing another widely shared view: that kidney transplantation is still experimental, with the exception of transplants between twins.[2] One reason kidney transplantation is judged to be less than routine therapy is that, in Dr. Jean Hamburger's words:

We know now that, six months or one year after transplantation, success or failure is predictable in many cases, *but not in all.* . . . Some of our patients are doing well after more than 4 years, despite a gross [tissue] mismatch; on the other hand, we have some poor results with no apparent mismatch. [Hamburger 1969]

In addition to survival figures, indicators that the profession uses to assess kidney transplantation include the predictability of outcome; funding; the extent and type of clinical service (the number of centers where transplants are performed and their university affiliation or lack of it, and category of surgeons doing the operation); and the amount of mass-media coverage. Some of the reasons given for assigning kidney transplantation a predominantly therapeutic status rely on these factors. Merrill wrote in 1968 that "kidney transplantation has become enough of an established procedure so that funds for patient support as a research venture are gradually being withdrawn" (Merrill 1968, p. 63). Walsh based his judgment that kidney transplantation is moving into the realm of "everyday therapy" partly on the grounds that "hitherto, most of this work has been done by the great pioneers in major research centers. Surgeons everywhere are now seeking to emulate the successes of the pioneers" (Walsh 1969, p. 78). In fact, though, Walsh exaggerates in saying that kidney transplantation is being done by "surgeons everywhere." According to a letter from the American College of Surgeons/ National Institutes of Health Organ Transplant Registry in August 1970:

There are 150 institutions performing transplants that are registered. As of now, there are 39 institutions which have performed more than 30 transplants, and 111 which have performed less. This is the basis for determining "large" and "small" centers. There are 54 university-affiliated centers and 19 are clearly not university affiliated [in the United States]. We are less sure of the foreign affiliations, but believe the breakdown is fairly accurate [16 university and 48 non-university-affiliated centers]. Also attached is a list of the chief renal transplant surgeons from the larger centers. The list reads like a *Who's Who* of transplantation.[3]

Many observers have claimed that kidney transplantation is no longer newsworthy because it has been absorbed into regular surgical practice. A particularly eloquent statement to this effect was made by Sir Peter Medawar in 1968:

In the long run, the best quantitative measure of the success of clinical transplantation is the degree to which it does *not* receive publicity, i.e., the degree to which we take its accomplishments for granted. Kidney transplantation is no longer reported in the papers unless some particularly macabre circumstance surrounds the act of grafting. People are beginning to take it for granted. . . .

In other words, it has been almost completely received into the ordinary repertoire of surgical practice. We shall have succeeded with liver and heart transplantations when they too are no longer news, and we all wait impatiently for that day to dawn. [Medawar 1969, pp. 666–67]

Although we agree that publicity might be a telling indicator, our own data do not support the belief that kidney transplantation has receded from attention to the extent that Medawar and others contend. A press clipping service provided us with articles on organ transplantation and artificial organs published in national and local American newspapers from January through May 1969 and January through May 1970. According to our count, 254 articles on renal transplantation appeared in the first period, out of a total of 2,215 clippings received, and in the second period, 219 out of 706 articles dealt with kidney transplants (excluding articles on hemodialysis). Another perspective on the status of kidney transplantation is provided in the final section of the Ninth Report of the Human Renal Transplant Registry, covering the period through 15 April 1971.

Although it is tempting to interpret certain data as showing increasingly successful transplant experience, analysis does not bear this out. There is no statistical difference between the results of patient survival and duration of function of grafts performed in any of the last four years. This fact was noted in the Eighth Report and is still true. It appears, then, that renal transplant results as a whole have reached a plateau of success at this time. [Ninth Report of the Human Renal Transplant Registry. ACS/ NIH Organ Transplant Registry, 1971. Preprint Copy, p. 25]

In trying to sort out and decipher the special phraseology that clinical investigators use to express their appraisal of kidney transplantation, we have concluded that the majority regard this procedure as in an intermediate stage between the poles of human experimentation and established therapy. We would term this a "postexperimental" or "pretherapeutic" phase.

Even a rough consensus on placing kidney transplantation in this middle range, however, has not resolved uncertainty and debate over exactly how experimental or how therapeutic the procedure is, and, concomitantly, on whom it may justifiably be used. A significant development in this continuing discussion has been that some investigators contend that kidney homografts should be applied to patients who are not terminally ill. In this way they are appealing to their colleagues both to acknowledge and to actively usher in a new stage. A prominent advocate of this has been Dr. John P. Merrill:

First of all I believe it is perfectly clear now on the basis of over 2,000 human renal allografts that the two year survival rate particularly for sibling donor recipient pairs justifies kidney transplantation as a feasible procedure at the practical thera-peutic level. The recent results of cadaver transplantation are equal to those for open heart surgery for acquired valvular disease. I think therefore that we may consider as candidates for a renal allograft patients who have not necessarily reached the point of terminal degenerative disease. Under optimum circumstances patients with renal failure should be considered for transplantation earlier than we had previously thought. . . . Furthermore, improvements in the techniques of intermittent hemodialysis for chronic renal failure allow the patient a reasonable alternative even should the transplant fail. Finally, it is evident that a second or third transplant may succeed where a first has failed. [Merrill 1969, p. 162]

In contrast to this position is a relatively "conservative" per-spective on kidney transplantation, weighting more heavily its uncertainties and therapeutic limitations. For instance in 1970 Thomas Starzl felt called upon to assert that he held the same assessment of kidney transplantation as he had in 1965:

At the April, 1965, meeting of the American Surgical Associa-tion, an account was given of the 36 patients of Series 1 who were still alive after followups of one to 2½ years. The chronic survival of so many (56%) recipients from an original group of 64 was an encouraging notion, particularly since it seemed likely that the majority of the homografts were going to continue functioning for a long time. Nevertheless, the opinion was offered that ". . . for the present it would seem most reasonable to regard homotransplantation as an effective, but incompletely characterized, form of palliative therapy."
Although 29 (45.3%) of the original 64 patients in Series 1 remain alive after an additional interval of 5 years, there is no reason now to change the foregoing point of view since late failures have continued to be observed. [Starzl et al. 1970, pp. 456, 460]

By any or all of the indicators that have been employed to evaluate the status of kidney transplantation, cardiac transplanta-tion is in an experimental phase comparable to the "black years" of renal homografts. The survival rate from a heart transplant is very low; it has proved extremely difficult to predict its outcome by criteria such as preoperative morbidity and tissue matching; and it is preponderantly funded through research grants. That heart transplants have been done in many countries and by a large number of surgical teams does not mean that the procedure has become significantly less experimental. For, as we will show more fully in chapter 7, a "bandwagon" phenomenon is involved, and many surgeons have done only one or two transplants. Finally, the coverage of heart transplantation by the press and other mass media has been so voluminous and dramatic that "surgeons and others close to the field of organ transplantation have expressed surprise, and some shock, over the fierce outpouring of public interest it has evoked" (Schmeck 1969, p. 670). We will have occasion to discuss later one of the major causes of this public fascination with cardiac transplantation: the special symbolic meaning of the heart.

To laymen and physicians alike, the most important of these experiment-therapy indicators is the primary measure of "success and failure"—the survival rate. Here is the National Heart Institute's "Summary of heart transplants as of survival September 1, 1970":

Total No. of Transplants 165
    U.S.:   103
    Foreign: 62
Total No. of Recipients: 162
Total No. of Deaths: 140
Number of Survivors: 22
    U.S.:   16
    Foreign: 6
Of Those Recipients Still Surviving:

6 months + : 19	15 months + : 14
7 months + : 19	18 months + : 11
8 months + : 18	21 months + : 10
12 months + : 16	24 months + : 2

The dispute over the status of cardiac transplantation involves several questions: whether it is too experimental to warrant further clinical trials; and if it should continue, at what pace, by whom, and under what conditions it should be done. Virtually no one denies that the surgical techniques for implanting a heart are well developed. At issue is what can be learned about managing rejection and other postoperative complications in the heart transplant patient that cannot be learned in animal studies or from the kidney recipient, for whom dialysis is available should the transplant fail.

The debate that began almost immediately after the first human heart was implanted has involved both oral and printed exchanges that reflect clinical investigators' strong feelings and ideological convictions about their work. These discussions have been reported in lay as well as professional media.

Dr. Christiaan Barnard's first human heart transplant was performed on Mr. Louis Washkansky on 3 December 1967. It immediately sparked a wave of concern and criticism as well as awe and acclaim. In response to some of the more critical reactions, Barnard committed himself to an extreme position in the experiment-therapy controversy: "I wouldn't like to call this operation an experiment—it was treatment of a sick patient. Although Washkansky died, I don't think we have any evidence that transplantation is not good treatment for certain heart diseases" (Quoted in *Time*, 29 Dec. 1967).

Dr. Barnard still ardently believes in the value of cardiac transplantation in "opening up some more months of life to the desperately ill patients on whom we did the procedure" (Barnard, personal interview). But he has somewhat moderated his original stance. For example, in his final summation of the session on 'the pathological findings in patients who have died," at the 1968 Cape Town Heart Transplantation Symposium, Barnard said:

I think this has been a very depressing sort of meeting, but I don't think it has shown anything that we didn't know before we started heart transplantation. It has shown . . . that we must accept heart transplantation as a palliative procedure at the moment, not as a curative procedure. Some of these patients we will keep alive for a few weeks, some for a few months and some for a few years until we can better control the immunologic attack of the recipient on the transplanted organs; so don't go away too depressed. [Shapiro 1969, p. 232]

Although Barnard has conceded that what heart transplantation "has to offer dying patients [is] not a new and healthy life, but only a prolongation of life and alleviation of suffering," he remains convinced that "to curb transplantation at this stage would be to strangle one of the most promising and exciting fronts of medical endeavor." He argues this position in the following way:

Critics complain that manpower and financial expenditures involved in transplants far outweigh the results obtained, and that other medical services have a more urgent and real claim to medical resources. But similar attacks were once leveled by similar critics at open-heart surgery. This criticism is extremely conservative and dangerously shortsighted.

We should note that there are recipients of heart and liver grafts who are in their second post-transplant year—and not without dramatic relief. . . .

To deny medicine its full thrust in this direction would be irresponsibly shortsighted. Indeed, it is difficult not to conclude that any withdrawal from this new frontier would be professionally unethical. [Barnard 1970]

Like Barnard, Dr. Denton Cooley has fervently argued in favor of cardiac transplantation, stressing that "it's done a lot more than lengthening the life of ten or twelve people for a year or more," and he has been preoccupied with "trying to show that the thing we are fighting for is worth fighting for" (Cooley, personal interview). Cooley too has emphasized the therapeutic benefits of the procedure in which he has pioneered. Seven months after human cardiac transplantation began, and after he had performed six such operations, Cooley told a press conference that "cardiac transplantation has reached the point where, if properly performed, it could be considered a therapeutic measure . . . and no longer an investigative procedure" (Quoted in *Montreal Gazette*, 26 July 1968). He expressed much the same opinion, albeit in a more circumspect tone, one month later in a professional paper on his team's heart transplant cases:

Until recently cardiac transplantation in man was considered to be primarily investigational and of limited practical value in treatment of heart disease. Four seriously ill and incapacitated patients underwent cardiac transplantation with restoration of adequate cardiac function and circulation in each. Two patients are alive and apparently well 6 weeks and 3½ weeks, respectively, after operation. . . . This experience suggests that human cardiac transplantation is feasible and deserves further clinical trial. [Cooley et al. 1968, p. 479]

A stand opposite to Cooley's and Barnard's is seen in the experimental heart surgeon who is reluctant to personally engage in cardiac transplantation because he feels it is so experimental that its risks outweigh its benefits and that he can make more meaningful research and therapeutic contributions in other ways. Dr. Dwight E. Harken is one such surgeon:

As we estimate a significant death rate from *biologic barriers* (rejection, lymphatic, and neurogenic factors), we must add the immediate surgical mortality which for properly selected recipients, often with poor lungs, livers, and so forth, would be a 20 per cent mortality, perhaps more. Thus, probable mortality rates, biologic barriers, surgery, and other complications rise to a level *precariously close to the probability* of medical prognostic error for the recipient who is to lose the heart that is currently sustaining his life.

The circumstances have not been defined in this perspective. Heart transplantation in an early experimental prototype form is here. Each man who contemplates entry into the field of cardiac transplants must arrive at his own decision by balancing the use of the considerable resources for a few transplants against his obligation to treat ailing people and extend heart surgery techniques in other ways. So far, I have elected the rehabilitation of a fair number of people while attempting to improve prosthetic valves, coronary circulation, and mechanically assisted circulation. I reserve the right to change tomorrow but today I am proud of our restraint in not performing heart transplantations yesterday. [Harken, in Blumgart 1970, p. 57]

Barnard's response to this point of view was expressed, half humorously, at a panel discussion in which both he and Harken participated: "I think it is very difficult to look into the future [of cardiac transplantation], but one thing I can predict is that in ten years' time, Dr. Harken will be doing heart transplants" (*First Annual Kennedy Symposium* 1968).

Midway between the zeal and activism of Barnard and Cooley and the caution and abstention of Harken lies the restrained, carefully planned way in which Dr. Norman Shumway has committed himself to heart transplantation. Shumway, developer of the surgical techniques for cardiac implants, has a twin perspective: "Heart transplantation is therapeutic from the perspective of the designated recipient. Heart transplantation continues, however, to be a field of clinical investigation from the viewpoint of the medical scientists involved" (Shumway 1969, p. 1033). One of the factors that motivates him to perform this surgery is the feeling that "when you get a very sick patient . . . it is very difficult to withhold something that can be at least attempted" (*First Annual Kennedy Symposium* 1968). At the same time, his involvement in "clinical transplantation of the heart" is what he considers to be the "logical conclusion of many years of intense laboratory research" that he has devoted to this field (*First Annual Kennedy Symposium* 1968). On these dual premises, Shumway has mounted a "*program* or clinical investigation of cardiac transplantation," one that involves "cautious clinical trials" and that has several well-defined objectives:

the evaluation of immediate and late post-transplant hemo-dynamics; the investigation of reinnervation of the homograft; the search for specific and sensitive parameters of homograft rejection; the evaluation of immunosuppressive agents in the control of rejection; and the establishment of criteria of selection of transplant recipients. [Shumway, Stinson, and Dong 1969, p. 739]

By spring 1970, Shumway's program had reached a point where he felt it was possible and responsible to publish an "initial appraisal of the therapeutic value of this procedure for selected patients with advanced heart disease." On the basis of their analysis of the postoperative course of their first twenty patients, the Stanford team arrived at what they termed an "optimistic estimation" of current one-year survival. This appraisal was based in part on a comparison between heart and kidney transplantation.

Despite the small size of this series, however, the current over-all 1 year survival rate of 35 per cent would appear comparable to the present results of cadaver kidney transplantation, as reported through the Kidney Transplant Registry, and significantly exceeds the early results in this field. In addition, our experience compares favorably with the limited trials of liver and lung transplantation which have been reported. The improvement in results suggested by separate analysis of the most recent year's experience, although limited, would tend to confirm these considerations. Indeed, this optimistic estimation of current 1 year survival after cardiac transplantation at 51 per cent closely approaches the results of kidney transplantation in selected series whose data are superior to those noted in the Registry. [Stinson et al. 1970, p. 318]

These are the two major role-positions taken by heart trans-plant surgeons arguing for continuing the clinical application of this procedure: on the one hand a zealous insistence that it is a meliorating, if not curative, treatment for cardiac patients other-wise doomed to die; and on the other the more moderately ex-pressed, but no less passionate, avowal that it is a significant and fruitful form of legitimate clinical investigation. Linking these two postures is a common underlying faith that medical knowledge and therapeutic efficacy eventually will be advanced by the cardiac transplantation trials:

A convincing case can be made . . . that the problem of organ rejection is yielding to concerted attack and that many of the costly and uncertain aspects of transplantation will be steadily reduced as the drawbacks and complexities of this form of treatment yield to further progress. With the advances that seem feasible in the near future, it is safe to anticipate rich rewards for medicine—rewards in knowledge ranging from better cardiac-assist devices to a better definition of possible autoimmune diseases of the myocardium. The early round of heart transplants should be considered a success in that they have provoked the kind of concentrated effort that, in these circumstances, is sure to bring valuable progress. [Stinson et al. 1968, p. 802]

This at once affirmative and hopeful perspective on cardiac transplantation is by no means uniformly shared within the medical profession or among the lay public. Although it "has attracted a degree of interest . . . seldom equalled by any new development in medicine . . . [the] interest has taken the form of a continuing debate and discussion as to the medical, ethical, moral, and legal aspects of heart transplantation" (American Medical Association's . . . statement on heart transplantation 1968). Various medical professional groups have felt obliged to make formal pronouncements on the current status of cardiac transplantation. Among the statements issued have been those of the House of Delegates of the American Medical Association, the American College of Cardiology, the Special Task Force appointed by the National Heart Institute, and the Board of Medicine of the National Academy of Sciences.[4] Some points of consensus emerge from these documents. It is agreed that sufficient "basic and developmental research in the laboratory" has been conducted to warrant cardiac transplantation's "extension to man." It is also contended that "the spectrum of success . . . in human cardiac transplantation . . . ranges from short-term restoration of circulation to complete physical recovery with return to gainful employment in a previously incapacitated patient." It is nevertheless pointed out that although "a qualified physiologic success, limited to restoration of circulatory capacity by the transplanted heart, has been accomplished in more than 90 per cent of patients who have undergone cardiac transplantation . . . the goal of full restoration to a useful and satisfactory life has been achieved for short periods of time in but a few patients." Still, it is contended, "success in human cardiac transplantation has . . . been sufficiently impressive to encourage further trial." However, the admonition is given that "the procedure of total cardiac replacement is so formidable and uncertainties about the duration of life after replacement are so great that physicians may be expected to be conservative about recommending it for an individual patient." For "it cannot as yet be regarded as an accepted form of therapy, even an heroic one. It must be clearly viewed for what it is, a scientific exploration of the unknown, only the very first step of which is the actual surgical feat of transplanting the organ." For this reason, it is maintained, "it may reasonably be assumed that imminent death will be the basic criterion for total cardiac replacement, at least in the near future."

The overall judgment on the current status of cardiac transplantation that these position papers collectively render is that, "the procedure is a scientific investigation and not as yet an accepted form of therapy," and that "the primary justification for this activity in respect to both the donor and recipient is that from the study will come new knowledge of benefit to others in our society." In the light of this view and also in recognition of the fact that "theologians, lawyers, and other public-spirited persons, as well as physicians are discussing with deep concern the many new questions raised by the transplantation of vital organs," what are termed "guidelines" are recommended on matters such as the proper treatment of donors and recipients, the types of medical centers qualified to undertake the operation, and appropriate reporting of a transplantation both in medical journals and in the mass media.

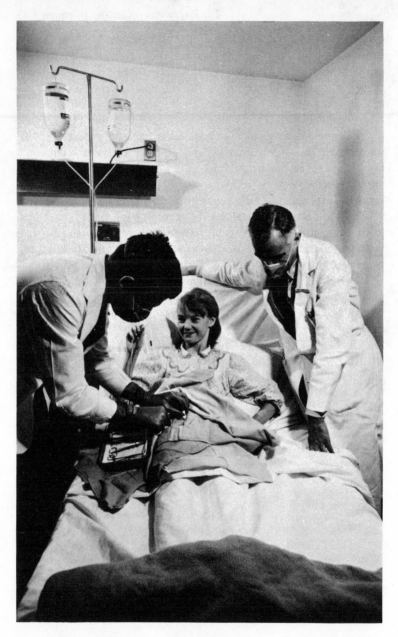

Photograph by Lee W. Henderson

2

The Courage to Fail Ethos

4

The Physician-Investigator and His Patients

The public image of the research physician is that of a cool professional, carrying out his activities with effortless detachment and equanimity. Many people, including medical professionals, believe that because the clinical investigator's patients are also his research subjects, he is less emotionally involved in the doctor-patient relationship than is the "pure clinician." Such onlookers would contend that the "use" of patients as human subjects implies a relatively impersonal, instrumental association.

In their professional publications and utterances, research physicians do little to change this impression. They seldom write or speak in public about the everyday realities of their medical responsibilities or about how they are affected by them. By and large, the closest they come to doing this is to discuss the ethics of human experimentation, where they focus on such abstract issues as the problems of abiding by the principles of informed, voluntary consent and the protection of privacy. Occasionally clinical investigators write post facto accounts of particularly heartening or disheartening periods of work in their research unit (see, for example, Moore 1965; Means 1958; Shorr 1955). Or in the course of a technical exposition they may allude to the many ups and downs through which they, their colleagues, and their patients passed while developing new treatments.

Despite the downplaying of emotion in their published work, our observation and interviewing of research physicians have affirmed our belief that the problems they characteristically face —uncertainty, limitation, and the reconciliation of the experimental and the therapeutic—subject them to considerable strain. The primary reason these aspects of their role are stressful is summarized in the telling phrase: " A great deal of what we know . . . was learned at the expense of this . . . patient" (Scribner 1967, p. 190). The special difficulty of the research physician, distinguishing him from all other scientific investigators, is that the "material" on which he works is the disease-stricken human being. The research physician's patient-subjects are suffering individuals who have come for help with serious, often terminal illnesses that lie outside the easy understanding or control of present-day medicine. Thus he experiences less frequently than other physicians the therapeutic satisfaction of "being able to make patients really well."

The relationship that may exist between the physician-investigator and his patient is epitomized by the eleven-year association between Dr. Belding Scribner, developer of the cannula-shunt apparatus that made chronic hemodialysis feasible, and Mr. Clyde Shields, the first patient on whom this device was tried. In an interview with the *Seattle Times* science editor, published four months after Shields died from a heart attack in March 1971, Scribner highlighted some of the special qualities of their long relationship. He emphasized the desperate nature of Shields's condition when they met; his fortitude, courage, trust, and professional collaboration and expertise; his commitment to the success of the dialysis enterprise as well as to his own survival; his sentimental attachment to the medical team, particularly to his physician and "old friend" Scribner, and to his artificial kidney machine, the "minimonster." Scribner's admiration and affection for Shields are patent in this account, as well as his gratitude to him for all that he and his colleagues were able to "learn on Clyde" and apply to the benefit of other dialysis patients.

Clyde was in and out of the clinic [in 1960]. We knew he was within two or three weeks of death, although he didn't know it. He said later he suspected it. . . .

Clyde was the guy who was there when we were ready, and who needed it most. It was purely an experiment. We had no idea that we would still have Clyde alive a month or even a week later. . . .

It was totally a chance thing that he became our first patient. And that's what made it so great because he turned out to be the ideal patient in dealing with these unknowns and the terrible emotional strain of not knowing what was ahead. He lost all his own kidney function in the spring of 1960, which made him much more prone to complications than the other early patients.

As a consequence, during the course of the first two years, he developed five or six diseases that we now know how to control. But we had to learn on Clyde.

He could instinctively sort out from all his problems the things that were really important to tell us. . . .

We were grappling with what now seems like a terrible technique. But Clyde didn't panic when things went wrong. There was something special about him that is hard to describe.

Time after time he was either the victim of a new problem or the observant patient who put us onto a new solution. For some reason, despite all his suffering, Clyde was very secure throughout. He had confidence that he was going to survive.

In the spring of 1960, he was going blind because of severe high blood pressure that we didn't know how to control at that point. Yet all through this he never showed despair. He just seemed to know we'd find a solution. He had enormous confidence that we'd see him through. [H. Williams 1970]

Research physicians are very much aware of the human consequences of the state of their art, the innovative treatments they administer, and the experiments they conduct. The uncertainty, inadequacy, and fallibility associated with their role are continually personified for them in their patient-subjects, and they are likely to have more intense and, in cases like that of Mr. Shields, more prolonged relationships with them than with "ordinary" patients. The seriousness of their illness and the ever present possibility of their imminent death deeply involve physicians in their care. The oscillations and development of their complex disease states are likely to result in repeated hospitalizations during which they are in daily contact with research physicians. The study units on which they are hospitalized are typically small, so that research physicians give them concentrated investigative and clinical attention. And when their medical conditions permit them to be discharged these patients are closely watched by the same research group, generally through closely spaced outpatient visits.

Research physicians tend to believe that to be too openly expressive about the "human problems" they experience as clinical investigators would be inappropriately "unscientific" and "emotional." Even in the intimate setting of daily meetings with their own teammates, they only occasionally make outright statements about how "disturbing" the special role of the clinical investigator can be: "If you listen for it, you'll hear one or another of us saying, 'How long can I live this laboratory life anyway? I've just got to get back to *real* medicine'!" (Fox 1959, p. 27). As we shall see, a more acceptable way of "sounding off" to one another is through highly patterned in-group joking about the most troubling aspects of their "laboratory life."

Given the informal norms restricting overt, seriously expressed reactions to their role strains, it is surprising how much research physicians reveal about their feelings in their scientific publications. Perhaps they are not conscious of doing so, partly because many of the affect-laden words they use to describe their clinical research have become "standard" in the medical literature. But some of the vocabulary they commonly employ in professional articles and monographs evokes a striking picture of a group of at once expectant and embattled medical men, winning some victories and undergoing many defeats as they grapple with intriguing, elusive, and dangerous unknowns that often threaten the lives of their patient-subjects. For example, the medical publications that we have cited in the three preceding chapters collectively portray the "dark days" and "black years" these physician-authors have known, when the "risk imposed [on patients] is extravagant" or "exorbitant"; "hazards" and "obstacles" that "have to be overcome" are rampant (such as the occurrence of "bizarre organisms . . . in an unexpectedly militant state in the tissues of . . . patients rendered passive by constant immunosuppression"); efforts both to advance knowledge and to help patients are not only "beset with difficulties," but also with "tragedies" and "catastrophes." "Repeated failures" to penetrate the "mysteries" of basic biological mechanisms, to avoid the "striking array of . . . complications" following experimental therapies that are "exceedingly troublesome at best and lethal at worst," and to "improve survival" are "keenly disappointing." The "outlook" is "grim," the "picture . . . dismal," results are "disquieting . . . discouraging . . . bleak." And an "air of hopelessness" prevails in an atmosphere "doomed to failure." The same publications also depict more "encouraging" periods. These are times when "despite the disappointing outcome of [particular] cases," the prospect of "success" seems closer. "Exciting procedures" are being developed, new insights and "breakthroughs" are being attained, and some of the "hurdles of transplantation" are being surmounted. Despite self-admonitions about the importance of "sober deliberation," "prudent consideration," and "avoiding overoptimism," the general feeling is one of "a remarkable change . . . in outlook," so that "the previous air of hopelessness" seems to be "dispelled almost overnight." Through the use of such evocative language, research physicians inadvertently document the heights and depths of their emotional involvement in the gratifications and strains of their work.

It is our impression that although clinical investigators are themselves reluctant to describe in detail what their work is like and how they feel about it, they generally are not resistant when others attempt to do so. In our own experience over the years as participant observers in the "daily round" of a number of such research teams, physicians have reacted positively to our presence and to our interest in their activities and attitudes. Furthermore, when they have heard us speak of our findings, or have read publications based on the research opportunities they provided us, they have usually expressed surprised gratification over being "understood so well." From this we conclude that research physicians are not so much opposed to public expression of the social and psychological aspects of their professional lives as they are normatively inhibited from personally communicating this information. They consider such communication not only beyond their own competence, but also unseemly behavior for physician-investigators who are supposed to be "objective," "composed," and relatively unconcerned about themselves.

One Recipient: The Case of Mr. K

The case of Mr. K, a kidney recipient, provides a glimpse of the concrete problems faced by research physicians working with transplant patients.

On 10 March 1969, Mr. K, a thirty-year-old salesman with a wife and child, received a renal transplant from an unrelated cadaver donor. The kidney came from a fifty-seven-year-old man who had been found on the street by police and brought to the emergency ward of University Hospital in a comatose state owing to a major head injury. He received intensive treatment with blood, epinephrine, steroids and antibiotics, but despite all efforts to revive him, he continued to be without reflexes and to make no spontaneous movements. Nor could spontaneous respiration be started. Repeated electroencephalograms (graphic recordings of the electrical currents developed in the cortex by brain action) showed "flat" brain waves. On the basis of these criteria physicians determined that he exhibited the characteristics of a permanently nonfunctioning brain and that "brain death" had occurred. Permission was obtained from his family to remove his kidneys for transplantation. Although the match between the donor (who was of blood group O+), and Mr. K (blood group B+) was not optimal, Mr. K became the recipient of one of these kidneys. From 10 March through 15 March, Mr. K's "clinical course" was described as "very good," and after surgery his blood pressure seemed to be better controlled without hypertensive drugs.

However, a few days after this encouraging outcome had been recorded—eight days posttransplant—Mr. K began to show signs of a rejection reaction. He ran a low-grade fever for several days, his urine output decreased, and his BUN (blood-urea-nitrogen level) rose. His steroid dosage was increased to "combat" this reaction. When this latest turn of events in Mr. K's condition was discussed by the transplant group, Dr. S, a surgeon and head of the team, expressed considerable "disappointment" over the fact that the ALS given to Mr. K had not succeeded in preventing this rejection episode. It suggested two possibilities to him, he said: in the future, the team ought not to carry out a cadaver transplant unless the tissue match was somewhat better than Mr. K's had been, or higher doses of ALS might be indicated, or both. And yet, Dr. S pointed out, increasing Mr. K's dosage of ALS might well prove more dangerous than the rejection reaction itself. Dr. T, an internist, reminded the group that Mr. K had already experienced at least four different sorts of reactions "following ALS, but not necessarily due to ALS." These included shaking chills on several occasions, diaphoresis (especially profuse perspiration), low back pain, and hives. The team could only speculate on the extent to which physiological and biochemical factors contributed to these reactions and to what degree psychological factors might have played a role. There was some talk about doing a kidney biopsy on Mr. K (removing a small amount of tissue from his kidney and examining it under the microscope), because it was virtually the only way to determine whether a rejection reaction was in fact taking place. No decision was made in this regard.

With the help of extra prednisone, Mr. K recovered so rapidly from his rejection episode that he was discharged from the hospital on 27 March. He was seen on a weekly outpatient basis in the transplant clinic. His condition remained stable with normal kidney function. By 9 April, he had been taken off ALS completely, and his prednisone dosage had been lowered. He was described by Dr. S as "bouncing around with his salesmen friends, and eager to get back to work." Before he returned home from his outpatient checkup on this particular day, Mr. K paid a surprise visit to the meeting held every morning by the transplant team. Everyone present showed great pleasure and a certain pride in "how well he looked, how good his color seemed to be, how alert he seemed, and how emotionally stable."

Three weeks later, Mr. K's entire medical picture had changed for the worse. At the usual morning transplant rounds, Dr. C, the team's chief renologist, bluntly declared that Mr. K was now "the most seriously ill patient" the group was treating. He had been hospitalized again because of a falling white blood count, the development of diabetes, and skin lesions possibly caused by *Staphylococcus aureus*. Over the past 36 hours his condition had become "considerably worse," accompanied by the stoppage of urine output and a marked increase in abdominal tension. Two tentative diagnoses were made: a rejection reaction and a gram-negative septicemia (a septic infection caused by a bacterium that becomes decolorized by alcohol when Gram's method is used to stain it). Treatment was initiated, consisting primarily of administering antibiotics and increasing his dosage of steroids. Dr. C reported the next morning that Mr. K was improved: he was "alert" and his urine output was better, though he still had muscle tenderness. "This is a remarkable tribute to the magic bullet of chemotherapy. I think we have made a shoestring catch with him." In the lengthy discussion about Mr. K's condition that followed, team members agreed that one of the primary factors that had made him susceptible to infection was that his immunosuppressive therapy, most particularly the Imuran he was receiving, had drastically reduced the number of leukocytes in his blood. They expressed "cautious optimism" about his prognosis.

Mr. K continued to improve over the next two weeks. The physicians of the transplant team were "relieved" and went so far as to say that he could probably go home as soon as his skin lesions started to heal. The group felt relaxed enough to admit that although Mr. K's infection "looked and still looks like a gram-negative sepsis, we never got a gram-negative culture from him, and we're still not really sure what caused his infection."

This encouraging interlude of respite did not last long. When the transplant team met on 28 May, a rapidly dying Mr. K was the chief subject of their anxious and troubled conference. Dr. N, the senior surgical resident, reported that Mr. K had developed a lung lesion, which was getting progressively larger and seemed to be unresponsive to all treatment. Mr. K was much weaker, and "obviously losing ground." His BUN and creatinine levels had risen sharply, and the night before his white blood count had been only 1,300. His temperature had spiked to 104 degrees, but came down after he received a new antibiotic. With bitterly ironic humor, Dr. N commented that this was probably "lysis (gradual abatement of the symptoms of a disease) due to getting his white blood count taken," rather than from

the drug therapy he was receiving. The group was particularly
concerned about the fact that Mr. K's lung lesion seemed to be
due to a pseudomonas bacteria. A patient on the burn unit of the
hospital had died of pseudomonas pneumonia the week before,
and it was suspected that this bacteria had also been responsible
for the infection from which Mr. E, another posttransplant
patient, had died several weeks before. The worried remark
was made that Mr. K's course seemed to be "closely mimicking"
Mr. E's. Dr. C interjected the macabre observation that the
second night after Mr. K's most recent readmission to the
hospital, "just when Mr. E was beginning to go down the slot,"
Mr. K's blood pressure had suddenly dropped, and he became
"cold and clammy" too. The group felt that there was just enough
circumstantial evidence to suggest that Mr. K had contracted a
hospital-borne infection, and a "deadly" one at that. Dr. N
suggested that if Mr. K did not respond to chemotherapy, a
surgical excision of his lesion should be considered; for if nothing
effective was done for him soon, his lesion would rapidly get
bigger, he would develop septicemia, and he would die. Dr. S
was concerned about the dangers of a surgical approach. If in the
course of surgery the contents of Mr. K's lung lesion spilled
into the pleural space, he said, this could be lethal in a man with
virtually no white blood cells for defense. He suggested that an
alternative procedure might be to try and drain Mr. K's chest.
But it was quickly pointed out to him that there was really no
fluid to draw out; the lesion seemed to be completely filled with
air. In a distressed and stymied tone of voice, Dr. S replied,
"Well, I suppose in a situation like this, if we've tried everything
else, we step off into the unknown, because probably we'll be no
worse off." At this point, Dr. R, another surgeon, spoke up.
"I may have a minority viewpoint," he said, "but I think we
should excise the lesion, and the sooner the better." He likened
the drug regimen Mr. K was receiving to "trying to treat
gangrene with topical antibiotics. If we don't treat him rapidly,"
Dr. R concluded, "we'll soon see a chest plate like the one
Mr. E had a few hours before he . . . "—here Dr. R paused,
then finally added the word "expired." Dr. S promptly agreed
with Dr. R. He ruefully added, "There just seems to be nothing
going for him, with a pseudomonas infection, the thin walls of
his lesion, a hematocrit of 19, on steroids, and a very low blood
count. There aren't too many around like him!" Dr. C admitted
that "at this stage of the game, I guess I have the attitude of a
medical man who has failed. I see surgery as the great white
hope. Basically," he mused, "there is no one more aggressive
for surgery than a medical man who has failed in all of his
treatments." Mr. K's condition is "tragic," Dr. S lamented, and
all the more so "because his kidney is so good." Dr. N now
expressed personal guilt, as well as regret over not having treated

Mr. K earlier, when he first came into the hospital and was still in an afebrile condition. "We made a mistake." Dr. G, an expert in infectious disease, tried to allay Dr. N's feelings on this matter. "We just don't know enough about pseudomonas and drugs with which to treat it," he said. He added that the appropriate drugs that are available at this time are all so toxic that they present a host of other serious problems. Dr. N, unbudging and inconsolable, stood his ground: "When we see pseudomonas, under any condition, we should treat it, no matter what the circumstances."

At the end of the meeting, the group decided to continue drug therapy for another 24 to 48 hours, and if there was no improvement in Mr. K's condition, to excise his lung lesion. They also decided to inform Mrs. K of the gravity of her husband's condition.

Mr. K died from his massive infection before the transplant team had a chance to make a last, desperate surgical effort to "save him."

Many Recipients: Western Medical Center

It is not an exaggeration to say that one case like that of Mr. K could easily consume the major part of a transplant team's emotional as well as intellectual and physical energy. But at the same time that a Mr. K is passing from one phase of his illness to another, such a team is caring for many other transplant patients. Some of them, like Mr. E, may be going downhill; others may have an ambulatory, outpatient relationship with the team. Yet no matter how encouraging the progress of a transplant patient may be, most will undergo numerous rejection reactions; all (except those few who have received a kidney from an identical twin) eventually will reject the donated organ; every one will suffer from some adverse side effects of immunosuppressive therapy; many will have recurrent symptoms of their underlying disease; and more than a few will have difficulty in coping with psychological and social problems that serious illness and a transplant have amplified.

Physicians keep a close watch over all their transplant patients —chiefly for these clinical reasons but also for followup research. For as long as the transplant recipient lives, both he and his physicians must bear the emotionally draining and time-consuming burden of constant surveillance of his condition. During one morning at the post-renal-transplant clinic of Western Medical Center, for example, we observed members of the transplant unit grappling with the wide array of problems presented by twenty-two patients whom they examined and whose cases they then met to discuss.

The patients' most common medical difficulties involved the threat of rejection, a range of complications associated with their immunosuppressive medications, such as infections, ALG reactions (including a possible de novo malignancy), and the effects of steroids on their weight and facial appearance. Although the changes in the recipients' appearance, such as the development of a moon face, often were the least serious of their problems medically, they seemed to be particularly disturbing both to the patients and to their physicians.

In many cases, the physicians frankly admitted that they could not pinpoint the cause of their patients' difficulties or prescribe a remedy for them. Of Mrs. R's continued complaints of malaise and weakness Dr. W could only say: "She just looks and feels like she has the blahs. I don't know how much of it is due to her medical condition, to the side effects of her drugs, or to the demands made on her as a forty-one-year-old wife and the mother of six children." When one physician rhetorically asked why seventeen-year-old John J, nineteen months after his transplant, had a constantly elevated temperature, another physician ritualistically intoned, "We don't know."

The problems of many patients were as much psychological and social as medical. In addition to handling Mrs. K's diabetes and joint pains, her physicians and social worker had to consider that she had "experienced overwhelming marital problems since her transplant a year ago and had already made one attempt to commit suicide." Twenty-five-year-old Mrs. G, who had a cadaver transplant four years before, became pregnant. After much soul-searching, she decided that in the light of her medical condition she should have a therapeutic abortion. Although the abortion was physically uneventful, it had had severe psychological repercussions from which she had not yet fully recovered. Dr. A said that she was "still in a state of mild depression"; Dr. C jokingly suggested that Mrs. G be reinforced in her decision and given emotional support "by telling her that her kidneys will come back since the abortion has taken place."

The complications presented by child recipients are particularly difficult and painful for a medical team. The retarding effects of steroid therapy on a child's growth and development and on his weight and appearance, for example, produce psychological and social stresses that the physicians can do little to resolve. Jimmy H, a fourteen-year-old boy, seemed to be "doing well medically." "But," his physician reported, turning to the team's social worker for counsel, "he's an extremely small boy for his age, with a high, squeaky voice. He's the star pitcher for his school's baseball team. But he's terribly upset because he's much smaller than his classmates and his voice hasn't changed."

The Cadaver Donor: Mark's Case

The impersonal professional vocabulary that members of a transplant team generally employ in their formal accounts of the donation-recipient process mutes the inherent emotionality of what actually takes place.

Cardiac donors used at Stanford have most often been emergency cases receiving their initial medical care at another hospital. . . . The patient (possible donor) is brought to the emergency room of that hospital critically ill. The family is informed within a limited amount of time that there is no hope for the patient's survival—or family members may take this presumption independently. . . . Serious thought about donorship usually begins slightly following the impact of pending death. Although family members still must struggle with their decision about donating, little question typically exists for them that the potential donor is dying or dead. . . .
Stanford transplant team members seek to develop or reinforce this feeling by trying to separate the pronouncement of death from the decision for donorship (the determination and pronouncement of brain death is made by three physicians who have no connection with the transplant team); by offering help to the donor family in dealing with the death and grief process; and by immediate exploration of signs that the family might be thinking of the recipient as a substitute family member (the latter is always discouraged).
If the family decides that the patient is to be used as a donor, good-byes are essentially said at that time. If the donor is at another hospital, the body is then brought to Stanford, but the family rarely accompanies it. If the donor is at Stanford, the family typically leaves some time prior to transplantation.
Although the family has contact with the transplant surgeon and social worker, the family's energy is directed primarily toward coping with the death and funeral arrangements. Transplantation occurs within hours after the decision is made. [Christopherson and Lunde 1971*a*, pp. 34–35]

The use of such uncharged vocabulary meets the norms of objective, dignified medical reporting. It also serves the more latent function of encouraging transplanters to conceptualize what they are doing, to themselves as well as to others, in terms that enhance their equanimity in the at once life-saving and death-ridden situation in which they function. Hidden behind the carefully controlled presentation is the highly stressful affective reality of what the members of a medical team (nurses and social workers as well as physicians) actually experience when they undertake responsibility for a transplant.

The protective screen of professionalism lifted for us one weekend in February. It began when the chief social worker of a transplant group received a telephone call in the midst of a dinner party, informing her that a prospective heart donor for Mr. Olaf L had just been admitted to the University Medical Center. Over the next twenty-four hours we shared the physical and emotional demands that preparing for and performing a cadaver transplant make on medical professionals, as well as on the patient-recipient, his family, and the relatives of the donor.

On a Saturday night in February, twenty-six-year-old Mark J was brought to the emergency room of a local hospital after a serious motorcycle accident. Mark was conscious, but agitated and confused, when he entered the hospital, and he soon lapsed into a comatose state. Surgeons performed a craniotomy to try to relieve the pressure on his brain, but he did not recover consciousness. He required artificial respiration, was unresponsive to stimuli, and showed a flat EEG tracing. All signs indicated massive brain stem damage. On Sunday night, with the permission of his next of kin, Mark was transferred to the nearby University Medical Center as a possible cadaver organ donor.

Several kidney patients were awaiting cadaver transplants at the Medical Center. In addition, the cardiac transplant team was ready to operate on Olaf L as soon as a suitable cadaver heart became available. Miss A, the transplant team's chief social worker, was called at her home Sunday night, shortly after Mark's admission, to alert her that a prospective donor had been admitted to the hospital.

At 11 P.M. that Sunday, Mark L was pronounced dead by a neurologist unaffiliated with the transplant team. Miss A later told us that this neurologist "tends to be skeptical and uncomfortable about heart transplants. I think this is a positive control over the possible tendency of physicians to declare a patient dead when they know that someone is awaiting a transplant from him." As soon as Mark's brain death had been pronounced, a cardiologist-member of the transplant team began a night-long vigil over his body in the intensive care unit, keeping his heart beating by mechanical means until the transplant surgeons were ready to excise it and place it in Olaf L's chest.

We arrived at the Medical Center at 9 A.M. Monday, with Miss A. Other members of the renal and cardiac transplant teams had been there for hours, preparing for the three transplants that would take place that day. Mark J, we learned, was to be a multiple organ donor: both kidneys, as well as his heart, were to be transplanted. The renal transplant team told us that the transplant probably would not take place before 11 A.M. because Mark's organs could not be removed until the two kidney recipients had been adequately dialyzed. Although Mark's heart would be removed before his kidneys, Dr. Y explained, the multiple transplant procedure involved "split-second timing" to ensure that the organs would retain maximum viability. As Dr. Y and his colleagues left the nursing station we heard him ask, "Who's going to take the heart out?"

We returned to Miss A's office, where she began trying to reach members of Mark's family by telephone. After failing to reach Mark's stepfather, she called his sister Susan, a young single girl with whom Mark had been living before his death. Both Mark and Susan, Miss A told us, were estranged from their family, and Mark had spent most of his time with friends in his motorcycle gang. Miss A had a brief conversation with Susan, who was "very emotional" about her brother's death and his role as an organ donor. Moments after their talk ended, Susan called Miss A back to ask about funeral arrangements for Mark, wondering whether she would have to make the arrangements or whether it would be handled by other family members or by his motorcycle gang.

Miss A then took us to the intensive care room, where the potential recipients of Mark's kidneys were completing their dialyses. The husband of one recipient was standing by her bed, watching her undergo these final preparations for what was to be her second transplant. "If I'd gone through fifteen years of suffering like my wife has," he told us, "I'd rather be dead than have to face another transplant. But if there's any justice in such things, my wife should do well this time." On an adjacent bed lay the second recipient. His arm was bleeding profusely, and he was thrashing agitatedly on the bed. The renal transplant team, we were told, had debated at length about accepting him as a transplant recipient, in part because he had been a heroin addict.

It was now early afternoon, and Miss A was paged by the main reception desk. The receptionist said that a young man who identified himself as Mark's brother urgently wanted to talk to her. We accompanied her downstairs to greet Joe, a tall, lanky boy in his early twenties, with long, neatly combed hair, dressed in slacks and a colorful sports shirt. With him was another boy, similarly dressed and wearing one small gold earring and a blue stocking cap. Joe explained that he was Mark's "motorcycle-gang brother," not his sibling. He had rushed to the hospital as soon as he learned about Mark's accident, and until Miss A talked with him he knew nothing about Mark's being a cadaver donor. He pleaded several times to be allowed to see his brother. She gently explained that this would be impossible, since Mark was now in an operating room and that after his heart and kidneys had been removed his body would be sent to the coroner for autopsy, a legal requirement when a person dies in an accident. Joe several times requested reassurance that everything possible had been done to keep his brother alive and asked exactly when he had been pronounced dead. Miss A explained in detail the process by which the medical team gradually and reluctantly decides that nothing more can be done for a patient like Mark. Both Joe and his companion were deeply moved and grief-stricken as they talked with Miss A, although they kept their composure throughout the interview and indicated their sympathy for her difficult job of dealing with the bereaved family. During the conversation, Joe and his friend indicated that they, rather than Mark's biological family, would probably want to arrange his funeral. Saddened, stunned, but still dignified, the two young men thanked Miss A and departed, saying they would go to Susan's house to see if they could help her.

At 3:30 P.M. Miss A called the hospital's publicity office to inform them officially that the heart and kidney transplants were in progress. She told them that the family of the heart recipient, Olaf L, had requested as little publicity as possible, but that

Mark's family wished to have the fact that they had offered his organs mentioned at least in the local paper.

Throughout the day, we repeatedly saw Mr. L's wife and mother, seated in the corridor outside the surgical wing waiting for news of the operation. Miss A stopped to talk with them each time we passed by, telling them various details of what they should expect once Mr. L returned from the operating room. Earlier in the day, before Mr. L was taken to surgery, we had visited his room briefly and met his mother, wife, and personal physician. Mr. L looked pale and drawn, but his manner was cheerful and expectant. Mr. L's physician was permitted to be in the operating room during the transplant, and at the end of the day, around 5 P.M., we found him sitting in the main nursing station of the intensive care unit looking weary but relieved that Mr. L had successfully completed surgery.

Mr. L's wife and mother were also waiting outside the intensive care unit where Mr. L had been brought after surgery. Both women had carefully controlled their emotions throughout the day, although they were close to tears. They now thanked Miss A repeatedly for her "goodness" to them during the long day, for spending so much time with them and briefing them so carefully on how Mr. L would look when he emerged from the operating room. Mrs. L asked whether she would be allowed to hold her husband's hand when she visited him in the intensive care unit "because," she explained, "I'm a toucher."

As the day ended, we made rounds with the kidney team and Miss A, visiting patients in their rooms on the clinical research unit and in the intensive care unit. The recipients of Mark's kidneys, recuperating from surgery in the intensive care unit were "doing well." The almost tearful husband of the woman who had received a kidney from Mark was standing close to her bed, holding her hand tightly and now looking not at all ambivalent about his wife's transplant. The renal team was exhausted. They had done three transplants in one day and were also handling a large caseload of critically ill pre- and post-transplant patients.

We left the Medical Center about 7 P.M., weary and emotionally drained. Two images continued to haunt us: Mark J lying in the intensive care room attended by nurses, though officially dead; and the face of his brother Joe when he was informed that Mark was lying on the operating table having his heart removed so that a fifty-one-year-old salesman might live.

How Research Physicians Cope with Strain

The clinical research in which the physician members of a transplant team are engaged is one of their primary means of coping with the uncertainty and therapeutic limitation that their patients continually present. Although advances in medical knowledge and technique do not typically occur in giant steps, the organized process of searching is for most research physicians an effective mode of doing something about those problems. It is a pragmatic commitment that is in part an act of faith. "One of the most important defenses in working with an experimental team is that of relying, when all else fails, upon 'science' and 'research.' A key part of the ritual when a patient dies is for the family to say, 'But did you learn from this? Was science advanced?' And the team replies, 'Yes, we learned a great deal. Future lives will be spared because of it'" (Christopherson 1971b).

Transplanters also find compensation for what they do not know and cannot offer their patients in the exhilarating challenge of moving beyond what is comfortably established in medicine. Dr. Eugene Dong, a cardiovascular surgeon on Shumway's heart transplant team has said with satisfaction, "I've done no routine open-heart work in six years." Characterizing cardiac transplants as "routine miracles," he says that when they become a firmly institutionalized, standard procedure he will probably "go on to something else" (Quoted in Astor 1970, p. 43). For many of the physicians involved in the transplant endeavor, the search for the unprecedented, the extraordinary, the still undiscovered or untried is closely associated with the desire to achieve more than ordinary professional status and recognition. This kind of ambition to achieve a great "first" helps galvanize transplant physicians to move forward with their work and to persist in spite of stress.

Transplant physicians derive a great deal of support from each other, as well as from their relationship to nonphysicians on the transplantation team. That transplanters may seek to establish what Gerald Holton has termed "companionship with a team" does not imply that they never disagree or work at cross-purposes

(Holton 1970, p. 933). In chapter 6 we will explore the confrontation between surgeons and internists that occurred at the Montreal Heart Institute, and analyze the moratorium that eventually resulted from it. In chapter 7, "The Case of the Artificial Heart," we will document a dramatic conflict between two heart transplanters in Houston, Texas, and trace its far-reaching implications. But by and large the members of a transplant unit share the demands, satisfactions, and frustrations of their daily activities, with the demonstrable mood swings and the ebb and flow of gallows humor that punctuate the group conferences and rounds we have recorded here.

The characteristic joking of transplant physicians turns primarily around their uncertainties, limitations, and experiment-therapy dilemmas. Laughing at their scientific and therapeutic inadequacies, at those aspects of their patients' predicaments that epitomize what medicine does not yet know and cannot do for them, and at their own chagrin at not being "a bunch of Sir Galahads" who can "rescue," "save," or "cure" helps physicians to come to terms with these stresses. Their humor is at once counterphobic, impious, defiant, and cathartic. It enables them to express a wide range of what they would consider negative emotions—anxiety, guilt, disappointment, anger, grief—in a way the group can accept. The jokes they make not only are self-mocking, they also affirm what these physicians believe clinical investigation ideally ought to do and someday will. Nowhere is this more evident than in the recurrent tendency of transplant physicians to use "game of chance" vocabulary when talking of their research or their patients' prognoses. When they refer to an experiment as "quite a gamble," for example, speak of "ten-strike" findings, or of making a "shoestring catch," they are using the same genre of humor. By comparing their professional activities to a gambling or sports event, they express the degree of uncertainty, unpredictability, and risk-taking that they feel characterizes their work; they lightly ridicule their efforts to be scientific and therapeutic under these circumstances; and they assert their sportsmanlike determination not to abandon the "game," but to persist and try to "win" it.

"Celebrating" the Patient: The Case of Victor Y

Finally, as we have already implied, the relationship that transplant physicians and their colleagues tend to establish with their patient-subjects provides them with certain kinds of support, gratification, and meaning. Transplant physicians, like clinical investigators more generally, are inclined to treat their patients as valued collaborators and colleagues, "friends," and "members of the family." They draw close to them, and, in the words of one physician, "celebrate" them in numerous ways.

Victor Y, a sixteen-year-old boy with terminal heart disease, came to the United States from Central Europe, to have Dr. W perform heart surgery on him. He underwent a cardiac transplantation, after which he was hospitalized for many months. When he was discharged from the hospital, he made frequent visits to the outpatient clinic, until the transplant team felt that he was sufficiently recovered to return to his country. During his stay in the hospital Victor, like many other cardiac surgery patients, was regularly permitted to spend time in the "dome" of the surgical amphitheater, watching Dr. W carry out heart operations. When he became an outpatient, members of the transplant team did such things as accompany him to a parents' evening at the school he was temporarily attending and take him to football games. When the staff gave Victor a party for his seventeenth birthday, he announced that he now had two birthdays to celebrate—his own and that of his heart. When he returned to his own country patients and staff together gave him a farewell party, complete with a cake and so many gifts that his baggage was four times overweight at the airport. His most prized gift was a handsome new coat, from Dr. W. At the airport, Victor was interviewed by TV newscasters. He gave them a very informative interview, replete with medical details. At the end of the interview he thanked his surgeon, the hospital staff, and the people of the city of X for all they had done. "My heart is now American," he declared. Before he boarded the plane, he gave his guitar to Dr. W's chief nurse, saying: "Don't ruin it; I plan to come back and play it." He also invited her to visit his country. "If I'm not there, come anyway," he insisted, referring for the first time to the eventuality of his death.

In certain respects, the case of Victor Y is special. Not only was he particularly young, but he also underwent this still dramatic operation in a foreign country, far away from his family and friends. For these reasons, and because of his engaging personality, he may have received particular attention and affection not accorded to every recipient. ("He was one of the joys of my life," said a nurse who felt very close to him. "There's a vacant spot that we need to fill now that he's home.") However, by and large, in the transplant situation exceptionally close personal and professional relations develop between patients, physicians, and the core members of the medical team. Here is the way Barnard wrote about his first heart recipient:

Shortly before noon I dropped in to see Louis [Washkansky]. I had come to know him in a way that had never happened with other patients. He had been there longer than usual, and our concentrated care had brought us into unusually close contact. As a result, he had become a friend as well as a patient. He was rough, an uncut diamond—and very real. Above all else he wanted no pity. As death was closing in on him, he gave no quarter—fighting back with growing impatience, generally directed at us. Every day he gave the same ultimatum. If we did not get him a donor he was going to get up and go home. He could no longer stand on his left leg nor even breathe while lying on his back, but this did not prevent him from threatening us with a walkout. [Barnard and Pepper 1969, p. 268]

Transplant patients come to be viewed as esteemed and heroic companions in a perilous but promising group endeavor that makes "front-line" kindred of all participants. They are accorded special considerations not usually granted "ordinary" hospital patients. Transplanters involve them, almost as professional peers, in the process of their diagnosis, therapy, prognosis, and clinical investigation. The opportunity that Victor Y was given to observe Dr. W at work in the operating room is only one example of such treatment. More common is the inclination of the team to give transplant patients a great deal of technical information about their disorders and the experiments in which they take part, as if they were working members of the medical group.

Shared "awareness of impending death" (Christopherson and Lunde 1971c, p. 40) also tends to increase the communication between the transplant team and patients (and family members) as well as to intensify the relationship between them. At Stanford, for example, "open discussion of death" with candidates for heart transplants and their relatives has been "encouraged and aided by team members for several reasons":

It helped to release the emotional energy of key family members for use in coping with the stresses of transplantation rather than in protecting tenuous patterns of denial; it helped family members continue their grief work if a patient died relatively soon after transplantation; it helped create an atmosphere of frankness about the transplant which included family members as well as patients; and it reflected our concern that the concept of

informed consent in clinical investigation be fulfilled. [Christo-
pherson and Lunde 1971c, p. 40]

Whenever a "fellow survivor" of a heart transplant has died, the
members of this transplant team have tried to notify other patients of the death before public announcement was made and to
talk over the causes and implications of the event with them.

Transplant physicians "celebrate" these patient-subjects they
know so well in many ways. They are treated as "stars" in the
innumerable conferences, rounds, and meetings at which the team
presents them to other physicians and medical professionals. They
appear as key cases in papers, articles, and monographs. They
are often told of their "appearance in print" in medical publications and thanked by the physician-authors for their "cooperation" and "collaboration" in the procedures and studies reported.
Transplant patients, especially those who receive heart implants,
are both privately and publicly extolled by physicians and their
colleagues for their outstanding "courage," "dynamism," and
"zest for life." In their tributes, medical professionals acknowledge that these particular attitudes and character traits provide
the team with the emotional support, as well as the ethical
legitimation, that they feel they need to conduct human transplants:

I'm enclosing a photocopy of a newspaper article on our latest
[heart] transplant patient which I think helps symbolize the kind
of person who wants a transplant and is able to handle it well.
. . . His World War II experiences, and those during the Korean
War when he was a B-52 bomber pilot give you a picture of
this well-integrated, daring, involved-with-life man who runs
great risks, and yet has never lost a challenge, and has great
confidence in himself. It would be inconceivable to him just to lie
down and die when there's another option available, and yet
he's not as "afraid" of dying as the average person. . . . He's a
complex sort of "historical" man, for whom this heart transplant
is almost an inexorable result of his previous life style. While
not all patients are this dramatic, all but about five (of twenty-
five) do meet the pattern in some way. [L. K. Christopherson
personal communication]

Because the recipients of organ transplants are "newsworthy,"
the mass media provide physicians with another way to call public
attention to these patients. Finally, as the case of Victor Y sug-

gests, the transplant team has a tendency to celebrate patients in an at once more literal and ceremonial manner. They give parties to mark rites of passage such as their birthdays, the anniversaries of their transplants, and their forthcoming discharge from the hospital.

As was already indicated, these distinctive features of the transplant team's relationship with patients are manifestly connected with their longer and more concentrated care, the proximity of death, and a collective determination to fight back. They are also associated with the ethical and pragmatic reasons why physicians feel that gravely ill patients who undergo an experimental procedure of the magnitude of an organ transplant must be as knowledgeable as possible about the nature of their illness, its probable outcome, alternative modes of treatment, and the potential benefits, risks, and discomforts of whatever tests, studies, or innovational therapy to which they submit. Conferring with patients and instructing them is essential to obtaining the kind of "informed, voluntary consent" that is mandatory for any experimentation with human subjects and to making patients sufficiently competent and motivated to care intelligently for their complex disease states.

Treating their patients as personal associates and professional colleagues, and according them special recognition and privilege, seems to have other, latent functions. It helps members of the transplant team to "feel better" about the adverse clinical implications of their uncertainty, therapeutic limitations, and experiment-therapy dilemmas. By involving their patients so totally and equally in their work, transplant physicians share the heavy burden of responsibility with them. By honoring them, they offer patients symbolic compensation for their suffering and for medicine's current inability to dispel it. And through their frequent party-ceremonies they thank patients for the ways their sheer survival has endowed the transplant undertaking with meaning and wish them Godspeed.

5

The Heart Transplant Moratorium

A clinical moratorium is the suspension of the use of a still experimental procedure on patients, which may last for weeks, months, or years. Moratoriums have occurred repeatedly in the history of therapeutic innovations. Typically, a moratorium takes place when the uncertainties and risks of a new treatment become starkly apparent and the patient mortality rate seems unbearable or unjustifiable. Pressure for a moratorium can come from physician-investigators' own reactions to the situation, from their colleagues, from the institution in which they work, or from patients and their families.

In this chapter we examine the course of human cardiac transplantation between December 1967 and the fall of 1970. During the first three years of cardiac transplantation, controversy over whether the procedure was developed enough to use on patients was repeatedly accompanied by the question whether a moratorium on heart transplants had already occurred. Both medical professionals and laymen seemed uncertain whether a moratorium meant the total cessation of human trials or if a slowdown or temporary halt in clinical application was also a moratorium.[1] In our judgment, the progressive decline in the number of cardiac transplants performed between December 1967 and the fall of 1970 constituted a clinical moratorium.

Heart transplantation in the first three years after Christiaan Barnard performed the "miracle at Cape Town" can be divided into four periods. (1) 1968 was heralded by the mass media as the "Year of the Transplant," when 105 were performed. (The total performed between 1968 and November 1970 was 166.) In November 1968, 26 operations were done, making this the peak month for heart transplants. (2) In January 1969 the Montreal Heart Institute decided to suspend cardiac transplantation. This helped bring about widespread discussion on whether a more general moratorium ought to be called. (3) By spring/summer 1969 the first enthusiasm over the promise of cardiac implantation had cooled, and those in the field were admitting to a "guarded outlook" about its present uses and future course. This was reflected by the decrease in the number of heart transplants performed per month. (4) Throughout 1970 the slowdown continued. It was now generally acknowledged by the profession and was generally referred to as a moratorium; the benefits and problems of the procedure were discussed with less impassioned rhetoric. Cardiac transplants were not as extensively covered by the press as in "Year One," and the kind of story that attracted special journalistic attention was any "expert" statement suggesting that an overall moratorium was occurring. However, as the third year drew to an end attention was focused on patients who had survived cardiac transplants, especially those who had lived for as long as two years. And several transplanters publicly predicted that there would be a heart transplant renaissance in Year Four.

Phase 1. Years of quiet, intensive laboratory research preceded the first human-to-human clinical transplants in 1967. The move to patient trials was presaged on 23 January 1964, when Dr. James Hardy at the University of Mississippi Medical Center transplanted a chimpanzee heart into a patient. The recipient, a sixty-eight-year-old man, died two hours after surgery because the implanted heart was too small to pump an adequate supply of blood.

Norman Shumway has written that "not until each of [three crucial] problems was solved could human application be suggested even for the sickest patient" (Shumway 1969, p. 739). A surgical method that permitted consistent survival of the animal recipient had to be perfected. The performance characteristics of the transplanted heart, functioning without its normal nerve supply, had to be documented. And "successful control" of rejection had to be demonstrated by "long-term" survival of laboratory animals. These problems were judged to be at least partially resolved by 1960, 1964, and 1965 respectively. The hundreds of animal transplants done at Stanford, for example, had produced an "early survival" rate in which 85 percent of the dog recipients lived for 4 to 21 days, a figure that Shumway and his colleagues believed warranted the move from animal experimentation to clinical trials.

Barnard's initial human case underwent cardiac transplantation on December 3, 1967, and survival of the patient for 18 days was appropriately designated as the beginning of clinical homotransplantation of the heart. Following numerous experiments in puppies, Kantrowitz, also in December, 1967, transplanted the heart of an anencephalic [failure of major portion of the brain to develop] newborn to an infant with tricuspid atresia [closure of the tricuspid valve in the heart] in whom a prior systemic pulmonary artery shunt had offered little palliation. The baby died a few hours after the procedure, but the interesting prospect of heart transplantation for infants with lethal and inoperable congenital cardiac anomalies had been introduced. Barnard's celebrated second heart transplant [Philip Blaiberg] was performed on January 3, 1968, with long-term survival.

The first human heart transplant at Stanford was done January 6, 1968. . . . Performance of the transplant was adequate until anoxic arrest occurred on the fifteenth day. [Shumway 1969, pp. 734–40]

No sooner had these first heart transplants been performed than medical and lay commentators began to air the grave problems that rejection would probably pose for those who survived surgery. Thus in January 1968 Dr. Howard Rusk wrote with some acerbity on the number of heart transplants already done, the attention accorded them by the mass media, and the problems the procedure faced:

As a result of the international epidemic of cardiac transplants it was not only difficult but practically impossible last week for the average television viewer to get out of the operating room or the cardiac clinic. . . .
This writter has discussed the present status of transplants with more than two score experienced cardiologists and researchers in immunology during the last three days. The consensus has been unanimous. The technological advances and surgical techniques have completely outstripped the basic immunological knowledge needed to prevent rejection.
[Rusk 1968]

By November 1968, nearly a year of clinical experience and some 90 heart transplants had begun to provide a core of data on what were now considered to be the major postoperative problems that heart recipients faced: short-term, acute rejection and chronic rejection, coupled with the danger of massive infection under the immunosuppressive regimen. In addition, at a meeting of the American Heart Association Denton Cooley first reported on a new difficulty, that of myocardiopathy: a condition in which an individual develops "antiheart antibodies" against his own or a grafted heart. About one-third of kidney transplant failures are also attributed to this sort of autoimmune response. Such reports caused cardiologists, immunologists, and surgeons at the meeting to express a blend of "short-term pessimism" and "long-term optimism" about the clinical future of heart transplants. Said one immunologist, "Let us hasten, but let us hasten slowly," and he warned surgeons not to "jump into" the field without measures to keep recipients alive because "there is danger of the field slipping into disrepute" (Lyons 1968).

During Year One of cardiac transplants, then, there was a constant but low-level voicing of concern over the immune barrier and the attendant problems we surveyed in chapter 1. As a service to the medical profession as well as to the public, Mr. Arnold Fox, chief librarian at the Associated Press, kept detailed, systematic data on the first one hundred heart transplants (this record-keeping task was subsequently assumed by the National Heart Institute). "Box-score" reports on how many transplants had been done and how many recipients had survived for how long were regularly issued in the press and were regarded as highly newsworthy. The cumulative "story" they told was that of the very high mortality rate associated with early clinical trials. By the end of the first year only forty-three out of one hundred recipients survived. Of the forty-three, twenty-four lived for three months or more, two for six months or longer, and one for over eleven months.

Despite the problems reflected in these figures, however, 1968 was hailed in the mass media and in many medical publications as the year of the heart transplant. The transplantation of a human heart was depicted as the quintessence of the "daring adventure" that medical research could be, and it was equated with the feats of the astronauts who had made the first manned lunar orbit in 1968. On 2 January 1969 the first anniversary of Philip Blaiberg's heart transplant was celebrated by the press, as well as by the patient himself, his family, and his close friends. His survival for a whole year was treated as a first birthday in *a* new life. To this day, the press continues to remember and report on any such "landmark" anniversary of a heart recipient.

Phase 2. Nineteen days after Blaiberg's first anniversary, on 21 January 1969, the Montreal Heart Institute announced to the press that it was suspending heart transplant operations. This public stand helped usher in phase 2 of cardiac transplantation. First accounts of the Montreal moratorium stressed that the institute's director, Dr. Paul David, was "completely satisfied" with the surgical techniques of Dr. Pierre Grondin and his transplant team. Rather, the press reported, the halt was "instigated" by Dr. Grondin when, during November 1968, five of the nine Montreal heart recipients, all of whom appeared to be recovering satisfactorily, died suddenly from rejection or massive infection. The institute declared that it would perform no further transplants until the high mortality rate accompanying the procedure could be lowered through a better control of rejection. To continue to operate under "the same conditions and problems that face us now would be immoral," Dr. David was quoted as declaring (Heart transplants halted in Montreal 1969).

Reaction to the Montreal announcement by others in the field was rapid, emphatic, and, perhaps most notably, publicly voiced. A United Press International survey the day after the Montreal statement reported that 39 out of 108 heart recipients were alive, and "doctors around the world said that they were not considering a moratorium" because "more knowledge resulted from every [transplant] done" (Heart transplants halted in Montreal 1969). One cardiac transplanter asserted he would "go ahead if the patient [had] no chances of survival without a new heart," and another stated that his center would not stop the operation but did "look at it with a more critical view than we [did] 3 to 4 months ago." Although transplanter Hassan Najafi objected to the introduction of moral judgments into the debate, he himself issued a moral injunction: "I take strong exception to the Institute raising the moral question in such a way. All a person has to do if he is troubled morally is to look optimistically at those transplant patients who are now living" (The heart-transplant debate 1969).

Several press accounts cited Grondin as the "instigator" of the moratorium. On 26 January he refuted any such intent at a press conference in Houston (where he had trained with DeBakey and

Cooley): "We're going to start doing transplants again as soon as we get back to Montreal. We simply wanted to thoroughly study what was happening before doing anything else. There was never thought of a moratorium" (Quigley 1969).

A meeting of the Society of Thoracic Surgeons in California on 27–29 January provided a forum for continuing the debate on the institute's decision while assessing the current status of cardiac transplantation. The cardiac transplanters themselves had divided opinions. Dr. Donald Effler, noted for his surgical treatment of coronary artery disease, criticized "the time, the effort, and the money" absorbed by cardiac transplants as well as, to him, the excessive and distorting publicity they had received. Countering Effler were surgeons such as Juro Wada of Japan, who held that the operation was at a "beginning" not a "stopping point," and that "you can't expect to have perfection from the very beginning." In more strident tones, his colleague Denton Cooley termed the moratorium idea "repulsive" and made the ideological affirmation that "one should not surrender to the enemy because he has lost a few battles." As is often done to justify a procedure that is under attack, Cooley said there might be valuable spin-offs such as a practical mechanical heart or a cure for cancer. He also invoked statistical morality to justify transplant attempts: 30 out of 108 survivors is a "remarkably good record" (Corbett 1969). Continuing these themes in a talk a few weeks later, Cooley declared that his "mission" in giving the talk was to "restore confidence in heart transplants and combat a wave of pessimism" resulting from the fully expected death of recipients.

By February 1969, in the wake of Montreal's announcement and the debate it stirred, the "doers" as well as the "doubters" were acknowledging more openly the magnitude of the difficulties that faced heart transplantation; and in light of the number of operations being performed (see fig. 1) they had to admit that an overall slowdown had occurred. Phase 3 of the reception of heart transplants was ushered in with newspaper headlines that declared: "Heart Transplant Future Looks Bleak"; "Heart Transplants Diminish: Better Conditions Awaited"; "Heart Transplants Halted at World's Medical Centers." These and other stories cited a variety of reasons for the drastic cutback in the number of transplants performed during December 1968 and January 1969. For example: recipients living more than two weeks had

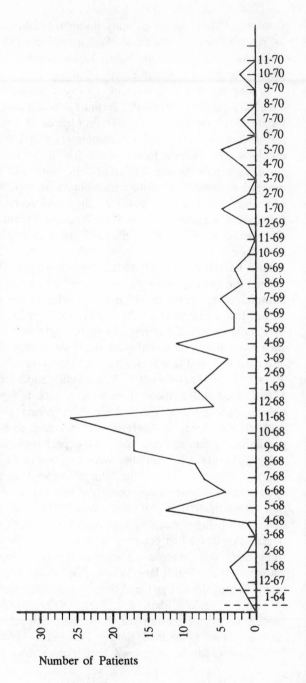

Fig. 1. Number of human heart transplants per month 23 January 1964 to 30 November 1970. Data supplied by the National Heart Institute. The total of 167 transplants reported through 20 November included 3 patients who received a second transplant and the use of two calf hearts, one sheep heart, one chimpanzee heart, and one artificial heart.

been found to develop atherosclerosis (thickening and narrowing of the arteries of their new hearts); the recognition that chances for survival were increased by better tissue matching made it harder to pair donors and recipients; some centers were busy "evaluating experience to date" but would continue with transplants "in the very near future."

In February 1970 we traveled to Montreal to learn the story of the Heart Institute's involvement in and disengagement from cardiac transplantation. One of our basic hypotheses was that before we could analyze why they had decided to stop heart transplants, we needed firsthand knowledge of why, and under what conditions, they had undertaken them to begin with. As we saw it, this decision was significant both symbolically and statistically. It was the first formal moratorium on human cardiac transplants called by any team or hospital. And it came from a group that had done nine cardiac implants, one of the largest numbers yet performed.

When Dr. Pierre Grondin and his team of twenty medical and surgical specialists assembled at the Montreal Heart Institute on 30 May 1968 to perform Canada's first and the world's eighteenth cardiac transplant, they established a milestone in the history of Canada's only specialized cardiovascular hospital. The institute is almost totally French Canadian, born out of many of the historical, social, and cultural factors that have shaped the French- and English-speaking communities of Quebec and also divided them from each other. Both its patients and its medical staff are overwhelmingly French Canadian.

The Montreal Heart Institute was founded in 1952 under the leadership of Dr. Paul David, an internationally recognized heart specialist and a man of more than medical prominence in Quebec. The Order of Grey Nuns at Maisonneuve Hospital collaborated with him, providing the institute with its original nursing staff. Dr. David, who became the institute's director, was convinced that it was morally and ethnically, as well medically, important that French Canadians should create, support, and have available to them the finest possible facilities for treating cardiovascular disease. He also believed that participating in such a scientific endeavor would be uplifting to them in several ways:

The Anglo-Saxon makes a cult of his institutions, the Frenchman has little respect for his and easily finds a thousand and one reasons to criticize them. The French-Canadian used to be poor, but for several decades he has been less so. Nevertheless, he retains the attitude of being poor, as becomes evident when he is solicited [for funds]. . . . Must we continue to be content with a strictly humanitarian and routine medicine and leave it to the more fortunate to be the forerunners of progress? I do not think so, convinced as I am that even in our poverty it is possible to reconcile the duties of charity with the obligations of science. . . . We lack confidence in ourselves and in our institutions. . . . Our history has subjugated us while at the same time we remain proud of our language, faith, and institutions. . . . In order to enrich ourselves on the spiritual plane of research, we must unite, and have confidence in our own people and Institutions. [David 1955; the account of the institute's development was also drawn from Snyder 1968 and from personal interviews]

The Montreal Heart Institute is now operated by a lay corporation and is affiliated with the Faculty of Medicine of l'Université de Montréal. Nevertheless, it proudly and gratefully acknowledges its former relationship to the Grey Nuns in its brochures. Furthermore, among the many photographs that line the walls of Dr. David's office is a personally inscribed picture of the cardinal of Montreal. These all indicate that the personnel of the institute still feel a historical identification with the Catholic church that is traditional for the French-Canadian community.

One is quickly impressed by the special atmosphere of the institute. It is gleamingly modern, but still seems intimate in its atmosphere. Its relatively small size (at the time of our visit 110 beds and a total staff of 300, including 50 physicians), along with its ethnic homogeneity, give it the feeling of an extended kinship system.

Pierre Grondin, tall, Gallic in appearance and manner, and cyclonic in activity, is proud of his rural origins and of the fact that he is a third-generation physician who once practiced as a country doctor. He became chief of surgery at the Montreal Heart Institute in 1963 after training in cardiovascular surgery with Michael DeBakey and Denton Cooley in Houston. By 1965, Grondin feels, the institute had become "the most active center of cardiac surgery in Canada, partly because we adopted the Cooley and DeBakey attitude": doing as much work as possible, for its own sake and as a means of attaining greater excellence.

The foundation for the institute's venture into human cardiac transplantation was laid in 1963 and 1964, as part of Grondin's efforts to establish a center known for its fine surgery. In that period he and his colleagues did some forty canine heart transplants, "more or less as a technical exercise," but judged "that there was no future in the procedure, for there were no survivors." In 1967, however, the transplant group began to reconsider the possibilities of cardiac transplantation, under the impetus of research reports from other centers, the development of renal transplantation, and a lung transplant carried out in Montreal in 1964. By 1968, Grondin believes, the institute had everything needed for a program of human cardiac transplantation, including a tissue-typing program and supplies of ALS and other immunosuppressive agents.

Although Grondin now believed that heart transplants were technically feasible, he felt he would like to see some "promising and worthwhile survival rates" before initiating his own clinical program, and he decided he might consider starting if Philip Blaiberg lived for at least four months. By April 1968 Blaiberg had reached this milestone, and Cooley's first two patients also appeared to be doing well. Thus Grondin made his "final preparations": a trip to Houston, where he watched Cooley perform his third heart transplant in May 1968. He recalls with pride that he was the only person present who was not a member of Cooley's team.

The decision to launch cardiac transplants at Montreal was formally made after Grondin returned from Houston. A ten-member transplant committee was created, "and when we all felt ready to go ahead, we did our first transplant" (in May 1968).

Grondin believed that the team was "extremely well prepared" to undertake heart transplants. However, at least one member of the staff disagreed, on the grounds that the institute "simply is not equipped to do clinical research, so heart transplantation has no place here." In his mind, the primary justification for performing cardiac implantation in its early development would be the contribution to medical knowledge a transplantation team could make. This same physician was also critical of the degree to which the Montreal Heart Institute was emulating the work of one of Grondin's mentors: "Right now we're just a factory doing surgery on a Cooley model." To him, "nothing would come out of" the institute's involvement in human heart implants "except temporary glory," and he did not consider the desire for professional and public recognition either an adequate or a worthy motivation.[2]

According to Grondin, the primary reason for undertaking human cardiac transplants was therapeutic, an attempt to extend a "period of worthwhile survival" to patients who seemed hopelessly ill. "Here is something we can offer these people," he was convinced during that summer of 1968.

In November 1968, after nine cardiac transplants, Grondin stated, "we quit because of what we saw happening elsewhere," particularly the high mortality rate Cooley was experiencing with his heart recipients. "For a while," Grondin recalled with pride, "we had the best world results. At the time the decision to stop was made, seven of our nine recipients were still walking around" (see table 1).

Montreal's ninth and final heart transplant was done on 29 November 1968, the day before the moratorium was decided

Table 1.   Summary of Cardiac Transplantation at the Montreal Heart Institute

Case	Date of Transplant	Date of Death	Reported Cause of Death
1	5/31/68	6/1/68 1 day	Low-output heart failure
2	6/28/68	12/1/68 156 days	Asphyxiation following indigestion
3	8/30/68	9/10/68 11 days	Stroke
4	9/11/68	1/6/69 117 days	Pulmonary infarction
5	9/19/68	11/19/68 62 days	Herpes viremia and cerebral pseudomonas abcess
6	10/20/68	12/19/68 60 days	Acute rejection crisis
7	10/25/68	12/18/68 54 days	Rejection
8	11/11/68	12/19/68 38 days	Bacterial pneumonia
9	11/29/68	3/14/69 105 days	Cerebral thrombosis

30 November 1968: decision to call moratorium made by institute staff
21 January 1969: existence of moratorium reported in lay press

SOURCE: Heart transplant data supplied by the National Heart Institute.

upon. This close timing, plus the fact that Grondin had a tenth recipient and a potential donor ready, suggest some conflict within the institute. According to Dr. David, he alone, as director of the institute, made the decision. He discussed the issue extensively with other staff members, both individually and at group meetings, but did not ask people if they personally would stop heart transplants because "that would have been passing the buck." The responsibility David assumed for decision-making was based as much on the charismatic authority he exercised in the institute and in the larger French-Canadian community as on his formal authority as director. Because he was widely esteemed for his medicomoral leadership, his judgment was likely to be highly respected.

However Grondin, the surgeon, was at first in less than full accord with David's decision to halt transplants and maintains that he would have gone ahead with the tenth operation had the candidate been as sick as the previous recipients. Grondin pointed out to us that the surgeon is apt to have a different perspective from the internist. In his own office is a sign that he feels typifies the stubbornly determined and dogmatic mentality of many surgeons: "There are two sides to every argument, but I don't have time to listen to yours." Another member of the institute, a cardiologist, noted that the surgical staff's opinions generally prevailed when things were going well, but that the medical men's views predominated when there was a difference of opinion and things began to go badly. This seems to have entered into the dynamics of the institute's cardiac transplant moratorium.

In the end, Grondin was dissuaded from proceeding with a tenth heart graft by a meeting with the other members of the transplant committee. Among the considerations the committee stressed were the problems and losses being experienced by Grondin's former chief, Denton Cooley. One of the remarks that had a special impact on Grondin was phrased as a rhetorical question: Dr. Cooley is incurring a very high mortality rate with the heart transplants he is performing. Do you think you are a better surgeon than he is? A somewhat chastened Grondin, in all honesty, answered, no. In light of the subsequent course of most heart recipients, Grondin now feels that it was "fortunate we did not do a transplant on the tenth case we considered, because he lived quite long without it." This kind of hindsight is one of the only ways the experimental surgeon can know "for sure" how well a candidate for an innovative procedure would have done without it.

Within a few weeks of the institute's decision to call a moratorium, Grondin had also decided that a halt was in order. "We reached the other side of the wave; now [in December 1968] patients started to die." He and his colleagues felt helpless against the twin threats of rejection and infection. "There was nothing we could do; any medication we used looked like water." The third recipient succumbed to infection, because "we gave him too much cortisone to try and forestall rejection. It was at this point that we decided, aah, it's not worthwhile unless we find something new. The procedure will be worth resuming only if we go back to the laboratory and find some new way to induce tolerance."

One of the interesting facts gathered in our interviews in Montreal was that the decision to call a moratorium was made at the end of November 1968, nearly two months before it was announced in the lay press. Dr. David recalls that he and several of his colleagues at first preferred to halt transplants without any public announcement, but finally decided that this would not be honest. He noted that cardiac transplantation at the institute had been extensively and continuously covered by the press when it seemed to be a "triumphant procedure," and it would thus be dishonest not to report the decision to suspend the operation because of the high mortality caused by rejection and infection. A second reason for making a public announcement, Dr. David acknowledged, was "to prevent any further transplant attempt." Accordingly, he revealed the institute's moratorium in an interview with a reporter from the *Gazette*, Montreal's major English-language morning newspaper.

Dr. David also expressed with some pride and gratification his belief that the Montreal Heart Institute's willingness to make its decision public may have encouraged other centers to slow the pace of heart transplants or to stop the procedure altogether. In Grondin's judgment, however, the institute's decision has had little direct influence on other centers. Rather, he attributes the general slowdown in cardiac transplants to expense; inability to establish a reliable prognosis in patients with advanced coronary artery disease; and the short survival period of most heart recipients, coupled with the fact that "we don't know why long-term survivors have survived."

Despite the course his institute chose to take, Pierre Grondin was optimistic about the future of cardiac transplantation when we talked with him in 1970. "I think heart transplants will eventually make it. We had to go through the era that we did." And he believes that his fellow cardiac transplanters respect Montreal's decision, even though the press has reported negative reactions by colleagues.

The Montreal Heart Institute's collective decision to withdraw from the field of cardiac transplantation was the most formal and manifest instance of a clinical moratorium occurring in phase 2 of the first three years of human heart transplants. As figure 1 indicates, this moratorium occurred just as the number of heart implants done per month, nationally and internationally, took a sharp plunge from the peak it had reached in November 1968— a high point it has not attained, or even approached, since. September through November 1968 represents what might be called a "bandwagon" period in the history of heart transplants. It was a time of high enthusiasm and hope about cardiac transplantation, among surgeons and lay persons alike. Furthermore, what Dr. Irvine Page has called "the circus trappings and glitter created by the first human transplant" had still not been "slough[ed] off," and heart transplanters were being treated as heroes. The promise and the prestige that surrounded the operation generated, in Page's words, "what appeared to be an international race to be a member of the me-too brigade" (Page 1969*b*, p. 109). Sixty implants were done over the course of these three months. Although certain cardiac surgeons led the field in the number of transplants performed, there were thirty surgeons at nine medical centers in the United States and in twenty-one other countries who did at least one such procedure. In dramatic contrast, only six transplants were carried out in December 1968, at four centers in this country and at two foreign institutes. No surgeon performed more than one transplant during this month. Of the eighteen surgeons who had done a total of twenty-six transplants in the previous peak month (November), fourteen never undertook one again.

Looking back over the three-year period, we find that of the sixty-four teams that had engaged in heart transplants through 1970, two teams (Shumway's and Cooley's) had done more than 25 percent. Fifty-four teams had done no more than one to three operations: thirty-eight had done one cardiac transplant, thirteen had done two, and three teams had performed three. Together, these fifty-four teams accounted for seventy-three of the total of 167 transplants recorded by the National Heart Institute as of 1 December 1970. In other words, a recurrent phenomenon that seems to have significantly contributed to the downslope after November 1968 was a "jumping off the bandwagon" by teams that "went on the record" by performing a transplant or two and then rapidly exited from the field.

The major reason more than half the teams did only one transplant is probably that they were discouraged by the short time the recipient survived. The kind of experience many such groups underwent is satirically portrayed by a science writer commenting on the five-hour survival of Czechoslovakia's only heart recipient:

As the international heart transplant bandwagon careens onward —Czechoslovakia being the latest country to leap aboard at the time of writing, and as quickly to topple off in the now unhappily familiar manner—it is becoming tragically clear that those Jonahs who have been warning that the time is not yet ripe for such operations are being proved tragically right. [Chedd 1968, p. 122]

Although apparently quite different in its dynamics from the halt called by the Montreal Heart Institute, this pattern might also be considered a subtype of the clinical moratorium.

Phases 3 and 4. After the decline in December 1968, heart transplants were performed at a slower rate, with a high of eleven operations in March 1969 and a low of no operations in November 1969 and March 1970. One of the major factors contributing to the decelerated pace was the departure of so many teams from the field.

Many surgeons and medical centers maintained their stand on not engaging in heart transplantation. Dr. Dwight Harken has been cited previously as one representative of this position. The prominence of these physicians and hospitals helped deter others from "leaping aboard the bandwagon." Their outlook not only was conveyed to their colleagues, but was also transmitted to the public in feature news stories, of which the following headlines are examples: "University [of Washington] Rejects Heart Transplants;" "Barnes Hospital Cool to Heart Transplant;" "MGH Will Continue Waiting, Won't Do Heart Transplants;" "Cite Insufficient Study for Heart Transplants" [to be done at the Peter Bent Brigham].

Over this period, various persons and organizations of status in the medical profession issued warnings to slow down on heart implants. The arguments were similar to the ones offered by cardiac surgeons announcing their decision not to enter the field at all. For example, Dr. Helen Taussig, a past president of the American Heart Association and co-developer of the "blue-baby" heart operation, made a particularly important and comprehensive declaration of this sort. As she saw it in February 1969, the problem of rejection, the "extremely high" late mortality rate, the pain and discomfort of the procedure, and its cost in terms of dollars and manpower were some of the reasons why a slower, more judicious approach to heart transplantation was indicated and was in fact beginning to occur.

far from endorsing Dr. Christiaan Barnard's hope that three times as many transplants will be done in this coming year as were done in the previous year, our hope should be that physicians and surgeons will proceed with extreme caution until such time as a cardiac transplant will not announce the imminence of death but offer the patient the probability of a return to a useful life for a number of years. [Taussig 1969]

As a more cautious perspective on cardiac transplantation gained ascendency, surgeons became more hesitant about implanting a poorly matched donor heart. They also gave increasing attention to other new surgical techniques for treating advanced coronary artery disease, such as procedures for replacing portions of diseased artery with a graft from part of the leg's saphenous vein.

The high mortality rate connected with cardiac transplantation continued unabated in phases 3 and 4 (see table 2). This high mortality rate notwithstanding, however, by the end of the third year as many as ten of the twenty-three surviving recipients had lived for more than two years. Despite a growing pool of what transplanters viewed as "long-term" survivors, the mortality rate, more than any other factor, contributed to the mounting skepticism and concern felt by both physicians and laymen. One of the most evident signs of this mood swing was the growing shortage of heart donors. As early as February 1969, the then most prolific heart transplanter, Denton Cooley, complained in a press

Table 2.   Heart Recipient Survival and Mortality through
           30 May 1970   N = 162

Time (months)

	0–3	4–6	5–9	10–12	13–15	16–18	19–21
Patients alive 30 May 1970	3	3	2	1	0	2	7
Patients dead after surviving to interval	104	20	5	3	7	3	2

SOURCE: Data supplied by the National Heart Institute.

NOTE: The 162 patients include 3 retransplants and 1 artificial heart–human heart transplant, for a total of 166 operations.

interview that the "stream of donors [had] dried up."[3] Six months later, in a review of the status of cardiac transplantation, *Newsweek* reported that Cooley now also faced a lack of potential recipients.

> Just a few months ago, as many as a dozen desperately sick patients lay in the wards of . . . St. Luke's Hospital anxiously waiting for heart transplants. . . . Last week, not one patient was waiting for a new heart at St. Luke's. "People are choosing to stay at home," says . . . Cooley. . . . "Either they have lost their interest or their courage. And whether it's negativism or loss of confidence, doctors don't refer patients to us." Everywhere, it seems, heart transplant surgeons are beset by distrust and doubt. [Transplants: Guarded outlook 1969]

The death of the world's most celebrated heart recipient, Dr. Philip Blaiberg, occurred on 17 August 1969, nearly two years after his operation. He died of "heart failure due to smoldering coronary artery insufficiency traceable in turn to chronic rejection. The autopsy did not show any of the ordinary changes in the heart muscle associated with acute rejection of the heart. Instead, there was marked narrowing and hardening of the coronary arteries, much more so than in the aorta and femoral arteries, the large arteries of the abdomen and the leg" (F. Moore 1970, p. 274). Blaiberg's death was a chastening reminder that medicine has not begun to overcome a problem intrinsic to cardiac implants, the latent development of coronary artery disease in the recipient's new heart.

Blaiberg's death could have been expected to sharply increase the number and intensity of enjoinders for a halt to cardiac transplantation. But this did not occur. Although his death was covered prominently and extensively by the press, we found only one article that asked for an in memorium stoppage. The medical correspondent for the London *Times* dramatically declared that: "What is certain . . . is that Dr. Blaiberg must not be allowed to have died in vain. The heart surgeons of the world must show their respect for this gallant soul by vowing to carry out no more heart transplantations until the full lessons of those already done have been absorbed" (Blaiberg's death a signal . . . 1969). Most statements about the implications of Blaiberg's death simply advocated "moving ahead . . . with a renewed sense of caution." Some doctors—who asked their *New York Times* interviewer not to identify them—expressed hope that "an era of 'me-tooism' had now come to an end" and felt that heart transplantation might now enter a second stage of a more cautious, limited approach (Blakeslee 1969). In retrospect, we can see that Blaiberg's death created only a mild stir in the press because it was expected by most persons who had followed the course of cardiac transplantation and because a more conservative outlook on heart transplants had taken root.

In June 1969 a second world symposium on heart transplantation convened in Montreal. This time the participants were in a less ebullient frame of mind than at their Cape Town conference a year earlier. According to one physician who attended the gathering, although the surgeons present felt it imperative to reiterate for the public that "they would continue doing heart transplants as usual . . . in reality, everyone left with the decision to do cardiac transplants at a slower pace." For some centers "a slower pace" came to mean cessation. For example, in mid-February 1970 Dr. Donald Effler, president of the Society of Thoracic Surgeons, made it known through the *Journal of the American Medical Association* that after performing two heart transplants he and his colleagues at the Cleveland Clinic had decided to do no more for the time being. He was very careful to suggest that a moratorium should not be called lightly and that he did not wish to unduly influence other centers. "I don't favor a blanket moratorium because I'm against prohibition in principle. But we have declared a moratorium of our own on organ transplantation, except for kidneys" (Quoted in *JAMA*, 211 (1970): 1112).

The number of heart transplants has also been limited by controlled and planned programs to which surgeons like Shumway have committed themselves. One of Shumway's few pronouncements on the moratorium issue came in September 1969 at a Chicago symposium, when he declared that the Stanford program would maintain the same even pace it had kept for one and one-half years. Commenting on the reduction in both the number of transplants being done and the number of centers doing them, he said: Now that the procedure has "lost some of its geopolitical attractiveness, those programs that have been oriented to the solution and identification of anticipated problems are moving along" (Stanford heart transplant team plans few changes 1969).

On the third anniversary of human cardiac transplantation, a few grafts were still being performed. The records of the world's most active cardiac transplanters indicate the status of the field at the end of its first three years.

As table 3 shows, in 1970 only Shumway's team was doing heart transplants regularly. Between January and 1 December 1970, eight of the seventeen transplants done were by the Stanford group; the other nine were done at seven different centers. Furthermore, as it was expressed during discussion of a report on their first twenty patients,

The world experience is quite different from that of the Stanford group, as would be expected. The fraction of patients

Table 3.   "Box Scores" of Cardiac Transplanters

Surgeon	Number Performed	Number of Survivors	Date of Last Transplants (as of 30 Nov. 1970)
Lower	5	1	February 1970
Barnard	5	1	April 1969
Kahn	6	1	July 1970
Grondin	9	0	November 1968
Lillihei	10	0	December 1969
DeBakey	12	2	January 1970
Cooley	23	0	September 1969
Shumway	27	9	October 1970

surviving at 6 months with [the Stanford] cases excluded shows a figure in the world experience of just over 21 per cent. The fraction surviving at 1 year with those cases excluded is just over 6 per cent. [Bergan, in Stinson, Griepp, et al. 1970, p. 319]

In terms of numbers of transplants performed, Shumway's and Cooley's teams led the field. In spring 1970 they had conducted an equal number of heart implants. But, as Cooley himself conceded, their results stood in sharp contrast:

Our series is the same size as that of Drs. Shumway and Stinson, but the results have not been nearly as good. We have performed cardiac transplantation on 20 patients, and at the present time none are surviving. Our first operation was performed on May 2, 1968. The last patient died on March 28, 1970. [Cooley, in Stinson, Griepp, et al. 1970, p. 320]

Since September 1969 Cooley has done no heart transplants. Shumway's program has continued at a deliberately slow pace, averaging one transplant a month. The dramatic contrast between the results obtained by Shumway's team and those obtained by all other transplant units epitomizes the degree to which the clinical investigator must live with uncertainty. For as of December 1970 Shumway and his colleagues did not feel they could yet identify the factors that positively distinguished their work.

At the end of Year Three, two new variants in the outlook on cardiac transplantation were visible. Several prominent cardiac transplanters implied that "the medical community may see a resurrection of interest in transplants in the next year or so" (Drake 1970). For example, in a press interview on the third "anniversary" of the first human implant, Shumway predicted a "reawakening of interest" in the operation in 1971. His prediction was based on two major factors. First, cardiac surgeons were increasingly using the saphenous vein bypass graft on patients with severe heart failure. Shumway felt that after this operation, the patient's condition would improve for a time and then severely worsen, necessitating a second radical procedure, cardiac transplantation. Second, he believed that as knowledge of Stanford's research and clinical achievements was disseminated through professional publications and mass media accounts a number of other centers of medical excellence, perhaps ones that had not yet engaged in cardiac transplants, would undertake clinical programs (Shumway, in Altman 1970*a*; and personal communication, Lois Christopherson).

The other factor was the far greater attention accorded to this anniversary than to the previous one. The *New York Times* carried a first-page headline, "3 Years of Heart Transplants: 23 Live." It focused primarily on the recipients who survived, and on Shumway's group in particular because its results were the best. The "ordinary" quality of life that many recipients reportedly enjoyed was emphasized. "They move about as ordinary citizens, attending to ordinary tasks, filling their lives with plans for now and for the future" (Blakeslee 1970).

These variants seem to constitute new kinds of petitions "for there to be more co-operation within the profession and a return of the goodwill and charity of the public toward organ transplantation, which suffered so severely following the unfortunate and often inaccurate publicity surrounding so many of the cardiac transplantation operations" (Calne and Williams 1970, p. 427).

These petitions were triggered in part by a very specific type of shift in the mortality/survival figures for cardiac transplantation. Although the death rate continued to be high, a small number of recipients (ten) had lived for more than two years. To at least some transplanters and commentators this fact, plus the assumption that some patients might live even longer, "cast a more favorable and hopeful light on cardiac transplantation," potentiating a new stage in its evolution from experiment to therapy (Stinson, Griepp, et al. 1970, p. 320).

The Clinical Moratorium: Causes and Attributes

The cardiac transplant moratorium is not an idiosyncratic event. Moratoriums have been common in the process of therapeutic innovation, and they are generally related to the dynamics of clinical investigation.[4] Many of the factors that may induce, deter, or end a clinical moratorium are manifest in the four phases of human heart transplantation that we have depicted.

Every medical and surgical procedure, even the most established, carries some uncertainty about its efficacy and safety. Gaps in knowledge, technical inadequacies, and the problems of uncertainty that stem from them are inherent in medical research and practice, particularly during a period of therapeutic innovation, creating intensive strains both for research physicians and for their patients. This is one reason why a moratorium is likely to occur during the early phases of clinical trial and error and evaluation. The investigator continually weighs the known and probable risks and the benefits of a new procedure and makes and remakes decisions about when and on whom a new treatment may justifiably be used.

The most immediate and manifest reason for suspending a therapeutic procedure is that the mortality rate associated with it is judged to be "too high." However, as we have seen, there is no simple definition of therapeutic "success" and "failure" and no ready answer as to what constitutes an "acceptable" mortality rate at different points along the experiment-to-therapy continuum or with various kinds of patients.

There were pioneers in cardiac transplantation who had the commitment and drive to go on. In the words of one such transplanter, "You don't solve a problem by desisting. It's obvious that heart transplantation is here to stay. I'm very optimistic myself. You're bound to have some problems, because you can't travel an unknown road and expect to find it paved." For other physicians, the "prohibitive" mortality rate associated with heart transplantation—largely created by the nonsurgical problem of rejection—evoked stricken, helpless feelings that moved them to initiate a moratorium.[5]

As we saw in chapter 4, physician-investigators have various patterned ways of coming to terms with their professional stresses, which may either push them toward a moratorium or pull them away from it. From a certain point of view, their research constitutes a primary intellectual and moral mechanism for coping with uncertainty and the unknown. It enables them to try to do something about gaps in knowledge and about therapeutic limitations and to express their belief that their efforts will eventually bring clinically relevant medical advances. This has inclined certain physicians to continue performing cardiac transplants in what may seem a self-propelled way.

Since the turn of the century, most clinical research in medicine has been conducted in hospitals, and it has increasingly been done by teams. A significant proportion of such work now takes place in university-connected hospitals which are committed to the advancement of medical knowledge as well as to the care of patients, the training of medical professionals, and, in recent years, more generalized community-oriented health functions. Affiliation with a hospital that can provide the complex facilities, highly trained personnel, and kinds of patients necessary for his work is indispensable to the research physician. His work is also directly affected by a relatively recent development in modern hospitals: human experimentation review committees made up of his medical peers.

Membership in such a collectivity may provide investigators with a way of sharing responsibility, and with the kind of day-by-day counsel, support, and release of tension that helps them continue their research despite its strains and frustrations. However, because the solo investigator pattern has largely given way to a team model, research physicians are more immediately subject to being criticized, contradicted, or overruled by their collaborators. Thus group feeling may compel an investigator to agree to a moratorium on clinical trails.

This kind of group pressure, for example, was brought to bear on Pierre Grondin at the Montreal Heart Institute. He had every intention of continuing his heart transplant program until he was subjected to counterpressure by the director of his institute, his internist-cardiologist colleagues, and the transplant committee of which he was a member. Through his dialogue with the committee, Grondin came to feel that a moratorium was indeed indicated. The subsequent deaths of all nine of his heart recipients confirmed him in his assent.

A clinical investigator's relations with colleagues that are more distant than his own research team or hospital may also help determine whether he continues a line of experimentation, especially if such "outside" colleagues have high professional prestige. The opinion a high-ranking physician has of his work can affect an investigator's professional reputation and as a consequence both his morale and the facilities at his disposal. Denton Cooley exerted this long-distance influence on Grondin. Initially, Grondin's desire to emulate Cooley was so strong that one of his teammates at the Montreal Heart Institute felt that their heart transplant program was a "Cooley model." Subsequently, however, the high mortality rate of Cooley's heart recipients became a potent factor in Grondin's assent to halting the Montreal program.

A research physician's "social circle"[6] within the medical profession may also stimulate him to undertake and continue certain forms of clinical trials, or may lead him to abandon them. Both these stimuli operated in the relationship between Grondin and

Cooley. As we saw in chapter 5, the professional backgrounds of transplant surgeons are so similar and overlapping that this entire group might be considered a social circle. Over the years, in a complex of medical institutions and in various professional roles, they have had ample opportunity to exert both manifest and latent influence over each other's transplantation endeavors. Heart transplant surgeons form an even tighter social circle. In September 1969 Crane and Matthews indicated that "almost one half (10) of the 23 heads of surgical teams performing [heart transplants] in the United States and Canada for whom biographical information was available (no information = 5) had been associated, either as teacher or as student, with two institutions, Johns Hopkins University and the University of Minnesota" (Crane and Matthews 1969).

The course of an innovative procedure like cardiac transplantation is shaped not only by scientific and professional factors but by the public's general attitude toward medical research and innovation and by its response to a particular development. The great amount of popular attention accorded to medical science reflects a high cultural value attached to health, longevity, relief of suffering, and the "conquest of disease" and public interest in the medical researchers who are trying to achieve these goals. To an increasing extent in modern societies, the mass media reflect and shape lay attitudes toward medical innovation, in ways that may either aid or impede it.

The press and other media have given extensive coverage to organ transplantation, especially heart implants.[7] Dr. Irvine H. Page has characterized it as "instant reporting" and contended that "there has never been anything like it in medical annals" (Page 1969b, p. 109). At the outset of cardiac transplantation, the media accounts were flamboyantly positive. Some surgeons have acknowledged that this attention encouraged them to undertake and continue heart transplants. The media gave the surgeons involved public recognition and support, and in some instances catapulted them to fame. Publicity about heart transplants also facilitated their work by emphasizing the need for donors as well as the promise the operation held for desperately ill patients. However, in certain other aspects the mass media undermined rather than reinforced the continuance of heart transplantation. Medical spokesmen have said that the "too optimistic" impression the press gave of the state of cardiac transplantation had a boomerang effect on the public. In addition, newspapers kept a "box score" on all heart transplants and their outcomes, demonstrating the typically high mortality rate for a therapeutic innovation in this very early stage of development. Furthermore, as some physicians have pointed out, the "transplanter" has often been presented as a taker of organs rather than as a healer and the patient's guardian. Debates about the pros and cons of cardiac transplantation have taken place as much on the pages of daily newspapers as within the medical profession. And to some extent the spectacular way some heart transplant surgeons have been presented has subjected them to criticism from their colleagues because such publicity violates professional norms of privacy, modesty, and disinterestedness.

The evolution of heart surgery, including cardiac transplantation, also demonstrates that concepts and beliefs deriving from the cultural tradition of a society may latently influence whether a moratorium will occur. The fact that in Western society the heart was considered to be so delicate and vital by physicians as well as by laymen was long an impediment to cardiac surgery. The Judeo-Christian conception of the heart as a mystical organ, where the soul and the most noble motives and sentiments of man reside, has also forestalled attempts to manipulate it. These underlying ways of thinking about the human heart surfaced in earlier innovative periods of cardiac surgery and receded once the operative techniques had been sufficiently perfected to demonstrate their practicability and therapeutic benefit. In the more recent era of cardiac transplantation, these same conceptions have again manifested themselves.

Moratoriums may occur for one or more of several reasons: after a series of clinical trials, some physicians may cease to use an experimental procedure; other physicians may try it once or twice and then stop; physicians working in a particular institution may collectively withdraw from further clinical trials; some pioneer physicians may continue, but at a slower pace. The moratorium period is usually one of reflection, reevaluation, and study. During this time the physicians often return to laboratory experiments to try to solve some of the problems that led them to suspend human trials. A therapeutic innovation may sometimes be permanently abandoned, either because it has proved to be unfruitful or noxious or because, in the natural flow of medical advance, it has been superseded by a better one. But such an abandonment, as we have seen, does not constitute a moratorium.

The question whether a slowdown should be considered a moratorium has been particularly raised in connection with human heart transplants. It has been suggested that the drop in the number of implants done per month was simply a leveling off to a pace that is "normal" for early clinical trials of a radical surgical procedure. The research physicians who take this position seem to be reacting primarily to the possible accusatory implications of the label "moratorium." For many people the word connotes a permanent stop to something that should not have been started in the first place; the debates over calling a moratorium on the war in Vietnam have contributed heavily to this connotation. At a scientific meeting in December 1969, we personally had an experience that bore out these apprehensions about how a "heart transplant moratorium" would be interpreted. During a press conference on organ transplantation we were asked by a number of journalists to make statements indicating that our research indubitably showed that a moratorium on cardiac transplants was in effect. The stories they were mentally preparing (some of which were subsequently printed) implied that clinical investigators had been "caught in the act" of abandoning a "failure" which had been medically improbable and morally dubious to begin with.

Clinical moratoriums take place only when the pressures on the research physician to desist from certain trials on patients are stronger than the pressures to continue generated by what would ordinarily be his scientific and therapeutic obligations. Here we return to an essential attribute of the clinical moratorium. The physician who commits himself to clinical investigation must conduct research with patients. His goal is to advance medical science and practice in ways that he hopes will benefit his subjects and other patients with similar or related medical problems. Within the limits of the ethics of human experimentation, the research physician has an obligation to contribute to ongoing investigation. Through these research activities, he is bound to apply the latest developments in knowledge and technique to diseases that cannot otherwise be adequately prevented or treated. If for some reason an investigator wishes to interrupt or roll back this process, as in calling a clinical moratorium on his own or his colleagues' work, the burden of proof falls on him.[8] In some way he must explain to colleagues and patients why he feels this step ought to be taken. For when he invokes a moratorium he challenges institutionalized values that work to keep clinical research going: "We have made a beginning; now it is time to proceed. . . . Why do we continue? Because if we don't, these people will die, and if we do, some will improve." A call for a clinical moratorium, then, entails seeking legitimation from significant others to temporarily halt an otherwise obligatory research activity, on the grounds that this suspension will ultimately serve the values of clinical investigation better than continuing the trials in question.

6

The Case of the Artificial Heart

The case of the artificial heart centers on the implanting of a total mechanical cardiac replacement, which remained for sixty-four hours, in a patient with terminal heart disease. This surgical event, on 4 April 1969, marked the first time in medical history that a complete mechanical substitute for the heart had been used in man. There have been no further attempts to place such a device in desperately ill patients. The man who received this cardiac device was Mr. Haskell Karp. The physician who implanted it in his chest was Dr. Denton A. Cooley, renowned heart surgeon, who at the time of the operation was clinical professor of surgery at Baylor College of Medicine in Houston, Texas, consultant in cardiovascular surgery at Saint Luke's Episcopal Hospital–Texas Children's Hospital, and surgeon-in-chief of the Texas Heart Institute. His principal collaborator was Argentinian-born Dr. Domingo Liotta, an assistant professor of surgery at Baylor and a full-time research assistant in the Artificial Heart Program conducted jointly by Baylor University and Rice University. Liotta's role chiefly consisted of the part he played in the development of the mechanical pump. A fourth major figure was Dr. Michael E. DeBakey, eminent cardiovascular surgeon and researcher, president of the Baylor College of Medicine, professor and chairman of Baylor's Department of Surgery, senior attending surgeon at Methodist Hospital, director of the Fondren–Brown Cardiovascular Research and Training Center at Methodist Hospital, and principal investigator of the Baylor–Rice Artificial Heart Program. Although DeBakey was not present when Mr. Karp received his implant, his roles as principal investigator in the Artificial Heart Program and president of the medical school centrally involved him in the surgical act and its repercussions. The complex relationship that had developed between Cooley and DeBakey over the eighteen years that these two titans of cardiac surgery had been associated quickened the emotional absorption of both men in the case. The origins and consequences of the implantation drew in not only a local Houston network of medical institutions, but also the Lawrence General Hospital in Massachusetts and the National Heart Institute in Bethesda, Maryland. The attention it received from the mass media was vast, dramatic, and prolonged; it reached a second crescendo when Cooley decided to remove the prosthesis and replace it with a cadaver heart transplant, and a third when a series of investigations into the medical ethics of the case were undertaken by Baylor, partly in response to inquiries from the National Heart Institute.

As researchers engrossed in a historical and sociological study of the implications of organ transplantation, we were struck by the case of the artificial heart and avidly followed its unfolding. But it was not until after our return from a field trip to Houston in March 1970, where we had been cordially received by Dr. Cooley and Dr. DeBakey and their colleagues, that we began to consider doing an analysis of this intricate case. As we thought about it and discussed it, we became increasingly convinced that this medical-surgical event involved some of the most important social and ethical issues that can affect therapeutic innovation.

In the fall of 1970 we sent letters to Dr. Cooley and Dr. DeBakey explaining our interest in the case and advising each man that we had written to the other. We said we hoped to write a carefully documented, fair-minded and nuanced account that would be edifying and useful to them as well as to readers of our book. We asked each of them if they would be willing to help us gather more firsthand data on the case and to gain better understanding of its significance and said we were ready to come to Houston to see them and any of their colleagues who might be relevant. Dr. DeBakey promised us his full cooperation. Dr. Cooley regretfully informed us that he could not help us with our project because another writer was already working on the material. He did not tell us the name of the writer or whether he was a journalist, a novelist, or an academician.

Despite this asymmetry, we decided to go to Houston in November 1970 to learn what we could, reserving judgment about whether we would be qualified to write a responsible chapter. Since we were precluded from seeing Dr. Cooley a second time we felt we did not have the right to make personal contact with Dr. Domingo Liotta, and we could not study Haskell Karp's medical records. Nor did we meet William O'Bannon, the engineer who designed and built the console that powered the artificial heart. However, beginning with Dr. DeBakey, we succeeded in interviewing an otherwise representative cross-section of physicians, nurses, engineers, laboratory technicians, and "pump" technicians (the pump is the heart-lung machine on which the patient is maintained during open-heart surgery), who were involved in the Haskell Karp case, its preliminaries, and its sequelae. We were also allowed to review key primary documents gathered for the various investigations that were conducted at Baylor. We already had an ample file of professional papers and communications on the development of the artificial heart and its clinical use. And we had a very large collection of news articles on the case. (The series of stories written by John Quinn for the *New York Daily News* and by Judith Randal for the *Washington Star* were the most richly detailed, accurate, and perceptive of these.)

When we returned from Houston, we once again took stock of our data and carefully evaluated their reliability and validity. Despite the gaps in our materials, we judged that they were adequate for the analysis we intended to do. Our aim was not to record the complete and definitive history of the case of the artificial heart or to resolve conclusively all debate about what ought and ought not to have been done. We wished to write a narrative that would serve as a base line for our analysis of the wide-ranging medicomoral issues the case seemed to epitomize. We hope that we have succeeded, without making either heroes or villains of those involved.

Members of the international transplantation fraternity, other medical professionals, and the public all learned of the clinical innovation through the same channels: "1st Man-Made Heart Inserted: Patient's Condition 'Excellent' "; "1st Artificial Heart Planted by Cardiowhiz"; "Total Artificial Heart Is Implanted in

Man"; "Artificial Heart Beats on for Skokie Man, 47"; "Artificial Heart Keeps Man Alive." On 5 April 1969, in first-page headlines, newspapers heralded the first use of a completely artificial heart (orthotopic cardiac prosthesis) in man.

The history-making patient was a forty-seven-year-old man from Skokie, Illinois, the father of three sons, who had worked as a printing estimator. Mr. Karp had been incapacitated for several years by a series of heart attacks. He had been hospitalized at Saint Luke's since 3 March, awaiting a decision whether his severely damaged heart could be surgically repaired.

Karp's medical saga was as brief as it was dramatic: The artificial heart was implanted on 4 April 1969—Good Friday. Recognizing that the mechanical heart would be viable only for a short time, the surgeons planned to transplant a human heart into Mr. Karp as soon as one became available. In newspapers and on television, Mrs. Karp made a nationwide plea for a donor to come forward.

> Someone, somewhere, please hear my plea. A plea for a heart for my husband. I see him lying there, breathing and knowing that within his chest is a man-made implement where there should be a God-given heart. How long he can survive one can only guess.
>
> I cry without tears. I wait hopefully. Our children wait hopefully, and we pray.
>
> The Lord giveth and Lord taketh. But the Lord also gave us gifted men—such as Dr. Denton Cooley and Dr. Domingo Liotta —who are instrumental in prolonging life.
>
> Maybe somewhere there is a gift of a heart for my husband. Please.

On 7 April Mrs. Barbara Ewan, a candidate-donor, was admitted to Saint Luke's. She had been flown to Houston from Lawrence, Massachusetts, by a chartered air ambulance. She had been in a coma at the Lawrence General Hospital since 19 March. Forty-eight hours before her trip to Houston, after a period of anoxic arrest, tests had shown her to be suffering from irreversible brain damage. After a telephone conference between physicians in Houston and Lawrence and a meeting of Mrs. Ewan's closest relatives, family consent had been given for her to be taken to Houston to donate her heart to Mr. Karp. Because Mrs. Ewan was a widow, her oldest child, a married daughter, had the ethical and legal responsibility of officially granting this permission. Ninety minutes after her arrival in Houston, Mrs. Ewan was formally pronounced dead from a stroke, by four doctors who were not members of the prospective transplant team. Her heart was immediately implanted into Mr. Karp. Thirty-two hours later, on 8 April Haskell Karp died from pneumonia and kidney failure.

The press hailed the use of the prosthetic heart in man as the third major. advance in cardiac transplantation. They ranked the implantation of a left ventricular bypass by Dr. Michael DeBakey on 21 April 1966 as the first such breakthrough and Dr. Christiaan Barnard's transplant on Mr. Washkansky on 21 December 1967 as the second.

Many members of the medical profession were surprised at the news. They had believed that the clinical use of an artificial heart was still many years away. Furthermore, they did not associate Cooley with work in this area. Only nine months earlier, on 3 August 1968, at a seminar in Long Beach, California, Cooley had made the widely quoted statement that "the mechanical heart borders on science fiction and wishful thinking" and had said that even as a temporary device one could not expect it to be used clinically for at least three to five years.

The first press releases on the operation stated that the heart had been designed and built by Dr. Domingo Liotta, in collaboration with Dr. Cooley at Saint Luke's.[1] Liotta reportedly had completed work on the heart itself, at a cost of $5,000, several weeks before the operation, but the external power device that maintained the unit's pumping action, built at a cost of $20,000, had been completed only three days before surgery. Liotta had joined Michael DeBakey's staff at Baylor College of Medicine in 1962 after several years of research on the artificial heart in Argentina, where he had achieved a certain priority in this new field. At Baylor, Liotta became a full-time researcher in the Artificial Heart Program, under the directorship of DeBakey.

The complex historical sequence of roles that DeBakey, Cooley, and Liotta played in the development and implantation of the artificial heart raised a number of factual questions with ethical import. Who was actually the principal developer of the unit in Mr. Karp's chest, and under whose auspices had it been financed and built? Had a heart developed by Liotta and other researchers in the Baylor laboratories actually been used? If so, how had the unit come to be employed clinically at Saint Luke's? Had Cooley or Liotta made their plans known to DeBakey, or to officials of the National Heart Institute, which funded the Artificial

Heart Program, as required by the public health guidelines on government-financed programs involving human experimentation? On the other hand, if Liotta and Cooley had indeed developed their own model—albeit in a remarkably short time and for very little money—how much testing had it received in laboratory animals and what were the results of those tests?

Careful reading of the first reports of the implant also elicited questions about the quality of consent obtained from Mr. Karp for this experimental trial. In his interview with reporters, Cooley emphasized that the device represented an infant stage in the development of artificial hearts. In support of his decision to use it on a patient, he affirmed that "a journey of a million miles can begin with only one step" (Plastic heart works 1969). But statements by Cooley and other hospital spokesmen about Mr. Karp's willingness to participate in this "journey" were frequently inconsistent. According to first reports on 5 April, the initial plan was to surgically reconstruct Mr. Karp's damaged left ventricle. In the course of this operation, Cooley discovered how badly diseased the entire heart was and ordered implantation of the cardiac prosthesis as an "emergency measure," although he had not planned to use the device clinically so soon. However, the press also stated that Cooley had obtained both Mr. and Mrs. Karp's permission to use the heart before surgery. This suggests that he had at least tentatively planned to perform the prosthetic implant. In an interview with the *New York Times* on 6 April Cooley said:

we had explained to him about the plan to repair and told him there was a 70% chance for success but a 30% chance it would fail. He also was told we would make every effort to keep him alive by using the device [the artificial heart] until we could get a transplant donor. And we told him we would make every effort to find a donor. [Texas plea made for heart donor 1969]

On 8 April, after Mr. Karp had received a human heart, his wife told newsmen that her husband had talked her into agreeing to a transplant because "he wanted to live as a man, not lie there as a vegetable. It was his decision." That same day, Cooley revealed that Mr. Karp had opposed a transplant. Four days before the operation, Cooley had "assured Mr. Karp he would not do a transplant as long as he didn't want one." But on 4 April, just before surgery, Cooley continued, Karp finally agreed to a transplant or use of the prosthesis, if necessary to save his life. When

Cooley was asked in a 6 April press interview why he had decided to use so new and unproved a device, he replied that the artificial heart implant was carried out "in an effort to save my patient's life. If there is any censure or criticism, I will lay myself at the mercy of the court" (Artificial heart patient's condition good 1969).

In addition to the issues of scientific priority, the justifiability of a human trial, and informed, voluntary consent, two other aspects of this case initially disturbed medical onlookers. First, the entire sequence of events, and the chief surgeon's comments upon them, were dramatically recounted by the lay press long before a reflective, scientific account was given to medical professionals. Second, many physicians had serious doubts about the propriety of flying a heart donor across the country to make her gift. As they saw it, such a journey might have encroached upon the dignity of her death and also deprived local candidate-recipients of needed cardiac or kidney transplants.

A more detailed history of the intricate events in the laboratory, the operating room, and the clinic is prerequisite to an analysis of the general implications of the case of the artificial heart. We will trace what we consider the key happenings: the development of the Baylor–Rice Artificial Heart Program; the collaboration between Cooley and Liotta that led to clinical use of a prosthetic heart; the events that took place in and around the surgical amphitheater at the time of Mr. Karp's implant, transplant, and death; and the various investigations conducted by Baylor College of Medicine and their sequelae.

Michael DeBakey's interest in developing a mechanical substitute to help patients with irreversible heart disease began in the late 1950s. He launched investigative work at Baylor and began efforts to persuade the government to fund artificial heart research. In 1962 he invited two surgeons—Dr. William C. Hall, who had been working on aortic valves at the University of Kansas, and Dr. Domingo Liotta—to join his staff. Liotta had already spent several years in artificial heart research. In 1960, he and Dr. Willem Kolff had independently made "the earliest successful laboratory attempts at replacing the heart with an artificial intrathoracic pump" (Hall et al. 1964, p. 685).[2]

The initial thrust of DeBakey, Hall, and Liotta's research was total cardiac replacement. In the course of developing a biventricular artificial heart, the first model they designed was a left ventricular bypass: a pump intended to assist the cardiac patient's failing circulation for several weeks while the heart's own major pump, the left ventricle, recovered function. In July 1963, as DeBakey and his colleagues later reported, "after successful use in over 100 dogs, an opportunity arose" to "try the bypass clinically."

The patient (G.W.), a forty-two year old Negro man, was admitted in severe congestive failure. After several weeks of intensive medical management, the patient became compensated. Catheterization studies revealed a severe aortic stenosis and regurgitation. At this time he was considered a reasonable operative risk and on July 18, 1963, an aortic valve replacement (Starr-Edwards No. 8) was performed. Eighteen hours post-operatively, the patient had a cardiac arrest. The chest was immediately opened and the heart resuscitated. After this procedure, the patient showed signs of damage to the central nervous system, renal failure, and rather promptly went into refractory left ventricular failure (evidenced by severe pulmonary edema). Because of the hopelessness of the situation, the patient was considered to be an ideal candidate for left ventricular bypass. On July 19, 1963, one of the experimental models of the artificial left ventricle was placed in the patient. Both clinically and radiographically, pulmonary edema subsided, respiration deepened and neurologic signs improved. The patient remained anuric and peritoneal dialysis was started on July 22, 1963. After nearly four days of continuous left ventricular support, the patient died although the artificial left ventricle remained functional. Postmortem examination showed chronic damage to the liver, lungs and kidneys, probably related to long-standing decompensation.

To our knowledge this represents the first attempt with an implantable artificial ventricle in a human subject. A human model has since been designed and is now awaiting clinical trial. [Hall et al. 1964, p. 688]

According to Dr. William Hall, Mr. W had a cardiac arrest several days after his aortic valve surgery.

His problem now was that of left ventricular failure. Dr. DeBakey was called in as a consultant on the case, and he suggested trying the left ventricular bypass pump that had been developed in the laboratory. The one that was available was only large enough for implantation in a dog. . . . That device is now in the Smithsonian Institution. . . . We had already done everything known to medicine, and still the patient was going downhill.

Furthermore, Mr. W did not have irreversible brain damage, so there was a possibility that he was a salvageable patient. . . . We knew the problems with the pump, but we felt that if we could just support him for a day or two, we could get on the front side of the curve. Once we accomplished this, then we could take the pump out. We knew, too, that this pump doesn't do permanent damage, so there was the possibility that we could do it without causing any harm. Of course, we may have done some damage, for the pump may have been one of the causes of the emboli. At the same time, we did manage to get the patient out of pulmonary edema by using the pump. So, at one and the same time, the patient died because of the pump and lived longer because of it. . . . It was able to help with his original problem of left ventricular failure. [Hall, personal interview]

By 1964 the Baylor group had developed and tested a second artificial heart model, this one designed to provide complete replacement of the ventricles. But the team encountered multiple problems that needed protracted research, and so they redirected their attention to the development of a left ventricular bypass pump, this time under companion grants to Baylor and Rice from the National Heart Institute. This marked the formal beginning of the Baylor–Rice Artificial Heart Program, with DeBakey as principal investigator, Hall as program director, and Liotta as full-time assistant. The program had its inception in 1963, soon after the clinical trial of the ventricular bypass, when DeBakey increased his efforts to persuade the government to sponsor a nationwide artificial heart program. Since the National Heart Institute was not yet geared for such a program, Hall was "loaned to them as an 'expert' for six months, setting up the contract mechanism for what was to become the artificial heart program" (Hall, personal interview). Hall has recalled with amusement the actual writing of the grant proposal that launched the Baylor–Rice program after he had returned from the National Heart Institute. He had never before written a grant proposal, and after setting down the kinds of work that he and his colleagues expected to do, he tallied up the costs and found they amounted to $25,000. He was quite proud of having put together the grant proposal and of requesting such a modest sum. But when DeBakey saw the proposals, "he almost threw them at me. In fact, I think he actually did. For Dr. DeBakey was thinking on a much bigger plane. He was considering a whole range of problems that might be studied in connection with the development of the artificial heart. He had decided to solve the whole problem, and not just build a little pump. When Dr. DeBakey got finished with the grant proposal, it totaled $4.5 million, which was awarded" (Hall, personal interview).

By 1966, the left ventricular bypass was judged ready for clinical trials, having "proved safe and effective in tests on a large series of animals." The pump's "clinical effectiveness" was then demonstrated when it was implanted in "a series of patients critically ill with heart failure" (DeBakey, Hall et al. 1969, p. 127). These trials were extensively covered by the mass media.

After the implants of the bypass pump, for a number of reasons the Baylor program again began to focus on a biventricular artificial heart for human orthotopic implantation. In their earlier work with the biventricular and left ventricular bypass pumps, the team had identified and resolved many of the problems in the use of synthetic materials, pump design, and pump control. Further, in Dr. Hall's words, "after several trials with the left ventricular bypass pump, it became apparent that this was a tremendously expensive procedure, and that we would be approaching the national debt if we tried to keep everyone in left ventricular failure alive" (Hall, personal interview). Then, "with the first human cardiac transplantation late in 1967, the need for development of an artificial heart at least for temporary use, became more urgent" (DeBakey, Hall et al. 1969, p. 127).

Thus in 1967, as principal investigator of the Baylor program, DeBakey authorized work on an orthotopic heart. When reevaluating the program in January 1968, he directed Hall, Liotta, and other members of the staff to submit all research proposals under the National Heart Institute grant to him for review and approval. Progress reports from Hall and Liotta to DeBakey throughout 1968 record the development of the double-ventricle pump as it evolved and was refined from modification of the left ventricular bypass. On 10 September 1968, a signed and dated diagram of the biventricular pump was prepared by a Baylor medical artist, Ben Baker, and "the experimental model was ready to be fabricated for study of the control mechanism required for maintaining proper balance of both pulmonary and systemic circulation and adequate cardiac output and perfusion during total mechanical replacement of the heart" (DeBakey, Hall et al. 1969, p. 129).

Calf experiments with the biventricular pump were authorized by DeBakey early in January 1969, "to test the technical feasibility of replacing the entire heart with this device, to learn what modifications in design were needed for proper anatomic attachment, and to obtain physiologic data for use in determining proper control of the driving mechanism of the pump" (DeBakey, personal communication).

Liotta conducted the first calf implant on 30 January 1969 (DeBakey, Hall et al. 1969, p. 137). But *the day before*, 29 January, he submitted an abstract entitled "Orthotopic Cardiac Prosthesis" to Dr. Vincent L. Gott, program chairman, American Society for Artificial Internal Organs (ASAIO), for presentation at the society's annual meeting on 21–22 April 1969. Liotta was senior author of the paper; he listed five coauthors from the Baylor program, including DeBakey. A footnote to the abstract acknowledged financial support from the National Heart Institute grant.

The abstract is significant for three reasons. First, according to DeBakey, it was written and submitted by Liotta "without [his] knowledge or consent" (DeBakey, personal communication). Second, the description of the artificial heart model it contains is identical with the one Cooley depicted when he reported on the Karp implant at the ASAIO meeting in April 1969. Third, the abstract described the results of animal experiments *that had not yet taken place*. Liotta's paper claimed that:

in 10 calves, total replacement of both ventricles was carried out for 24–44 hours with the animals standing normally.

These experiments revealed excellent new-endocardium formation at the blood pump interface, changes in blood cellular mass were not significant, and they evaluated the integration of physiological parameters into controlled systems.

Atrial pressures have been the main feedback mechanism utilized. The first clinical application is envisioned during open heart surgery in which cardiac function cannot be restored.

DeBakey apparently did not learn of the abstract until a few days before the paper was to be presented at the meeting, after the Karp operation. The advisory committee of the Baylor–Rice National Heart Institute grant, and DeBakey as its principal investigator, immediately requested that the paper be dropped from the program. A telegram to this effect was sent to Dr. Gott on 17 April, signed by DeBakey in his capacity as president of Bayor College of Medicine.

When the calf experiments anticipated by Liotta actually were conducted, the results were significantly different from those he had predicted. As reported by DeBakey and his colleagues in the April–June 1969 issue of the *Cardiovascular Research Center Bulletin*, only seven, not ten, calves had a pump implanted; none could "stand normally" after the operation; and all but one died far earlier than the twenty-four- to forty-four-hour period cited in the paper.

Table 4 summarizes the technical and physiological problems that beset the first recipients of a completely man-made heart.

Table 4. Results of Implantation of Biventricular Artificial Heart Pump in Seven Calves

Calf No.	Date of Implantation	Duration of Experiment	Fate of Calf
4578	1/30/69	59 min	Died on table; technical difficulties.
4576	2/3/69	67 min	Died on table; technical difficulties.
4582	2/13/69	47 min	Died on table; technical difficulties.
4583	2/20/69	50 min	Died on table; rupture of pump diaphragm.
4584	2/24/69	12.5 hrs	Some reflex movement, but calf unable to stand. Rupture of pump diaphragm. Renal failure; no urinary output during last 8 hrs.
4587	3/17/69	8 hrs, 25 min	Some reflex movement, but calf unable to stand. Renal failure; no urinary flow. Calf intubated and on resuscitator. Increasing anoxia.
4596	3/20/69	44 hrs	No reflex movement. No urinary output. Calf virtually cadaver from time of implantation. Calf heparinized and given artificial respiration.

SOURCE: DeBakey, Hall et al. 1969, p. 137.

As he wrote in his report of this work, DeBakey viewed the calf implants only as preliminary trials, yielding valuable data on technical and physiological aspects of the artificial heart but at the same time indicating the magnitude of the research and testing yet to be done before it would be ready for a clinical trial.

Results of these preliminary experiments suggest that a biventricular pump of this design can be developed to duplicate the functions of the two ventricles of the heart, but much work needs to be done before it will be possible to obtain proper control of the mechanism for adequate perfusion and viability of vital organs. Although two calves survived a short time, functional viability was inadequate. . . . Human experimentation must await unequivocal evidence of the safety and effectiveness of such a device in humans. [DeBakey, Hall et al. 1969, pp. 140, 142]

Heterograft valves had been used in the first three hearts, implanted on 30 January, 3 February, and 13 February. DeBakey had earlier anticipated and had told Liotta that these valves would not function satisfactorily, and he accordingly asked Liotta to discontinue their use. DeBakey also "instructed Dr. Liotta in further modifications in technical design of the pump for improved attachment, particularly atrial attachment. On 24 February, the fifth animal experiment was performed, this time with a prosthetic valve. [DeBakey] assumed that Dr. Liotta had purchased the Wada valve [a type of prosthetic valve], and only later learned that they had been obtained from Dr. Cooley" (DeBakey, personal communication).

The working relationship between Cooley and Liotta that led to the Karp implant began about the time the calf experiments were initiated, in January 1969. Over the next four months, Cooley later said, he and Liotta developed the heart that was used on 4 April (see note 1). In a private conversation shortly after the Karp operation, Liotta admitted to DeBakey that Cooley had approached him and suggested that they collaborate in the clinical use of the artificial heart. Liotta contended that Cooley persuaded him not to inform DeBakey of their plans. Liotta said that he assented to this secretiveness because he knew that DeBakey was not yet ready to approve clinical use of the pump, although as a full-time employee of the Baylor program, Liotta was required to inform DeBakey of his research plans and was not free to work on outside projects without DeBakey's consent.

A major component of the heart unit, the large power console that drives the pump, was designed by William O'Bannon, an engineer whose salary was paid by Rice University's portion of the National Heart Institute grant. On 17 January 1969 Liotta asked O'Bannon if he could build a duplicate of the console for Cooley. Although Liotta asked that the request be kept confidential, O'Bannon consulted his immediate superior, Dr. J. David Hellums, who advised him that the work could not be done at Rice because of the terms of the NHI grant. O'Bannon nevertheless agreed to build the console, working in his own garage during his spare time. He later said he had been "overwhelmed by the opportunity to work for Dr. Cooley," and also thought it was an interesting technical challenge to make the unit available at a relatively low cost, about $20,000. However, O'Bannon affirmed that the unit "was not designed for humans and had I known it was going to be used on a man, I might not have done it" (Randal 1969).

It was not until he had nearly completed the console that he began to suspect it was intended for human use. When he delivered the unit to Cooley on 2 April, he included a note stating that it was for use with experimental animals only and had not yet been fully tested (Quinn 1969b).

During the weeks when O'Bannon was constructing the power unit, Liotta was working in the Baylor Surgical Research Laboratories on fabricating and assembling the heart itself. The biventricular pump is constructed from hand-cast aluminum molds made in three sizes, small, medium, and large. The molds were fabricated by Mr. Louis Feldman, who is in charge of the laboratories' machine and plastics shops. Liotta told Mrs. Suzanne Anderson, a plastics technician, to have three "perfect" pumps ready for him by 20 March. Since no animal experiments were scheduled, this order, plus a further series of instructions, made Mrs. Anderson feel that "something was up." She began to suspect that the pumps were intended for human use when Liotta told her to line them with Dacron velour, use Silastic rather than elastic adhesive, and lengthen the tubing by several inches. He then announced that he would assemble the pumps himself, a task normally performed by the technicians. Mrs. Anderson noticed that Liotta seemed "nervous" and that he kept checking on her and her colleagues, pushing them to work faster than their normal pace and reiterating his demands for perfection. One day, for example, when he inspected a pump Mrs. Anderson had just lined and found it unsatisfactory, he exclaimed, "You're going to kill someone!" (Anderson, personal interview).

As the parts of the pump were manufactured and assembled, Mrs. Anderson entered them on a checklist, of which Liotta seems to have been unaware. At the time, she entered a note indicating that there was something "different" about these pumps. This was her shorthand way of referring to the many unusual events that she had observed during their construction.

Liotta inserted the valves and diaphragms into the pumps and personally assembled the units on 29 March. On 3 April, the pumps were gas autoclaved (sterilized) at the Baylor laboratories, once again making the technicians think that a clinical procedure might be planned. After that, Mrs. Anderson reported, the pumps "disappeared," and the next time she saw one of them was on a television program about the Karp operation. Liotta later testified that he had simply put the pumps into his briefcase and taken them to Saint Luke's.

While Liotta was assembling the pumps, William Hall, director of the program, was busy preparing to leave Baylor. On 1 April he was to become head of the bioengineering department at San Antonio's Southwest Research Institute. The technicians in the surgical laboratories assumed that Liotta had been authorized to take on some of Hall's functions and prerogatives. Partly for this reason, they discussed their uneasiness about why the pumps were being made only among themselves. "I didn't feel I could go to Dr. Liotta and say, 'I know you're up to something,'" Mrs. Anderson said. "He was acting head of the program, and besides, I wasn't going to take on any doctor" (Anderson, personal interview).

Final preparations for clinical use of the heart went forward swiftly once the pumps had been assembled and the power console had been delivered by O'Bannon on 2 April. On 3 April, the day the pumps were taken to Saint Luke's, Cooley called the medical photography office in the Baylor Department of Surgery to request that movies and still photographs be made the next day during the open-heart surgery scheduled for Haskell Karp.

That same day, O'Bannon called his chief at Rice, Dr. Hellums, to tell him that Cooley and Liotta were going to implant an artificial heart in a patient and wanted O'Bannon to assist in the operating room. Hellums gave three reasons for not approving the request: he had no evidence that the device had been adequately tested; DeBakey had not agreed to its use; and he did not want Rice "involved." The following morning, just before the operation itself, Cooley personally called Hellums to request O'Bannon's presence. Hellums again explained why he could not grant permission, and told Cooley that O'Bannon "has sincere doubts as to whether this pump has been properly tested" (Quinn 1969*b*).

When Liotta and Cooley were unable to obtain O'Bannon's expertise for the operation, they turned to Mr. Sam Calvin, an electronics engineer with the Baylor program. On the evening of 3 April, Liotta asked Calvin to come to Saint Luke's and "look over a new machine he had set up there" (Calvin, personal interview). While Calvin and Liotta were inspecting the pump unit, they were joined by Cooley. In the course of their conversation, Calvin recalls, Cooley mentioned that Mr. Karp might be a good candidate for an artificial heart, if things did not go well during the next morning's operation. "I was surprised," Calvin said, "because I didn't think we were ready for application of the artificial heart on the human level. I was reluctant to get involved, but Dr. Liotta told me it was my responsibility to check the pump unit, and I thought he was speaking as my chief."

Calvin spent some eight hours that night testing the pump unit to make sure that no unexpected problems would occur during an implant, and found that "virtually everything went well." Cooley and Liotta had completed their preparations for the first human implant of a totally artificial heart.

Cooley had five open-heart surgery cases scheduled on 4 April at Saint Luke's Hospital. Case number five was Haskell Karp, to be operated on for a ventricular aneurysm. A member of the "pump (heart-lung machine) team" remembers that the day unfolded "just like any other day, except that we did notice a great deal of equipment in the hall when we arrived in the morning." Just before case five was to begin, there "was sort of a holdup, and lots of people milling about. We didn't think too much about this, except to wonder if a transplant was going to take place. But when we got into the operating rooms, we decided that it was probably not a transplantation after all because there seemed to be no donor around."

The brief history of Karp's life with an artificial heart and then a human donor heart is outlined in a paper written by Cooley, Liotta, and their associates.

This report describes the emergency use of a total mechanical cardiac replacement for 64 hours in a 47 year old man with terminal cardiac disease who died 32 hours after cardiac transplantation.

[The patient] was admitted to The Texas Heart Institute on March 5, 1969, with advanced coronary arterial occlusive disease and complete heart block. Ten years previously, at age 37 years, he had experienced his first major myocardial infarction.

Complete atrioventricular block was identified in the electrocardiogram recorded on admission, and the ventricle was activated by the pacemaker impulse, thus obscuring any diagnostic configuration. Urinalysis, blood urea nitrogen and other blood chemistry determinations were normal. . . . Coronary arteriograms revealed severe narrowing of the right coronary artery 4 cm. beyond its origin; many collateral vessels, including one to the left coronary system; and complete occlusion of the anterior descending and left circumflex arteries, with small collateral arteries supplying the myocardium.

The patient was opposed to a cardiac transplantation, which was considered the operation of choice, and preferred a myocardial excision with ventriculoplasty—a procedure he knew of from news reports. After one month of intensive medical treatment without improvement, operation was performed.

First Surgical Procedure

On April 4, 1969, the heart was exposed under general anesthesia by a median sternotomy incision. . . . Little intact myocardium remained since scar tissue replaced over two-thirds of the left ventricular myocardium and almost the entire septum. An extensive area of fibrous transformation of the left ventricle and septum was excised and ventriculoplasty performed. Attempts at resuscitation of the heart failed, and cardiopulmonary bypass was continued while the heart was removed in the same manner used for cardiac transplantation. The cardiac prosthesis was placed in the pericardial sac after the atrial cuffs and arterial grafts were trimmed and tailored to ensure proper fit. . . . The patient remained in the operating room, which was converted into an intensive care unit providing the necessary equipment for monitoring, respirator support and isolation.

Postoperative Course

The patient regained consciousness within 15 minutes after the incision was closed. He responded to verbal commands and moved all limbs. . . . On April 6, 1969, the day preceding cardiac transplantation, leukopenia and moderate thrombocytopenia were evident, and the leukocyte count was 2,7000/cu. mm. Urinary output decreased progressively during these three days despite intravenous administration of mannitol and fluids. Dialysis was not attempted because the patient did not have significant azotemia or acidosis. His temperature was normal, and no signs of pulmonary or surgical infection were noted.

On April 7, 1969, at 5:00 a.m., a 39 year old woman was admitted to the hospital with irreversible brain damage after a period of anoxic arrest 48 hours previously. After blood and tissue compatibility was established between donor and recipient, both patients were placed in adjoining operating rooms.

Second Surgical Procedure

With the patient under general anesthesia, the sternotomy incision was reopened and the prosthesis exposed. . . . The prosthesis was removed from the pericardial cavity and replaced by the cardiac allograft by use of the technic described previously. . . .

Postoperative Course

The patient regained consciousness within one hour of operation, and peripheral circulation was adequately maintained with a slow infusion of isoproterenol. Urinary output was scant, but blood chemistry determinations did not reveal serious evidence of azotemia or hyperkalemia. A roentgenogram of the chest taken several hours later showed a localized area of atelectasis or consolidation in the right lower pulmonary lobe. During the subsequent clinical course this area increased in size until, 32 hours later, the entire lower lung field on the right was consolidated, and cardiac action ceased. [Cooley, Liotta et al. 1969]

Among the critical issues that the published reports of the case raise are the primary motivation for implanting the artificial heart and the degree to which it was premeditated. In both his professionally published accounts of the operation and his statements to the mass media, Cooley has avowed that his use of the heart was an emergency procedure, a stopgap measure to tide over a dying patient until a human donor could be found. He has implied that the decision to use the prosthesis was made only after a ventriculoplasty had been performed and Karp's heart could not be resuscitated. But the chronology of Cooley's and Liotta's activities shows that although the implantation may have been a response to an emergency, months of preparation had gone into readying the artificial heart used.

It seems evident, then, that the artificial heart unit did not just happen to be on hand and ready for use when Cooley was unable to resuscitate Karp's heart after resecting the ventricular aneurysm. This judgment was reached by many who, directly or indirectly, were involved in the case. For example, one physician we interviewed has evaluated the operation as follows:

There was too much forethought involved in the whole process of the implant for one to believe that Cooley had made a last ditch attempt to save a dying man's life. The artificial hearts were there, consent had been obtained from the patient, and the whole team was assembled. In addition, Cooley had taken enough aneurysms off enough ventricles to know in advance whether it was going to work. After all, Cooley has done more of these operations than anyone else in the world. I will never be convinced that he was not prepared to put in the artificial heart in the first place. He might just as well have scheduled it as an artificial heart implant. There was no need for him to go through the comical stage of resecting the aneurysm, and then dramatically saying, "This is not going to work."

It is also relevant that although Mr. Karp had been "opposed to a cardiac transplantation," which Cooley "considered the operation of choice," he finally gave consent for this procedure or an artificial heart implant on 4 April, the day he was scheduled for open-heart surgery. In principle, since Cooley reported no indication that Karp's condition had suddenly become worse, he could have postponed the ventriculoplasty and tried to locate a heart donor, now that the patient had agreed to undergo a transplant. Furthermore, implanting a mechanical heart to keep Mr. Karp alive until a donor could be found was at least as risky as simply waiting for a donor. It was known that the cardiac device could support the patient's circulation only for a limited period, and there was no way of predicting whether a heart donor would become available in time to save Mr. Karp. In fact, by April 1969 Cooley was already experiencing what he called a "drying up" of cardiac donors. All this circumstantial evidence strongly suggests that Cooley had an emotional vested interest in replacing Mr. Karp's heart with a cardiac prosthesis.

A second set of questions concerns what has been termed the "authorship" of the pump and the source of funds used for its development, construction, and testing. The first press releases issued by Cooley and by other "spokesmen" for Saint Luke's gave the public a clear impression that the unit had been pioneered by Liotta and Cooley.

Liotta and Cooley developed the artificial heart over the last four months. Liotta had used various models of the device over the last 10 years on experimental animals, including calves and dogs. [Total artificial heart is implanted in man 1969]

The hospital said that the artificial heart had been developed by Dr. Domingo Liotta. . . . Dr. Liotta was reported to have been working on the heart since 1959 when he was still in Argentina and to have been using the device in animals over that period. [Artificial heart is implanted in man 1969]

An unexpected breakthrough in refinements of the linings and valves three to five years ahead of schedule kept a 47-year old Illinois man's artificial heart pumping a rhythmic man-made pulse beat of life Saturday. . . . "We use what we consider a better valve, one which we began using clinically three months ago," Cooley said. "We're so enthusiastic that it gives good (blood) flow and so little blood destruction. It gave us the stimulus to move ahead with this device. . . ." . . . Dr. Domingo Liotta, . . . who designed the artificial heart, said 57 materials were tested before deciding on the right lining. "This is No. 29," Liotta said. [Artificial heart is performing well 1969]

The artificial heart differs from that developed by Dr. Michael DeBakey in that DeBakey's device was used only to bypass the heart's left ventricle. [1st artificial heart planted by cardiowhiz 1969]

In his statements at the Baylor hearings, Cooley vacillated about where and by whom the heart had been developed. According to John Quinn of the *New York Daily News*, who obtained transcripts of the hearings, Cooley at one point testified that:

What we wanted was a resuscitative type of pump which would give us time so we could secure a suitable donor. I talked to Dr. Liotta about this. Dr. Liotta brought the pump which he had designed in 1961, and I knew that Dr. Liotta was as well versed as anyone; so I talked to him about the possibility of helping me to develop such a device. Dr. Liotta expressed a willingness to do so. [Quinn 1969b]

"In his testimony," Quinn went on to report, "Cooley said he'd described for Liotta 'the type of pump I wanted' and 'I drew the design.' He later shifted ground to say he had simply made improvements in Liotta's 1961 design." These improvements, as we mentioned earlier, consisted primarily of incorporating Wada-Cutter hingeless valves into the pump, valves that were used in the fourth Baylor calf experiment after Cooley supplied Liotta with them. The other unexpected breakthrough that Cooley and Liotta had described to the press was the pump's Dacron lining, "no. 29" of the 57 materials they had tested. But DeBakey contended that this lining was a special feature of the pump developed at Baylor and had been conceived by him.

Cooley first said that he and Liotta made the pump unit during a four-month period, entirely at their own expense, with $25,000 supplied privately by his own Texas Heart Institute. Private funds do seem to have paid for the $20,000 power console built by

O'Bannon. Cooley testified at the Baylor hearings that when he asked Liotta to work with him on an artificial heart, he stressed that their project should be conducted without the use of NHI funds. He also reassured Liotta that it would be legitimate for them to collaborate if they worked outside Baylor. But under questioning Cooley wavered in his statements. He made less definite assertions about who had borne the costs of the pump's construction and testing. He still alleged that he had purchased the basic materials, but specified only the Wada-Cutter valves. He admitted that the heart had been built in the Baylor research laboratories, and that he knew Liotta was obliged to work full time for the Baylor Artificial Heart Program.

Although Cooley gave conflicting reports about the heart's authorship, Liotta made an unequivocal statement about its origin. He acknowledged that the model implanted in Mr. Karp had been designed at Baylor through research funded by NHI grant HE–5435, that the unit itself was fabricated in the Baylor Surgical Research Laboratories, and that it was essentially identical in design and function with the device tested in calves under DeBakey's supervision.

Liotta's assertion was corroborated by others affiliated with the Baylor–Rice program. However, the papers that Cooley subsequently published still maintained, at least implicitly, that the heart was a product of his and Liotta's work. His first report was made at the ASAIO's April 1969 meeting and subsequently published in the society's *Transactions*. Describing the cardiac prosthesis, Cooley wrote that "the same concept has been tested in earlier work (1959–1960)," citing Liotta's original work on an orthotopic heart, and went on to note that "Hastings et al. have tested a similar pump design." He then briefly alluded to "previous experimental work in this [Saint Luke's] laboratory" that had "demonstrated the validity" of the pump's concept. The extensive work by the Baylor laboratories on single and biventricular pumps was recognized only by two citations to 1966 and 1967 papers dealing with fabric linings (Cooley 1969, p. 255).

A second paper, published in November 1969, again cited Liotta's 1961 paper and referred the reader to the *Transactions* paper for "details of design and flow characteristics" of the pump. Cooley's short discussion of other work on artificial heart models is remarkable for the manner in which he passingly acknowledges that DeBakey had worked in this field:

Outstanding contributions have been made to the field of total heart substitution by the work of Akutsu, Nosé and Kwan-Gett and their co-workers in the experimental laboratory using a pulsatile flow mechanical device. Liotta et al. recorded the first clinical attempt at partial functional replacement of the left ventricle using an implantable pump in a human patient. E. Stanley Crawford implanted this pump in his patient on July 19, 1963, inserting the device in parallel with the left ventricle. The inflow connector was inserted into the left atrium and the outflow connector sutured to the descending thoracic aorta. DeBakey also referred to the clinical use of this left ventricular bypass pump. The clinical employment of a device for circulatory assistance in series with the left ventricle was reported by Kantrowitz et al. [Cooley, Liotta et al. 1969, p. 729]

Cooley's oral and written statements notwithstanding, the diagram of the artificial heart published in his paper for the *Transactions of the American Society for Artificial Internal Organs* was nearly identical to the schematic drawing prepared on 10 September 1968 of the biventricular pump developed by De-Bakey's team. The two diagrams are reproduced in figures 2 and 3. According to DeBakey, Liotta submitted the September 1968 diagram, with a few penciled-in changes, to a medical artist in the Baylor Department of Surgery on 17 April 1969. He asked that the drawing be prepared as an illustration for the paper on the Karp implant that he, Cooley, and Hallman were preparing for publication in the ASAIO *Transactions* (DeBakey, personal communication).

By the time *Life* reporter Thomas Thompson came to Houston to interview him, nearly a year after the Karp implant, Cooley admitted that he "took" the heart developed and built at Baylor, "used it," and would "use it again."

"Did you use Dr. DeBakey's heart?"
"Well," he answered slowly, not seeming to duck the question but searching for the way to answer it, "I guess, in effect, I took it. I didn't believe they were working on it. The staff had deteriorated. I knew Dr. Liotta was frustrated. I told him it would be a marvelous chance to develop one at our institute. I told him I would bear all the expenses personally. We proceeded with it, we did animal experimentation with increasing success, we felt we could keep a man alive for two days. When the time came, I used it. I just couldn't let another man die on the operating room table. [Thompson 1970, p. 74]

A third set of concerns relates to the uncertainties and incon-sistencies expressed in both the spoken and written accounts of the causes of Haskell Karp's death on 8 April. These statements, in the main, centered on the causal role of the artificial heart in Karp's death, although the possible role of a rejection of the human heart he received on 7 April is also unclear. In his report to the ASAIO two weeks after Karp's death, Cooley reviewed the pathologist's study of the donor heart and stated that "these findings were interpreted as revealing no absolute evidence of rejection or of an immunological response in the allograft material" (Cooley 1969, p. 255). But in a November 1969 letter to the public relations department of *McCall's* magazine, in connection with their publication of Barnard's autobiography, Cooley wrote that "we did a cardiac transplantation [on Mr. Karp] which resulted in the patient's death 36 hours later from rejection."[3]

From a strictly mechanical perspective, the artificial heart performed its pumping function well during the 64 hours it remained in Karp's chest. But almost immediately after the implant, physiological and biochemical danger signs appeared. In his write-up of the case, Cooley noted that Karp's urinary output had "decreased progressively" after the operation, but that "dialysis was not attempted because the patient did not have significant azotemia [retention of nitrogen, which may be a sign of uremia] or acidosis" (Cooley, Liotta et al. 1969, p. 727). By 7 April, the day of Karp's heart transplant, his renal problems had mounted, as was reflected by an alarming three fold increase in his BUN level. Some four hours after the transplant, a renal specialist was called in as a consultant. The report he later submitted to the Baylor faculty committee detailed Karp's critical condition and indicated that renal failure had ensued sooner and more severely than Cooley reported in the literature.

The renal specialist was told that Karp had been "virtually anuric" (had not passed any urine) since his cardiac implant, and he found the patient to be semicomatose and in need of continuous ventilatory aid. When he reviewed Karp's laboratory data and examined him, the consultant in part judged that he was suffering from virtually complete urinary failure, the cause of which he could not specify precisely, and from cardiogenic circulatory insufficiency, deterioration of brain function owing to lack of oxygen, and "immediately life-threatening" metabolic acidosis. Treatment was initiated that succeeded in reversing the metabolic acidosis. But until his death on 8 April Karp remained so anuric that the renal consultant was unable to obtain a urine specimen for further diagnostic evaluation.

Fig. 2. "Schematic drawing (Sept. 10, 1968) showing design of biventricular artificial heart" (DeBakey, Hall, et al. 1969, p. 128, fig. 1a).

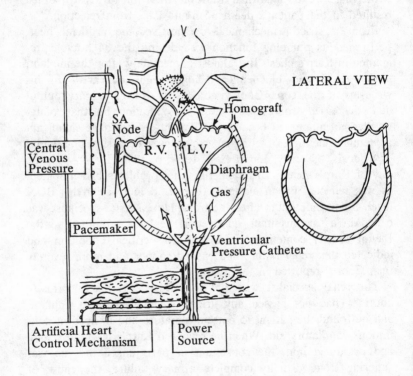

Fig. 3. "Schematic representation of the orthotopic cardiac prosthesis. A dual-ventricular pump was used in this first clinical case" (Cooley 1969, p. 256, fig. 1; by permission of *Transactions of the American Society for Artificial Internal Organs*).

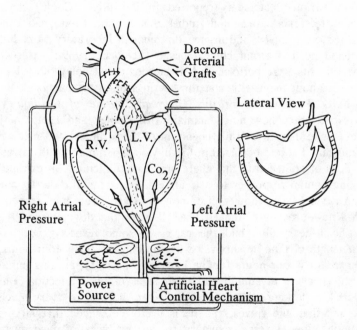

At the ASAIO meetings, Cooley maintained that Karp's "death from pneumonia and renal complications was not directly attributable to the mechanical prosthesis." Accordingly, he stated, "total replacement of the heart with a mechanical substitute may now be feasible for more prolonged periods" (Cooley 1969, p. 263). To those familiar with the Baylor animal experiments, however, Karp's downhill course seemed to closely parallel the fate of the calves that had survived the implant procedure itself. The pump's inability to maintain the viability of vital organs, as seen in the occurrence of brain damage due to oxygen deficiency and of irreversible kidney failure, had caused DeBakey to preclude human trials with the device.

In various statements reported in the press, Cooley made vague references to animal studies that he and Liotta had conducted on 9 calves, and argued that enough laboratory work had been done to warrant clinical usage (Schmeck 1969a). If such experiments were performed, it is curious that Cooley offered no details about them, either at the hearings or in his papers in the ASAIO *Transactions* or the *American Journal of Cardiology*. Irrespective of how much animal work Cooley and Liotta may have done, they were fully cognizant of the technical and medical problems that had occurred in the Baylor experiments with calves.

It is of course true that there are many difficulties in extrapolating human responses to a treatment from animal data; so one can never be sure how well or how poorly patients may respond to a new procedure. Indeed Haskell Karp did do better on the artificial heart than had the calves in some respects—such as the length of time he survived with the implant (sixty-four hours, versus forty-four hours for the longest-living calf), and his initial responsiveness to stimuli and other signs of brain function. But DeBakey, among others, feels that Karp did not do "very much better" than the calves, and he is firmly convinced that all the complications "were secondary to the problem of inadequate perfusion, due to the effects of the implanted pump." Nor does he believe that it "matters very much how many hours or even days that you keep an animal alive in the lab with an implanted heart. This is not the major criterion. You need evidence that it can maintain a viable, functioning animal. . . . There's a difference between prolonging death and prolonging life" (DeBakey, personal interview).

To DeBakey it seemed almost inconceivable that Cooley could use the pump in a patient knowing of its prior performance in animals. He frankly and scathingly denounced this aspect of Cooley's actions in a July 1969 letter to Dr. Harold Brown, chairman of the Baylor College of Medicine Faculty Committee on Research Involving Human Beings, in which he reviewed a research protocol submitted to Brown by Cooley for work on an orthotopic cardiac prosthesis.

If the procedure planned for clinical use is the same as that used in patient Haskell Karp, the progressive deterioration in that patient from the time of insertion of the orthotopic cardiac prosthesis until its removal for cardiac transplantation was obviously irreversible, and these irreversible changes precluded the patient's survival. In many respects, the changes in Mr. Karp resemble those observed in the animal experiments described in the article [DeBakey, Hall et al. 1969] in the *Cardiovascular Research Center Bulletin*. . . .

. . . The primary purpose of applying such a device is to provide recuperability, and no evidence has been presented that the device described will accomplish this purpose or that it "offers a chance of salvage." The ethical stipulation in the National Institutes of Health guidelines for human experimentation that "the risks to the individual are outweighed by the potential benefit to him or by the importance of the knowledge to be gained," which is generally accepted by scientists, is not here satisfied, since the benefits of research can be obtained more ethically from preliminary laboratory experimentation, without undue hazard, discomfort, or suffering to or infringement on the dignity of, human beings. . . .

In the case of the device described, the absence of evidence of the reversibility of the damage caused by insertion of the device not only challenges the use of the device as a stopgap measure until cardiac transplantation can be performed, but also violates medical and scientific ethics. In addition, a scarce donor organ is being used under circumstances of higher risk of failure than would be the case in a patient who had not previously been subjected to experimental implantation of the prosthetic device.

A series of inquiries into the Karp case began on 5 April, the day the implant was made public. Dr. Hebbel E. Hoff, Baylor's Associate Dean for Faculty and Clinical Affairs, called an emergency meeting of the Committee on Research Involving Human Beings. The committee began its formal investigation on Monday, 7 April, chaired by Dr. Harold Brown. Like most people, Michael DeBakey had learned of Karp's operation from a newscast while, ironically, he was in Washington attending a conference on artificial hearts. Although he was chairman of the department of surgery as well as president of the medical school, DeBakey did not participate in the investigations other than to testify, because of his close involvement in the case.

A second committee, which supervised Baylor's multimillion-dollar grant from the National Heart Institute, began its own inquiry on 8 April. On 9 April, the press related that Dr. Theodore Cooper, director of the National Heart Institute, had written DeBakey to ask whether NHI funds had been used to develop the heart, including payment of Liotta's salary, and if so, whether the Public Health Service guidelines for human experimentation had been followed. He also requested a summary of any data obtained from animal experiments performed under the NHI grant before the implant. The following day Mr. L. F. McCollum, chairman of the medical school's board of trustees, announced that he had appointed a special committee, chaired by Dr. Hoff, to examine the questions posed by Cooper.

It was in the midst of the Baylor investigations that DeBakey learned about the abstract on "Orthotopic Cardiac Prosthesis" that Liotta had planned to present to the ASAIO meeting on 22 April. In his capacity as president of Baylor College of Medicine, he telegraphed the program chairman of the meeting requesting its withdrawal. Although the paper was canceled chiefly because of the falsified animal data it contained, Cooley attended the meetings and "received a standing ovation" when he requested time to deliver an oral report on the Karp case (Quinn 1969b). In addition to publication of that presentation in the society's *Transactions*, Quinn has reported that "Cooley and Liotta later sent a formal scientific paper to the *Journal of the American Medical Association*. For reasons which the editor declined to explain, the journal refused publication" (Quinn 1969b). At the AMA's July 1969 meeting in New York, however, Cooley and his colleagues did display an exhibit that included illustrations of the artificial heart and data from Karp's operations. Although the exhibit carried Baylor's sponsorship, according to DeBakey it did not "have the approval of the chairman of the department as required by the college" (DeBakey, personal communication).

The DeBakey group's paper on the biventricular pump's development and testing, as we have noted, was published in the April–

June 1969 issue of the *Cardiovascular Research Center Bulletin*. In May 1969, the nine co-authors of the paper took the unusual step of placing the following signed statement on the title page of the already published manuscript: "This is a true and accurate account of the development and testing of the orthotopic cardiac prosthesis" (DeBakey, personal communication).

After the special committee's hearings, McCollum reported its conclusions to NHI director Cooper: Liotta's "salary and to a substantial degree his research is supported by grant HE–5435"; a protocol for clinical implantation had not been reviewed by the medical school's research committee because none was submitted, nor did the committee members, or DeBakey, or any other official of the college know of plans for the implantation.[4]

After receiving McCollum's letter, Cooper wrote again for further verification that the artificial heart had been developed with NHI funds and used clinically without peer review and approval of the plan. He also asked McCollum to specify what "stringent steps" Baylor was taking to "insure that all protocols of the National Heart Institute and of this college will be followed in the future." In his reply on 9 May, McCollum reiterated the committee's findings and reported that the medical school faculty had recommended that as a condition for membership on the Baylor faculty, all new appointees and present staff must sign a statement agreeing to observe the college's regulations and by-laws. Those regulations include following the NHI guidelines and submitting clinical protocols to the research committee. He added that failure to comply with these provisions would lead to a "consideration of disciplinary proceedings."

The consequences of Liotta's involvement were also reported to Cooper at this time. On the basis of the special committee's findings, his salary from the NHI grant had been discontinued as of 16 April and he was suspended and later discharged from the Artificial Heart Program.

The full record of the special committee's hearings has not been released, even to the NHI, despite a request by Cooper on 14 May. On 29 May, McCollum informed him that the report and supporting documents had been declared confidential and privileged communications by the committee, and so the "complete record of the investigation" could not be made available.

In June 1969, the new appointment form was distributed to all faculty members of the Baylor College of Medicine. The last two paragraphs of the form letter responded to the college's and the NHI's concern to avoid another case like that of Mr. Karp.

May I bring to your attention the revised rules of the Committee on Research Involving Human Beings, which were adopted as rules of the college of medicine by the executive faculty on June 9, 1969, and approved by the executive committee of the Board of Trustees on July 7, 1969. These rules are: all research, whether supported by the Public Health Service or by any source, must follow the regulations set forth in the public health document dated May 1, 1969, and entitled "Protection of the Individual as a Research Subject". . . . A copy of this document is enclosed.

I have been asked by the Board of Trustees to point out that your acceptance of this appointment affirms that you will abide by the revised rules of the Committee on Research Involving Human Beings as outlined above. Your signature on the enclosed copy of this letter will indicate your acceptance of your appointment and your willingness to abide by these rules.[5]

On 8 July 1969 McCollum sent Cooper a copy of the appointment letter, generated by the Cooley and Moore operations (see note 5), and said he would notify him whether any faculty members objected to signing it. In a statement to the press, McCollum quoted from a press interview by Cooper on 15 May:

We believe that Baylor is seeking to insure further compliance with the public health service guidelines, and to provide for appropriate disciplinary action against any faculty member who violates them. . . . The NHI believes that the action taken by Baylor in this matter is evidence of its intention and its ability to enforce these guidelines.

McCollum then went on to say:

It would be hard to overemphasize the importance of Dr. Cooper's statement to Baylor. Our college of medicine currently receives approximately $3,000,000 a year for its cardiovascular research, including the Artificial Heart Program. Not only were these grants in jeopardy, but other substantial Federal grants might have been endangered had Baylor been held responsible for this violation of the Federal guidelines.

Dr. Cooper has vindicated the present administration of the college. The Board of Trustees has asked me to express its gratification for Dr. Cooper's statement and wishes to express complete confidence in Dr. DeBakey and deep appreciation of the dedication of a faculty and staff who made Baylor a great medical school.

Denton Cooley declined to sign the new Baylor appointment form, and on 2 September 1969 he resigned his position as clinical professor of surgery at the college of medicine. His action, as he stated in his letter of resignation to DeBakey, was taken principally because the Committee on Research Involving Human Beings had not approved his clinical research protocol for "development and application of an orthotopic cardiac prosthesis as part of a two-staged cardiac replacement." The protocol had been submitted to the Baylor research committee on 25 June, after it had been accepted by the equivalent committee at Saint Luke's Hospital and the Texas Heart Institute. DeBakey was one of the members of the Baylor committee who did not approve Cooley's protocol.

As president of the college of medicine, DeBakey notified Cooley that his resignation had been accepted by the board of trustees. In a lengthy letter on 11 September 1969, DeBakey reviewed the reasons he had rejected Cooley's artificial heart research protocol and dwelt on the broader themes of medical ethics involved in Baylor's requirement that all faculty members adhere to its guidelines for clinical research.

Dear Dr. Cooley:

I have received your letter of resignation as Clinical Professor of Surgery, dated September 2, 1969. It was upon the recommendation of your peers, the Executive Faculty Committee of Baylor, that the Board of Trustees adopted the guidelines on human experimentation to which you object. Of our 1,350 faculty members, both full-time and clinical, who were required to sign the statement indicating their willingness to abide by the guidelines, you alone refused. . . .

It is difficult to understand the logic of the statement in your letter that "the directive from the Board of Trustees requiring that all members of the faculty must agree to accept the action of a committee on human experimentation places some members of the clinical faculty in an untenable position." As a highly esteemed institution dedicated to medical education, research, and health care, Baylor College of Medicine must discharge its responsibilities not only to science and the scientific community, but to patients who come under the care of its faculty members and to society at large. In so doing, it must establish and enforce standards of ethics and criteria for medical research for *all* members of the faculty. . . . To have dual standards, one for full-time faculty and another, more relaxed, for clinical faculty, would compromise not only the clinical faculty, but the College as well.

Nor can standards of human experimentation be altered, depending on the source of supporting funds, as you suggest. Such a flexibility would grant a degree of autonomy to every investigator who receives private research funds, which might render the school vulnerable to criticism for conduct for which it has abdicated responsibility.

. . . In the eyes of the scientific community and the world, [Baylor] is, in fact, held accountable for the activities and conduct of its own faculty, as illustrated by recent events. Should Baylor's Committee on Research Involving Human Beings ever perfunctorily approve every proposal for human research that has been approved by the research committees of individual hospitals and institutes, it would become a rubber-stamp body that had renounced its charge and therefore no longer had a raison d'être.

[DeBakey next reviews Cooley's research protocol.]

With the increasing complexity of experimental operations and the increasing concern of society with moral and ethical values of science, the ethical considerations of human experimentation become more critical and the responsibility of medical schools more serious to protect the patient and society, to maintain the integrity of science, and to prevent a semblance of permissiveness that might not only violate the rights of the patient but also alienate society. As a consequence, scientific research and medical education would suffer. Since the parent institution is ultimately responsible for the ethical conduct of its faculty, Baylor must exercise every precaution to insure that scientific experimentation is practiced within ethical and moral codes.

It is regrettable that you find it impossible to comply with the requirements for human research and medical ethics recommended by the faculty of the Baylor College of Medicine and accepted by all similar creditable institutions.

Yours, sincerely,
[signed]
Michael E. DeBakey, M.D.

The departures of Liotta and Cooley from the Baylor College of Medicine marked the formal denouement of the case of the artificial heart.

In dramatic form, the case of the artificial heart raises vital questions concerning human experimentation in medicine and the ways that social, psychological, and ethical factors can affect it. One of the basic considerations was whether the prosthesis had been sufficiently tested and perfected on animals to justify its use in a man. It might perfunctorily be argued that the seven calf experiments conducted in DeBakey's laboratory, plus those Cooley said that he and Liotta carried out, were inadequate in quality as well as number. So far as we know, the clinical outcome of these experiments was so unfavorable that those animals who did not die on the operating table succumbed soon after the pump was implanted, without ever sufficiently recovering from surgery to stand on their own feet. Nonetheless, Cooley's statement that sufficient animal research had been done must be understood against the backdrop of some of the inherent ambiguities of clinical investigation discussed in earlier chapters. Laboratory experiments on animals are technically and ethically prerequisite to clinical trials of a new therapy on human beings. But there are no absolute criteria for determining when it is proper to move from the laboratory to the clinic. In addition, the animal model only imperfectly anticipates how a human subject will react. In these senses, human experimentation is always both premature and perilous. Thus the pertinent question about the clinical use of the artificial heart is *not*, was it precipitate and dangerous, but rather, did it go so far beyond the unclearly defined normative bounds as to be illegitimate? In the case of the artificial heart, the answer probably is yes. Even if all the preliminary calf experiments had been successful, the small number of animals on which the device was tried was not statistically significant; and in fact their clinical outcome was fatal in every instance.

Cooley's stated rationale for trying the prosthesis on Mr. Karp is associated with another crucial aspect of human experimentation, one that can assume life-and-death proportions, as it did in this case. Cooley contended that his primary reason for implanting the artificial heart was to do everything that was medically or surgically possible to save the life of his patient. But it seems likely that his motivation was far more complex. If for the moment we hold constant other factors that entered into his surgical decision, we are confronted with one of the most troublesome and urgent sets of problems in modern medicine. How far should the physician go in trying to sustain life? When, if ever, should he cease to try? Are there any conditions under which he has the right or even the obligation to withhold an available treatment from a terminally ill patient, or offer him one that could relieve his suffering by speeding his death? Where precisely does the process of prolonging life end and that of prolonging death begin? And to what extent ought the physician to take into account the state of health and "quality of life" his patient will experience if he succeeds in "saving" him?

In a first clinical trial like the implantation Cooley performed on Karp, these dilemmas of "ordinary" versus "extraordinary" means are further compounded. It is only on a patient as desperately ill as Mr. Karp that a clinical investigator has the right to initiate such a procedure. And if there were not physicians and patients willing to collaborate in such a bold venture, certain forms of therapeutic innovation would never reach the human level of experimentation. Furthermore, clinical investigators are subject to pressures which tend to push them toward using desperate, pioneering means with a patient like Mr. Karp. Their characteristically intense emotional involvement with the suffering patient makes it difficult for them to stand by as death claims the person for whom they have been caring. In this situation, most American physicians have a cultural proclivity to deal with their patients' conditions energetically, on the determined, optimistic premise that intervention will make recovery more likely. Above and beyond this, the recurrent need to wage a personal battle with death may be more developed in the research physician interested in trail-blazing procedures like heart surgery, organ transplantation, and the implantation of vital artificial organs than in physicians engaged in more usual forms of practice.

The case of the artificial heart also makes it quite clear that along with these heroic therapeutic and existential motivations, the competitive drive for medical priority and recognition can galvanize a physician to attempt an intrepid and hazardous procedure. There is strong circumstantial evidence for this interpretation in the data indicating that Cooley's implantation of the prosthesis in Karp was not purely a last-minute, on-the-spot emergency decision. Three months earlier, he had recruited Liotta to ready a pump for imminent patient use, and he later enlisted Calvin's help in the project. The artificial heart unit they prepared was present in the amphitheater and primed for use the day Cooley performed the ventriculoplasty on Karp. Furthermore, there seems to have been no sudden change for the worse in Karp's condition that obliged Cooley to carry out this procedure if he was to keep his patient alive for an eventual transplant.

Without implying a perfect parallel, it is ironically significant that a number of the factors that led Cooley to place the prosthesis in Karp's chest—and several of the reasons he gave for doing so—also seem to have entered into DeBakey's pioneering use of a left ventricular bypass in his patient, Mr. G. W., six years earlier. In the DeBakey case, of course, this initial human trial had been preceded by extensive animal work in his own laboratories, where as many as one hundred dogs were considered to have experienced "successful" implants. But, like Karp, G. W. was considered to be an "ideal candidate" for the procedure because "everything known to medicine . . . had already been done . . . and still the patient was going downhill"; because in spite of the seeming "hopelessness of the situation," his doctors felt that "there was a possibility that he was a salvageable patient"; and because they hoped that the pump, although built for use in a laboratory dog, could provide just enough support to get him "on the front side of the curve" before it was removed. G. W. died four days later, but this was the experience out of which DeBakey and his colleagues were able to design a human model of the implantable artificial ventricle which now has life-saving importance in cardiac surgery.

Clinical trials in which the physician imposes his will upon patients who do not fully understand the situation are flagrantly unethical, according to the various national and international codes for human experimentation.[6] One of the core moral injunctions is that informed, voluntary consent be obtained from any person who acts as a subject. A further extension of this principle is the conviction shared by many researchers that the investigator-subject relationship ideally should be collaborative.[7] One of the more ambiguous aspects of the case of the artificial heart is whether in a lucid, unpressured way Karp had given Cooley permission for each of the three consecutive surgical procedures: the ventriculoplasty, the pump implant, and the heart transplantation. A number of elements make it difficult to evaluate this: Cooley's apparent desire from the outset to do more than conventional heart surgery on Karp, and the motives that contributed to it; the effect of these attitudes not only on Cooley's own judgment and decision-making but also upon the dying Mr. Karp and his grief-stricken wife; the at once encouraging and discouraging influence that the mass media's treatment of cardiac transplantation had on the Karps and their publicity-sensitive surgeon; and what may have been their wavering opinions about what they ought to do in their besieged, in extremis predicament. It is far easier to affirm the cardinal importance of informed, voluntary, collaborative consent in human experimentation than it is to ensure that these conditions will be met. In this case some of the primary factors that can cloud the question of whether agreement has been obtained in an acceptable way converged in a particularly troublesome manner.

Haskell Karp's transplantation involved another dying patient and her family, flown from New England to Texas expressly to donate a cadaver heart to a man lying in the operating room (now converted to an intensive care unit), where his own heart had recently been excised and replaced by a cardiac prosthesis. The conditions under which Mrs. Barbara Ewan became the donor for Mr. Karp pose another whole group of problems. For one thing, her family's decision to offer her heart was triggered by Mrs. Karp's piteous entreaty, transmitted coast to coast by television, radio, and newspapers. From a certain point of view broadcasting this histrionic message, as the mass media willingly did, could be considered an act that misinformed not only the Karp and Ewan families but the American public. At the same time that the media heralded the artificial heart as a great new fait accompli, their communiqués also proclaimed that cardiac transplantation was such a miraculously effective procedure that "a gift of a heart" for Mrs. Karp's husband could "save" him. As Dr. Irvine Page bluntly put it, "the public was certainly grossly misled" (Page 1970). Nothing short of the belief that Mrs. Ewan's offering could meaningfully prolong the life of another person led her children to send her to Houston. Another disturbing aspect is that although Mrs. Ewan was deemed to be suffering irreversible brain damage after a period of anoxic arrest, she had not yet been pronounced dead when she was accepted as a candidate-donor and began her trip to Texas. Technically and morally speaking, she was alive until an hour and a half after her arrival in Houston, when four physicians declared her dead from a stroke suffered en route. It is well recognized that in this early era of transplantation the supply of donor organs available is far less than the number of persons who might derive at least some temporary benefit from this type of implant. One could ask, then, whether it was justifiable to transport Mrs. Ewan thousands of miles to give her heart, when someone nearby might have been a suitable recipient. In fact, because he had undergone two previous forms of cardiac surgery in rapid succession, Mr. Karp was probably less likely to benefit from a transplant than a patient who had not been subjected to these prior surgical traumas and to the damage that the artificial heart may have inflicted on him during the sixty-four hours it remained in his chest.

Another fundamental ethical standard of human experimentation requires that the possible benefits of what is tried on a subject outweigh the risks and discomforts to which he is exposed. Given the uncertainties that characterize any piece of research, this is difficult to calculate. But nothing less than a reasonably long interlude of added life, out of the hospital, that was active, satisfying, and free of pain could have sufficiently compensated Mr. Karp for the danger and suffering he incurred through his two-stage experimental surgery as well as through his grave cardiovascular illness. Mr. Karp did not have this interlude. What is more, it is entirely possible that his death was made more intricate and was even accelerated by deleterious effects, comparable to those seen in laboratory calves, that the artificial heart had on his vital organs, particularly his kidneys and brain. In a man as debilitated as Karp, this too is hard to pinpoint.

Another range of issues derives from the relationship of Dr. Cooley, Dr. DeBakey, and Dr. Liotta to the intersecting professional activities in which they were involved, to each other, and to the specialized technical personnel who worked with them in the laboratory and the surgical amphitheater. One focal aspect of the case was certainly the complicated and bitter priority dispute between the three surgeons. Sufficient documentary evidence has already been presented to indicate that the device Dr. Cooley implanted in Mr. Karp was, except for minor modifications, identical to the orthotopic cardiac prosthesis designed and tested in DeBakey's laboratory under a National Heart Institute grant, awarded to DeBakey as principal investigator. In turn, this prosthesis had been developed from the original biventricular heart and the left ventricular bypass pump that DeBakey and his colleagues had developed and pioneered some years earlier. We need not pursue this further. What does need to be examined is what led Cooley and Liotta to covertly take the artificial heart model from the Baylor Laboratories to Saint Luke's Hospital, secretly work on it, and at first claim that the pump unit they implanted in Mr. Karp was made entirely by them, financed by private funds. Dr. Domingo Liotta had worked on developing an artificial heart in Argentina and subsequently at the Cleveland Institute; in 1962, along with Dr. William Hall, he joined De-

Bakey's staff. He was one of two physicians who in 1960 independently made the earliest successful laboratory attempts to replace the heart with an artificial intrathoracic pump. (The other physician was Dr. Willem Kolff, the inventor of the first clinical artificial kidney machine, who was associated with the Cleveland Institute when Liotta worked there.) After adding Liotta and Hall to his team, DeBakey was able to organize his long-standing interest in developing a mechanical form of total cardiac replacement into an extensive program of laboratory investigation. In 1963, largely as a consequence of the skilled medicopolitical efforts of DeBakey, Baylor University and Rice University received companion grants from the National Heart Institute to launch a collaborative artificial heart project, under the aegis of DeBakey. Hall was appointed program director and Liotta full-time assistant.

Although Liotta played an important role in the ensuing work on the orthotopic cardiac prosthesis, it is hard to ascertain exactly how autonomous and essential his work was. The collective nature of team research always makes it difficult to identify individual investigators' contributions. The task of objectively evaluating Liotta's input to the project is further complicated because there are no indisputable criteria for appraising the overall significance of the specialized kinds of technical knowledge and skills he introduced. At an early stage in the events that followed Mr. Karp's operation, both Liotta and Cooley claimed that in 1961 Liotta had designed the heart pump used in Karp. This would mean that he brought this pump to DeBakey's laboratory when he came to work for him in 1962, and that it was the basic model for the cardiac prosthesis that was developed there.

DeBakey's own formulation of Liotta's role was "technical assistance."[8] In a private statement made seven months after the implantation of the artificial heart, DeBakey depicted Liotta as "hardly more than a technician" (DeBakey, personal interview).

Hall gives Liotta credit for having an "interest in things artificial," like himself, "at a time when that evoked 'pooh-poohs' from a lot of people, with the exception of Dr. DeBakey" (Hall, personal interview). He also acknowledges Liotta's earlier work with Kolff, and his competence "as an experimental surgeon." However, Hall makes an invidious distinction between an experimental surgeon and a "clinical surgeon." He categorizes the former as a calling only for the "technician" skills involved in operating on laboratory animals, as compared with what he considers the more intricate judgment and responsibility that human surgery entails. Furthermore, Hall asserts that Liotta's main task in the development of the artificial heart was "implanting the devices into laboratory animals," rather than making "the actual design decisions," as he and DeBakey did (Hall, personal interview).

Mr. Louis Feldman, machinist-technician in charge of the machine and plastics shops in DeBakey's surgical laboratories, considers the artificial heart to be "the product of the work of many people, perhaps as many as 40 people." He does not regard Liotta's contribution as singularly important in this common enterprise. According to Feldman, Liotta played a minor role in designing the pump; is a "good plastics technician"; helped to construct some of the devices implanted in the calves; but never built any of these models completely by himself (Feldman, personal interview).

Each of these commentators on Liotta is intellectually and emotionally involved in the case of the artificial heart to a degree that may color his opinions. No conclusions can be drawn from their statements. But all these persons, and others in the Baylor-Rice program whom we interviewed, reported that Liotta himself was convinced that the artificial heart was "his." He believed himself to be the primary person who designed, fabricated, and conducted animal experiments with the heart, they testify, and as such felt he had the right to do with it what he wanted. That Dr. Cooley approached Liotta to work with him, conveying the message that Liotta was as "well versed as anyone" in these matters, seems to have greatly reinforced Liotta's image of himself as the chief "architect" and appropriate purveyor of the artificial heart. Cooley's approach also appears to have been sufficiently flattering to have led Liotta knowingly to break his contract with DeBakey and the National Heart Institute by secretly working for Cooley and to have gone so far as to take three pumps manufactured and assembled in DeBakey's laboratory at Baylor over to Cooley at Saint Luke's, where the Karp operation was eventually performed. Observers agree that part of the explanation for this is to be found in the high admiration, almost hero worship, that Liotta felt for Cooley—his "fantastic" surgical ability, personal charisma, and public presence. Liotta's "idolizing feelings" about Cooley, it has been said by one of their colleagues, lured him into "giving Cooley what he asked for on a silver platter." In addition, Liotta seems to have been eager to move from animal experimentation to clinical use of the cardiac prosthesis and to have been despairingly impatient because De-Bakey took the position that "certain technical and physiologic problems . . . need to be solved before a satisfactory total mechanical replacement for the human heart can be developed. Human experimentation must await unequivocal evidence of the safety and effectiveness of such a device in animals" (DeBakey, Hall et al. 1969, p. 142). One of our Houston informants remarked that "anybody who gets involved in the artificial heart has to be a very ambitious man . . . because if things work out well [it holds forth] the possibility of instant immortality." Liotta appears to have had his share of this sort of "big man" ambition. Only an unusually fierce desire to get ahead of others in his field could explain why it was that in January 1969, without DeBakey's knowledge or consent, he submitted to the American Society for Artificial Internal Organs the co-authored abstract in which he described the results of calf experiments that had been planned but not yet carried out.

Finally, in this attempt to make sense of the motivation that led Liotta to participate in the case of the artificial heart and to violate many norms of medical and scientific research in the process, it should be mentioned that his relations with DeBakey were far from ideal. There was irritability on both sides. Liotta found DeBakey a hard taskmaster, very difficult to please. On the other hand, it seems that Liotta did not take instructions easily. He did experiments and tried procedures in the laboratory against which both DeBakey and Hall had advised. Liotta would impatiently switch from one approach to another, making the technicians work overtime. And he was known to buy things on his own, bypassing the established procedure that all purchases had to be made through Hall and with his approval. Such "crisis of authority" elements are not uncommon in team research. They may have contributed to Liotta's willingness to put three pumps into his briefcase and carry them out of DeBakey's laboratories.

It was Denton Cooley, of course, rather than Domingo Liotta, who was the chief medical actor in the case. As might be expected, the factors underlying his involvement are complicated and far-reaching. We have already discussed Cooley's allegation that his decision to implant the prosthesis was an emergency, "stopgap" measure, initiated to save his patient's life. Despite the degree of premeditation that this surgical act entailed, such motivation should not be entirely discounted. In his role as organ transplanter, Cooley has been a prototype of the surgeon who virtually refuses to relinquish his patient to death.

Cooley's strong drive for achievement, success, and fame is a motive to which he himself unabashedly testifies. "It's the center ring of the arena, and that's where I like to be," he frankly stated in describing the satisfaction he finds in cardiac surgery (Cooley, personal interview). He has been equally forthright in admitting that he has enjoyed the public and professional attention his transplant activities have brought him, which he feels he deserves (Cooley, personal interview). At the same time, Cooley spoke out vociferously against what he saw as a "faint-hearted" tendency for many physicians, patients, and their families to retreat from human cardiac transplantation when the mortality figures began to mount. But he had also referred to the possibility of the imminent development of an implantable cardiac prosthesis as "bordering on science fiction." It thus seems more than accidental that Cooley's conversion to the artificial heart, and his historic operation on Mr. Karp, should have coincided with the period when all but three of his seventeen transplant patients had died, when the supply of donors, as he himself phrased it, seemed to be "drying up," and when speculation was rampant about whether a moratorium had been called on this procedure. Cooley has also said he wished and felt obliged to be a perpetual pioneer. "I'd be derelict if I didn't try something I felt should be tried"; "I have enough confidence in myself and enough support from my colleagues around the world to venture it. A failure may set me back, but it won't wipe me out the way it would a younger man without my reputation" (Cooley, personal interview). On another occasion, Cooley voiced his commitment to being "first" in more chauvinistic terms. In a press conference, he declared that the Karp operation aided "the development of a device and a technique that were sorely needed. . . . I felt it was partly my patriotic duty to see that this was attempted first in our country" (Cooley sees a permanent "built-in" heart 1969).

Along with this achievement orientation, Cooley seems to have been propelled into implanting the artificial heart by his conviction that "enough laboratory work was done to put this thing on in this manner" (Randal 1969). To what extent Cooley really believed this and to what degree it was an after-the-fact rationalization is not easy to determine. There is much room for personal motives and philosophy to color judgments on this perennial issue in clinical medical research, both because of the inherent uncertainties in the process of inquiry and because the criteria relevant to this question are not codified. For example, Dr. Paul S. Russell has stated the problem, and his own position on it, in the following way:

I guess one quarrel I have had with my colleagues is my feeling that they have not always taken scientific information fully into account before proceeding with clinical trials. In other words, I believe that at least on some occasions, the first foray into the clinical arena later followed by a retreat into the laboratory, should have been avoided. But opinions will differ on this. [Russell, personal communication]

In the case of the artificial heart, the actions Cooley performed and the attitudes he voiced were significantly less measured and more drastic.

Everything was delivered at once. Everything, and the patient was there. It was all there so we decided to try it. The whole thing. . . . In my opinion, enough laboratory work was done to put this thing on in this manner and I would do it again. I have done equally bizarre things. [Randal 1969]

In a defiantly eloquent way, he also made it clear that his ideological stance on this consideration, and on all matters pertaining to cardiac surgery, is one of extreme professional individualism and autonomy.

I have done more heart surgery than anyone else in the world. Based on this experience, I believe I am qualified to judge what is right and proper for my patients. The permission I receive to do what I do I receive from my patients. It is not received from a government agency or one of my seniors. [Quinn 1969a].

This last statement refers directly to Michael DeBakey, the senior colleague Cooley considered his chief antagonist in the case. Although press stories that depict Cooley and DeBakey as "Houston's two master surgeons . . . locked in a bitter feud . . . at war over the human heart"[9] both exaggerate and simplify their relationship, the nature of their association is an essential contributory factor. Denton Cooley, who is twelve years younger than DeBakey, came to the Baylor College of Medicine as a full-time faculty member in 1951, after completing his surgical residency at Johns Hopkins, where he worked under Dr. Alfred Blalock. His curriculum vitae states that he "associated himself" with DeBakey at this time. He was, in fact, the first such younger colleague to work with DeBakey in Houston. In the very hierarchical, master-apprentice world of surgery, Cooley became De-Bakey's protégé. Over the years, Cooley gained experience, skill, recognition, and status. But DeBakey's seniority, his official positions at Baylor and at Methodist Hospital, and some of the distinctive attributes of his career pattern were such that both formally and informally he continued to be Cooley's superordinate. Two such talented, vital, striving, work-driven men could not be expected to work placidly side by side. But venturing any statement about the degree of competition that has existed between them is risky and delicate. This is a matter on which both DeBakey and Cooley are sensitive, and it is also a focus of much gossip and mythicizing. One description of this aspect of their relationship that seems more judicious than most was offered by a fellow surgeon in Houston:

They are two guys who do the same thing extremely well, and are highly competitive, much the way boxers are. . . . They are both men with great surgical skill . . . fantastic energy and fantastic self-discipline. . . . Each tries to outdo the other as well as himself, and perhaps they spark each other along in the process. . . . But for many years, they have been working near each other, rather than together.

Cooley and DeBakey are by no means junior and senior replicas of each other. In critical respects, they have contrasting surgical styles, professional profiles, and political and social outlooks. Like their similarities, these differences are potential sources of conflict. One surgeon who has worked closely with both of them distinguishes their operating talents and emphases in the following way:

Cooley is probably the best cardiac surgeon in the world, and DeBakey is the best vascular surgeon in the world. . . . Cooley doesn't feel vascular surgery to be as much of a challenge. . . . For him, it is more exciting to work on the heart. It is something that is there, that beats. It is something that starts and stops, and it is intriguing in this respect, like a toy. . . . Cooley enjoys shooting for speed. . . . He's the kind of man who, if given the reins, can race. . . . Cardiac surgery permits this. . . . Cardiac and vascular surgery both require considerable skill and experience. But the heart can fool you more. There are so many different heart diseases, and any or all of these can confront a surgeon when he gets in there. . . . A good vascular surgeon has to be meticulous and careful. He is working with smaller structures that tear easily. Cardiac surgery gives you wider latitude for mistakes. You don't have to take stitches as carefully as you do in vascular surgery, with a few exceptions like sewing up septal defects, where there is danger of getting the sutures around the a-v bundle and causing a block. Aside from this, cardiac surgery is straightforward anastomoses. It calls for big stitches like the sewing up of a saddle. But in vascular surgery . . . in which DeBakey excels . . . you have to be careful and precise. For instance, in order to jump a bypass, you have to have a lot of skill and patience. A slight jerk can tear it all to pieces.

Despite the renown both surgeons have attained, there are senses in which DeBakey's orbit of activities and reputation is more cosmopolitan and Cooley's is more local. DeBakey's involvement in research is partly responsible for this. He has sponsored, done, and published vastly more laboratory research than Cooley, who is predominantly a clinical surgeon, albeit one who works with daring on the growing edge of the field. DeBakey would refer to surgeons of Cooley's type as "cutting surgeons," as compared with more research-oriented "surgeon's surgeons," to whom not only he but the academic medical world generally attaches higher value and status. Beyond this, DeBakey, unlike Cooley, has played a nationally important political and entrepreneurial role in research. In both formal and informal capacities (for example, as chairman of the 1964 President's Commission on Heart Disease, Cancer, and Stroke and as a notable member of the Laskerites, a health lobby group surrounding philanthropist Mary Lasker), DeBakey has significantly influenced the medical science policy of the federal government over the years, especially the priorities and budgets of the National Institutes of Health.

DeBakey's physician-statesman achievements have also included the activities in which he has engaged as principal builder and developer of the Baylor College of Medicine's clinical, research, and teaching capacities. For more symbolically political reasons, the fact that he has operated on royal figures like the Duke of Windsor has enhanced his national and international luster.

Cooley himself remarks that, at least "until cardiac transplantation came along," he was regarded as a more "obscure surgeon" than DeBakey, by the mass media and the lay public. "The mass media said DeBakey was the well-known one. He got the publicity" (Cooley, personal interview). At the same time, Cooley has always been both more prominently involved in the local medical and social community than DeBakey and in certain ways more appreciated. Cooley was born and raised in Houston (DeBakey grew up in Lake Charles, Louisiana). He is an active participant in numerous fraternities and clubs in the city, including the Rotary Club of Houston, of which he is an honorary member, and several country clubs. All these affiliations are listed on his curriculum vitae. Cooley was the organizer of the Heartbeats, a local orchestra that plays popular music, mainly to raise money for Houston-based activities pertaining to cardiovascular disease and surgery. The ensemble is made up of cardiac surgeons and cardiologists; Cooley is the most notable of these medical musicians. Cooley has also succeeded in soliciting enough private funds from citizens of Houston to finance a new building for the Texas Heart Institute (where he is surgeon-in-chief), so that it has not been necessary for him to seek outside public support of any kind.

Cooley's pride in his private enterprise way of proceeding reflects differences in social and political philosophy between him and DeBakey which in turn have influenced the shape and impact of their careers. Whereas Cooley is wary of government participation in medical research and care, DeBakey has advocated and promoted greater federal support, responsibility, and initiative, not only in the pursuit of new knowledge, but also in "providing health to all people" (DeBakey, personal interview). Cooley and DeBakey are likewise divergent in their own professional incomes. DeBakey has a "full-time" appointment at Baylor. He receives a fixed salary from that institution; beyond that, his medical and surgical fees go to the medical college and center. Cooley's pattern comes closer to a fee-for-service arrangement. He retains as personal income a much larger proportion of what he earns as a clinical surgeon. In a politically and economically conservative community like Houston, Cooley's orientation is better understood and appreciated than DeBakey's. Within the local medical profession, for example, and the social circles to which it belongs, DeBakey is seen by many as "a renegade of the AMA" (DeBakey, personal interview). However, on the national plane his stance has given him more political eminence than Cooley enjoys.

All the foregoing leads one toward the supposition that along with many other motives, there was an element of defiance against DeBakey and what he represented in Cooley's implantation

of the artificial heart in Mr. Karp. Several of Cooley's and De-
Bakey's colleagues whom we had occasion to interview suggested
that it was also an act influenced by Cooley's desire to outstrip
DeBakey:

> Cooley considers himself to be the greatest cardiac surgeon in
> the world. . . . And so, his attitude was, "If anyone is going to do
> it, it should be me. Why should I play second fiddle to anyone?"
> . . . Cooley felt that he had been playing second fiddle to DeBakey
> for too long.

> It was a supreme form of "one-upsmanship" . . . the greatest
> act of one-upsmanship that Cooley could possibly have per-
> formed. . . . What he did, in effect, was wait until his buddy had
> spent five years doing something, and then slipped it out of the
> laboratory in the middle of the night. That takes the cake!

Cooley himself has testified that he had not only the right,
but in a sense the obligation to bypass his "seniors," the Baylor
Committee on Research Involving Human Beings and "a government agency," as he did in conducting the implantation without
informing any of them. He has argued that his status at the
summit of cardiac surgery permitted this and that the nature of
the situation required such bold and secretive action. Responding
to Mr. Karp's emergency situation, he has contended, entailed
overcoming a number of "obstacles to optimum patient care and
[the] furtherance of clinical research."[10] As Cooley saw them,
these obstacles included DeBakey's stubborn insistence that human
trials with the prosthesis would be premature and his certainty
that, if consulted, the Committee on Research Involving Human
Beings would not have granted him permission to use the artificial
heart. He attributed the position he assumed the committee would
have taken largely to DeBakey's influence. "DeBakey runs the
committee and they would have automatically turned me down,"
Cooley has stated (Thompson 1970). He also has referred to the
impediments he was determined to surmount in more historical
terms. "Every medical advance has met with the same type of
criticism" (Cooley feared hospital would halt heart project 1969).
Even after Baylor had conducted its various inquiries into the
case of the artificial heart, Cooley refused to yield on the matter.
In the end, as he wrote to DeBakey, it was primarily because he
could not "in good conscience comply with the directive . . . from
the Board of Trustees requiring that all members of the faculty
must agree to accept the action of the Committee on Human

Experimentation at Baylor before proceeding with clinical investigation,"[11] that he resigned as clinical professor of surgery at the medical college.

In effect, Cooley's recalcitrant attitude and behavior with regard to the Baylor committee and the Public Health Service guidelines represented a refusal to submit to the most important types of social control that have been instituted in American society to monitor biomedical research that entails human experimentation. Cooley deliberately eschewed peer review procedure, through which research protocols are screened by a committee of colleagues explicitly chosen to evaluate the ethicality of the investigator's intended use of human subjects.

As William J. Curran has pointed out, "The need to identify and to develop acceptable standards of care for human subjects . . . began to receive limited but respectable support in the American clinical research community in the late 1950's and early 1960's" (Curran 1969a, pp. 545–46). This nascent support, a consequence of the "steadily growing magnitude of . . . medical and scientific research in the United States concerning the health and illness of man" (Curran 1969a, p. 542), was given impetus by certain concrete events such as the Thalidomide tragedy in 1961 and 1962, the 1959–60 Kefauver hearings that devoted much attention to drug research conducted with human subjects, and the subsequent passage of the Drug Amendment acts of 1962. Under the influence of these developments and others, two major federal agencies, the Food and Drug Administration and the United States Public Health Service–National Institutes of Health conglomerate, initiated controls to regulate the use of human subjects in medical inquiries in 1966.

These controls were of two sorts: the development of ethical guidelines, codes, and sets of procedures for clinical research; and the establishment of the requirement that before a research protocol is funded (and more recently, before it is even submitted for funding), it be ethically evaluated by a review panel of peers at the institution with which the investigator is affiliated. The broad guidelines and the major concerns of the review committee were expected to focus on the proper protection of the rights and welfare of the human subject; appropriate methods of obtaining an acceptable degree and quality of informed, voluntary consent; the potential risks and benefits of the investigation; and the overall balance between them.

According to Bernard Barber, peer review committees are "probably universally established" (Barber 1970, p. 10)[12] in medical institutions throughout the country today, wherever clinical research is conducted. Barber frankly states that the fact that the National Institutes of Health not only require such systems of assessment and surveillance, but also "supply some 35% of all funds for bio-medical research," has played a major role in their creation and spread. For, "no institution with a research program could afford not to apply for these funds" (Barber 1970, p. 2).

As Cooley's outlook and behavior with respect to the Baylor committee suggest, the problem is not just whether such a peer review group exists in a particular medical school, hospital, or research institute, but how effectively it operates. A criterion of effectiveness particularly relevant to Cooley's actions is what Barber calls the "scope of control that peer review committees now exercise," using the proportion of enacted research projects reviewed and those not reviewed as primary indicators.

Barber and his co-investigators conducted a questionnaire survey of the peer review committees of a nationally representative sample of biomedical research institutions. Their sample of these institutions was drawn from the 3 March 1969 list of those receiving Public Health Service grants who had filed assurances that they would comply with the PHS guidelines. Two hundred and ninety-three institutions out of a possible 523 returned the questionnaires, a response rate of 56 percent. Barber reports that 86 percent of the institutions that answered said that "all clinical research" carried out there was reviewed; 9 percent responded that "only clinical research which involves a formal proposal for funds from whatever source" was reviewed; and 4 percent replied that "only formal proposals to do clinical research which involve requests for money from the Public Health Service" are reviewed. "Clearly, a small but perhaps important minority of research proposals" are still not being examined and evaluated by review committees, Barber concludes (Barber 1970, pp. 10–11).

Cooley's plan for implanting the artificial heart in Mr. Karp would fall into Barber's category of nonsurveillanced research. Barber and his associates found that one of Cooley's main reasons for evading the Baylor committee also constituted a more general "structured source" for bypassing the review process. "Research-

ers racing to establish priority of discovery or those who feel that
some case or situation presents them with 'now or never' opportunities to do research may both feel that this is an unacceptably
long time to wait . . . Instead of waiting, they go ahead without
submitting a protocol for review at all or, alternatively, submit a
protocol but go ahead before it is approved" (Barber 1970,
pp. 11–12).

The implantation of the artificial heart in Mr. Karp raises
critical and troubling questions about the involvement of not
only the surgeon-experimenters in this case, but also the engineers and technicians who worked with them. From our interviews with Suzanne Anderson, Sam Calvin, Louis Feldman, and
Gary Cornelius (a member of the Baylor pump team that operated the heart-lung machine for cardiac surgery both at Methodist
Hospital and Saint Luke's Hospital), a remarkably consistent
perspective emerged. Along with several of their colleagues who
directly or indirectly aided Cooley and Liotta, they either suspected or actually knew that they were participating in preparing
the artificial heart for a human trial. All believed that it was
probably "too soon" for it to be used on a man. At the same
time, none of them felt that they had the competence or the right
of the physician-investigator to offer a judgment on this issue.
What is always "ambiguous" in their situation, they pointed out,
is how a particular apparatus on which they are working under
the authority and supervision of doctors is eventually going to be
used. The most effective way of coping with this uncertainty, they
affirmed, is under all circumstances to "do the best possible job"
in designing, building, and assembling a device, without making
distinctions in quality between apparatus destined for animals and
those presumably intended for human subjects. All of the technical personnel were acutely aware of the "chain of command"
under which they worked. They considered themselves subor-
dinate to the physicians, in ways that made them disinclined to
challenge Dr. Liotta or Dr. Cooley, to refuse to do what they
asked, or even to honor the validity of their own apprehensions
and doubts.

William O'Bannon, the engineer who built the console that
powered the pump implanted in Karp, has testified that he was
"overwhelmed by the opportunity to work for Cooley" as much
as he was interested in "helping the cause along by getting this

into another investigator's hands at a damned reasonable price—
about $20,000" (Randal 1969). Cooley's charisma as a surgeon,
and the combined technical and business opportunity he offered,
overrode O'Bannon's concern that although the console "was not
designed for humans," Cooley might be planning to use it "on a
man" (Randal 1969). Suzanne Anderson was convinced that
Liotta's order to her to line the three pumps with Dacron velour,
and the subsequent disappearance of the pumps from the laboratory, meant that they were being readied for human trial. Nonetheless, she did not feel that she could "go to Liotta and say, 'I
know you're up to something.' He was the acting head of the
laboratory at the time, and besides, I was not going to take on
any doctor" (Anderson, personal interview). Liotta explicitly told
Sam Calvin that it was his "responsibility" to collaborate with
Cooley and himself in getting the artificial heart ready for use
should things not go well in the course of Mr. Karp's operation
(the scheduled ventriculoplasty). Calvin was "surprised because
I didn't think we were ready for the application of the artificial
heart on the human level." He also thought that a "shady deal"
might be pending, because the "secretiveness" requested of him
by Cooley and Liotta suggested, among other things, that De-
Bakey might not be aware of what was happening, or might not
have authorized it. Calvin did not know that a Committee on
Research Involving Human Beings existed at Baylor and should
have been consulted. He learned about it later, through the chain
of events that the case entailed. In spite of his inner questioning
and "reluctance," Calvin "had the impression" that Liotta was
"talking as my chief, and so it was my obligation to do what he
asked." Furthermore, he was "convinced that a man's life was at
stake, and that I could not refuse the physicians who were trying
to save it" (Calvin, personal interview). Both the life-and- death
reality and the mystique of the cardiac surgeon's work helped
push Calvin into conducting an all-night series of tests with the
artificial heart on the eve of Mr. Karp's operation, into being
present in the surgical amphitheater the next day (along with
two other engineers, John Mannis and John Juergens of Saint
Luke's Hospital), where he ran the control unit of the prosthesis,
and into the around-the-clock "on call" service that he and his
fellow engineers performed during the ensuing weekend.

The members of the pump team for the Karp operation were
not told that they might be carrying out their usual tasks for other
than a routine, though serious, form of cardiac surgery. They

felt that the preparation for Karp's procedure resembled that for a heart transplant. However, Cooley avoided the questions about "what was going on" that the head of the pump team asked him. According to Gary Cornelius, when they entered the amphitheater "all we knew was that there was now a man on the operating table, and that probably a transplantation was not going to take place after all, because there seemed to be no donor around":

The team went on the pump, as Mr. Karp's operation took place. Everything seemed to go fine. Dr. Cooley took the aneurysm out, and closed the heart up. We could see the patient's heart beating on the monitor. There were some peculiar things about what followed next. For instance, there were 2,000 cc's of blood in the pump which was unusual. This meant there was volume in the pump, but not in the patient. Next, Dr. Cooley gave an order to hold the blood. Then, the anesthetist gave no drugs. The next thing we knew, an artificial heart was put on the table and opened up. [Cornelius, personal interview]

The "secrecy" surrounding the operation was "not too disturbing" to Cornelius and his teammates. Heart transplants had accustomed them to working in a locked amphitheater, with a guard at the door, to forestall premature news coverage. It occurred to Cornelius that the artificial heart Cooley was about to implant in Karp resembled the model developed in DeBakey's laboratory, and he remembers thinking to himself, "I wonder if Dr. DeBakey knows this is happening." However, in his opinion the members of the pump team did not think at the time that "anything really wrong was being done," and once the implantation began they were caught up in the "excitement" of being present at such a medicosurgical first. We were interested to know if a pump technician like Cornelius felt that it was ever justified to refuse to work with a surgeon, or to carry out something he requested, on the grounds that he thought the physician in question was wrong or engaging in wrongdoing. Cornelius replied that he and his colleagues would not "walk out" on a surgeon if they "didn't agree with him," primarily because the refusal of the pump team to cooperate "would kill the patient faster than the surgeon could" (Cornelius, personal interview).

As can be seen, one of the most striking patterns that emerged from our discussions with some of the engineers and technicians involved was their collective view of themselves as being under the command of physicians in general, and surgeons in particular, in a way that obliged them to conform to what was asked of them by their medical superiors. In this regard, their definition of the authority structure into which they fit is comparable to a military model: technicians and engineers, like soldiers of lower rank, are expected to follow the orders issued by officers. The medical technologists believed that this arrangement was appropriate because surgeons had greater, more general competence than their own, as well as primary responsibility for the care and welfare of patients. In addition, they felt that because they were working in pioneering and crisis medicine, it was especially important that the surgeon be a real "captain," forcefully and effectively telling his subalterns what to do in the many unprecedented and urgent situations that confronted his laboratory and operating-room teams.

Although the technicians and engineers were aware that the devices on which they worked were ultimately destined for human use, their professional education had not included any training or socialization to prepare them for the issues with which they had to deal in the case of the artificial heart. Apparently, the ethical ramifications of their activities, and what these implied for their comportment in various work contexts, had never been discussed with them. One telling indicator of this hiatus was that until this case occurred, these medical technologists did not know about the peer group review mechanism for research with human subjects. There is a sense in which their involvement in the artificial heart episode provided them with more training in professional ethics than they had ever previously received.[13] If anything, the technicians and engineers expected to do whatever the surgeon ordered, on the assumption that even though they might have questions about its moral advisability, noncompliance would constitute insubordination.

Finally, this case raises serious questions about the appropriateness and adequacy of the regulatory mechanisms through which the medical profession is expected to insure ethical concern and practice in the conduct of clinical research. It has become apparent that although the "internalized controls of conscience" (Jaffe 1969, p. 409) ought ideally to provide basic safeguards, a number of the principal actors in the case of the artificial heart had not been properly socialized for such inner-directed ethicality. They were also subject to various kinds of social, cultural, and psychological pressures that pushed them toward behaviors that were borderline or deviant by the norms of the profession.

Formal peer group review, one of the major institutionalized arrangements for overseeing the morality of research with human subjects, was successfully bypassed while Haskell Karp was still alive. Only after his death, when the case was already in the public domain, was the Baylor Committee on Research Involving Human Beings sufficiently aware of what had occurred to call what amounted to a retroactive emergency meeting and investigation. At this juncture, two other bodies began to inquire into the case: the National Heart Institute, principally through the questions that its director asked Baylor Medical College to answer; and a special committee, composed of faculty and trustees, set up by the board of the medical school, whose primary goal was to account satisfactorily to the institute.

In the end, what sanctions were actually taken by Baylor, and by the medical profession more broadly, and what did these sanctions accomplish? Domingo Liotta was dismissed from the Baylor–Rice Artificial Heart Program; but he promptly was offered, and accepted, a full-time position working for Denton Cooley at Saint Luke's Episcopal Hospital. Cooley himself was not subjected to any disciplinary action by Baylor. He was permitted to take the option of resigning from his professorship at the college of medicine, on the grounds that he could not "in good conscience" sign the formal promise to abide by the Public Health Service guidelines for human experimentation that the board of trustees (as a consequence of their inquiry into the case of the artificial heart) made a precondition for appointment to the medical school faculty. Since November 1969, the heart-lung pump team has ceased to work at Saint Luke's Hospital. Ostensibly this action was initiated by Cooley rather than imposed on him. When the pump team received a collective raise in fees and salaries that fall, Cooley told them that he would no longer be able to afford their services. He subsequently assembled and trained his own pump group. Except for O'Bannon, the engineers and technicians who played key roles in Mr. Karp's operation still work for the Baylor–Rice Artificial Heart Program.

Because of the norms that prevent undue invasion of privacy and the infringement of privileged communication, the complete record of the Baylor committee investigations into the case has never been released.

In December 1969 the Harris County Medical Society of Houston informed the chiefs of staff of local hospitals that it had censured Cooley. Most probably the censure was a response to

Cooley's actions in the case of the artificial heart, but the president of the medical society would not publicly state the reasons. This was "internal business" of the society, he said, thereby implicitly invoking the norms of privacy and of professional self-regulation. A small Associated Press news release on the censure was issued. It took up only fifteen lines in the 10 December 1969 issue of the *New York Times.* Cooley was "not available for comment." At one point the American College of Surgeons also claimed to be investigating the case, but their findings were never revealed.

Michael DeBakey answered the letters addressed to him by Theodore Cooper, director of the National Heart Institute, regarding the use of NHI funds in the Baylor–Rice work on the artificial heart, the source of Liotta's salary, and the observance of ethical guidelines. He also testified in the medical college's investigation of the case. But because he felt he was "too closely involved" in the events and was likely to be viewed as "self-seeking" if he were actively implicated in its sequelae, he removed himself from all other aspects of the inquiry. It was not until 19 October 1970, in the course of an extended presentation at a National Academy of Sciences meeting held at Rice University, that DeBakey made the slightest public allusion to the case. He offered an overview on the present state of research on cardiovascular disease, including the relative merits and demerits of various heart assist devices and of cardiac transplantation. According to the 20 October 1970 *Houston Chronicle*, when "a picture of an artificial heart was flashed on the screen," DeBakey said in passing:

This is, of course, the experimental pump. Some of you may recall this was publicized on television as having been put in a patient. But of course it was the same pump that was developed in our experimental laboratory. It was just simply taken from our laboratory without our knowledge and done the way it was.

This quotation appeared in an article on page 1 of the *Houston Chronicle*, under banner headlines that read, "DeBakey Says Artificial Heart 'Taken' from Lab." The article also reported that "DeBakey's office issued a statement this morning saying the Baylor surgeon did not accuse Cooley of taking the pump." So far as we know, this local news story was not carried by papers around the country.

The only other time DeBakey has made formal reference to the case was as editor of *The Year Book of General Surgery, 1970*. In the section on "Transplantation and Artificial Organs," after reporting on "preliminary experiments" in animals with a biventricular artificial heart that he and his colleagues conducted, DeBakey inserted the following note in the text:

[The biventricular orthotopic cardiac prosthesis described in this report is the identical artificial heart that was covertly taken from the Baylor Laboratories to St. Luke's Hospital in Houston, where it was used in a human experiment on April 4, 1969 (see Tr. Am. Soc. Artificial Int. Organs 15:252, 1969; Am. J. Cardiol. 24:723, 1969), without prior approval of the institutional human research committee or by the responsible investigator of the project under which the device was developed. In the published reports of the human experiment, no scientific acknowledgement was made of the historical development of this artificial heart, as documented in this report of animal experiments. As may be observed from the conclusion drawn from the observations on the only seven preliminary animal experiments performed with this device, it was not ready for human implantation, and this conclusion was substantiated by the ultimate result in the human experiment—Ed.] [DeBakey 1970, p. 72]

By and large, the national medical community of clinical investigators has kept its silence about the case. One of the few censurious statements by a research physician that has appeared in print is that of Dr. Francis D. Moore, Mosley Professor of Surgery at Harvard Medical School and surgeon-in-chief of the Peter Bent Brigham Hospital. In a chapter on heart transplantation in his 1972 book *Transplant* Moore wrote:

Desperate measures like the interim substitution of a machine heart . . . call up for consideration a special ethical question: does the presence of a dying patient justify the doctor's taking *any* conceivable step regardless of its degree of hopelessness? The answer to this question must be negative. . . . There is simply no evidence to suggest that it would be helpful. It raises false hopes for the patient and his family, it calls into discredit all of biomedical science, and it gives the impression that physicians and surgeons are adventurers rather than circumspect persons seeking to help the suffering and dying by the use of hopeful measures. . . . It is only by work in the laboratory and cautious trial in the living animal that "hopeless desperate measures" can become ones that carry with them some promise of reasonable assistance to the patient. The interim substitution of a mechanical heart in the chest . . . had not reached this stage, for the simple reason that animal survival had never been attained. [Moore 1972, p. 275n]

On 2 April 1971 an unexpected sequela to the case of the artificial heart began. Mrs. Haskell Karp filed a medical malpractice suit against Denton A. Cooley, Domingo S. Liotta, Sam Calvin, and Saint Luke's Episcopal Hospital. Under the Texas Wrongful Death Statute, she asked four and a half million dollars in compensation for damages sustained by Mr. Karp, herself, and their three sons.[14] Such a case falls under tort law, the law of personal liability. And liability suits occur frequently in our legal system. But the kind of suit Mrs. Karp filed is uncommon. For, although in American society "the ethics of many experiments have been challenged by professional and lay critics . . . there have been . . . few lawsuits concerning the legality of experiment" (Jaffe 1969, p. 408). This may be because the subject is "caught up in the dynamic of medical research and be indisposed to harass the experimenter by a lawsuit." Furthermore, he is "normally not aware nor in possession of the evidence to demonstrate that his interests have not been properly protected. The medical profession resentfully clams up when one of its members is attacked and is not easily persuaded to testify against him" (Jaffe 1969, p. 408).

In count I of the "Plaintiffs' Original Petition" to the court, Mrs. Karp claimed that:

On or about April 8, 1969, Haskell Karp died as a result of surgical experimentation performed on him by Dr. Denton A. Cooley, Dr. Domingo S. Liotta, and others in St. Luke's Episcopal Hospital in Houston, Texas, on or about April 4, 1969. . . . On April 4, 1969, after Haskell Karp had been hospitalized for almost a month, Defendants, using devices approved only for animal experimentation, after removing the human heart of Decedent from his body, implanted an experimental mechanical device in Haskell Karp. The experimental mechanical device, commonly known as a mechanical heart, which was an invention of Defendants Cooley and Liotta, had been designed for animal experimentation only. The mechanical heart, in fact, had not been tested adequately even on animals, had never been tested on a human being, and Haskell Karp was the unfortunate victim of human experimentation. The mechanical heart caused Haskell Karp's condition to begin a process of irreversible deterioration from which he could not be saved.

Count II of the same petition alleged that Cooley and his colleagues had "induced" Mr. Karp to "submit himself to heart surgery":

The Defendants failed to inform Haskell Karp that the experimental mechanical heart, which was implanted within Decedent's body, had not been adequately tested, and further failed to inform him that each of the animals in which the device had been implanted had died shortly following the implant, and further failed to inform him that irreversible damage to his condition was the probable medical result of the implant. In addition, Defendants further led Haskell [sic] to believe, falsely, that unless the experimental operation was performed immediately, he would die.

It was also alleged that Dr. Cooley and the others "by their actions, have shown that they did not intend to repair [Mr. Karp's] heart, but that they intended at the outset, and in advance of the operation, to use [him] for human experimentation by implanting within his body the experimental mechanical heart." In addition, count II alleged, "Defendants further informed Decedent and Plaintiff that there was on hand, at a nearby hospital, a donor for a human heart, which was false, and Defendants knew this to be false at the time such representations were made."

Count III of the petition alleged that after the mechanical heart was implanted into Mr. Karp, his wife was informed that "a donor human heart was needed for her husband immediately, and that none was available to the knowledge of Defendants, although [Mrs. Karp] had been told prior to said operation that a human heart was in fact readily available for [her husband], should it be needed." Subsequently, Dr. Cooley and his colleagues "urged and requested" Mrs. Karp to "participate in a news conference for the purpose of making a public plea over television for a donor human heart." After her husband's death, the petition continues, Mrs. Karp was "persuaded by Defendants to issue a public statement vindicating and supporting" Cooley and Liotta, which she did, "although at such time [she] was in such an overwrought condition that she was unable to comprehend adequately what was occurring."

In the words of the district judge before whom the case was eventually tried, the major charges made against Cooley and the others could be summarized as follows:

Plaintiffs allege among other things: that the consent to the operation was fraudulently obtained; that it was not an "informed consent"; that under the circumstances the defendants were negligent in performing the corrective surgery, implanting the mechanical heart, and submitting the patient to the surgery for inserting the human donor heart; and that by fraudulent deceptive practices Mrs. Karp was used by defendants to secure a human heart donor.[15]

The case of *Karp* v. *Cooley* was tried over a period of ten days, from 19 June to 29 June 1972, in the United States District Court of Houston, and was presided over by District Judge John B. Singleton. The expert medical testimony that Mrs. Karp was able to mobilize was deemed insufficient in quality and weight to support her allegations. In the judge's opinion, "since there was no expert evidence that defendants performed any act negligently or that any of their acts were a proximate cause of patient's death, both surgeons were entitled to a directed verdict."[16] This means that, in the eyes of Judge Singleton, Mrs. Karp and her lawyers failed to present sufficient proof of their allegations for the case to be tried before a jury. Thus, the case was withdrawn from the jury's consideration by reason of the entry of a directed verdict. After nine days of hearings, he ruled that the medical malpractice, negligence, and fraudulent misrepresentation that Mrs. Karp alleged had occurred could not be legally established, primarily because they were not attested to by "medical doctors of ordinary knowledge and skill of the same school of practice of that or a similar community."[17] In Texas, as in almost all the states of the Union, such expert medical testimony is necessary to establish proof.[18] On close reading, the district court decision cannot be construed either as approving Dr. Cooley's conduct or as holding that he conformed with the ethical and legal standards required in cases of human experimentation. The final outcome of this case is still not determined. Mrs. Karp has appealed the decision to a higher court, and eventually the case will be heard in the United States Court of Appeals, Fifth Circuit, New Orleans.

In his brief on appeal, Mrs. Karp's lawyer makes claims about various errors the district court may have committed in its handling of this case, which underscore some of the most controversial aspects of the trial:[19]

POINT NO. 8
The Court erred, and abused its discretion, in quashing the subpoena for Dr. Hoff and the records of Baylor College of Medicine

relative to the Cooley-Karp incident, and refusing counsel the right to examine such records and to make a bill of exception to such ruling, where such records contained statements and affidavits of defendants and other witnesses constituting material evidence in the case.

POINT NO. 9
The Court erred, and abused its discretion, in quashing the subpoena of Dr. Michael DeBakey as a lay and expert witness for petitioners, thereby refusing petitioners the right to call such witness in "open court," he having previously given testimony by deposition concerning the use of the mechanical heart in Mr. Karp and his experiences with the same or similar device, together with his medical opinions concerning the standards of care relating to patients under the same or similar circumstances.[20]

In his decision on the case, Judge Singleton explained the grounds on which he decided to confine the interrogation of Dr. DeBakey to the privacy of his chambers:

Plaintiffs subpoenaed Dr. Michael DeBakey to testify. Defense counsel argued to the court that the previously publicized alleged friction between this witness and Dr. Cooley would be highly inflamatory and serve no purpose except to introduce issues into the case before the jury that were not properly before the court. Counsel took this position because Dr. DeBakey had indicated at his deposition that he would not give any medical opinion on the Karp case or willingly answer any hypothetical question developed from the Karp case facts. . . . Therefore, in order to minimize the increasing publicity of the trial, the court had Dr. DeBakey questioned in chambers with all counsel present and a court reporter. The record will amply reveal that Dr. DeBakey had not been employed to give any expert medical opinion; that he would not accept any employment in this case; that he had never examined Mr. Karp; that he had never seen Mr. Karp; that he would refuse to express any medical opinion concerning the treatment of Mr. Karp; that he would not express any medical opinion based upon hypothetical questions even if asked to do so; and in connection with the Cooley-Liotta mechanical heart used in Mr. Karp, he would refuse to express an in-court expert opinion concerning that device. Accordingly, this court concluded that Dr. DeBakey had no evidence of any probative value to present to the jury. Accordingly, to allow the plaintiffs' attorney to call Dr. DeBakey as a witness before the jury under such circumstances would in all reasonable probability result in creating a highly prejudicial and inflamatory situation that would serve no useful purpose.[21]

Before Dr. DeBakey testified, his deposition was taken. That
private deposition and the records of Baylor College of Medicine
"were ordered sealed during the trial."[22] In effect, they were impounded by the judge. He ruled that "no part may be reproduced
and given to any person in pursuance of the appeal, and the contents of the records shall not be given out for publication."[23]
Thus, the judge not only decided that it would "serve no useful
purpose"[24] for DeBakey to appear as a witness before a jury, but
he also made it impossible for Mrs. Karp's lawyer to have access
to the records that the court took into legal custody.

The judge's holding that DeBakey's testimony was not "evidence of any probative value to present to the jury"[25] is hard to
understand or justify. DeBakey surely was a singularly important expert witness. Personally and professionally, he had intimate and perhaps unique knowledge of many facets of the case.
Furthermore, the brief on appeal filed by the plaintiff contains
extensive verbatim materials from DeBakey's "excluded testimony" that seem highly relevant to what Mrs. Karp's lawyer was
attempting to argue, and appropriate for a jury's impartial determination:

Dr. Michael DeBakey's excluded testimony indicates that "the
pump was not ready for use in human beings" because in reasonable medical probability its use "will jeopardize the life of the
individual," and on that basis it was not acceptable medical
practice in April of 1969 to use a mechanical heart of this kind in
a patient. As of date of trial, he "still would not recommend it
on the basis of our experimental observations." His review of the
Karp surgery indicated a deterioration of renal functions and
"this is a pattern of part of the picture of the terminal events that
take place in animals" from their experiences with the mechanical heart.

On deposition, Dr. DeBakey stated Dr. Cooley was subject to the
rule requiring prior approval of the Human Research Committee
of the College, and that if he did not have approval of this
committee he would violate this rule in using the heart device. In
connection with repairs of the heart, he states:

"Q. If the heart does not, during fifteen or twenty minutes
    after surgical repair of an aneurysm—does not go back
    into at least normal function, how long would you work
    on this patient in effort to restore that heart before you
    totally remove the patient's heart?

A. Well, I wouldn't say—Let me say I wouldn't remove the patient's heart unless I were going to do a transplant. If I had a donor available, then I might plan to do that, but if I didn't have a donor I would never totally remove a patient's heart. There's no basis for it.

   But to answer your question—One part of your question —How long would we work on that heart, we have worked on hearts as long as several hours. Sometimes we are successful in getting the heart to take over at the end of that time and sometimes we are not. . . . We have had this experience, that patients with high risk procedures explained to them . . . and if they wanted to accept that risk we were willing to go ahead. But once it failed . . . that if it failed, there was nothing else to do and we would not take the heart out.

Q. In other words, you simply let the patient die naturally?

A. Exactly. We have had this experience unfortunately more times than I would like."[26]

According to the plaintiff's brief, DeBakey also stated that "based on the articles published by Cooley" about the Karp surgery and on his own experiments, he concluded that the artificial heart was not ready for human implantation. In his opinion, this conclusion was substantiated by the ultimate result of implanting the device in Mr. Karp. The pattern that takes place in animals was duplicated in the Karp case, DeBakey asserted, and "as far as I'm concerned, this pattern is progressive deterioration towards death. There's nothing that's going to reverse it."[27]

As the foregoing suggests, the vital nature of the testimony that DeBakey presented in a private hearing raises serious questions about the grounds on which the court decided that his evidence had no probative value. Furthermore, the judge's ruling that he would not require DeBakey to take the stand in the public court-room is problematic in other ways. Before the conference in chambers, Judge Singleton is reported by Mrs. Karp's counsel to have said that, "Because of the international reputation of the witness he would determine whether to require Dr. DeBakey to testify."[28] After the conference, he decided that due to the "previously publicized alleged friction" between DeBakey and Cooley, "to call Dr. DeBakey as a witness before the jury . . . would in all reasonable probability result in creating a highly prejudicial and inflammatory situation that would serve no useful purpose."[29]

One might ask why a physician—because he has an "international reputation," and because a potentially "inflammatory situation" exists between him and a fellow physician who is the defendant in a case—should be granted the option of refusing to testify in open court. This would not have happened with any ordinary citizen, or probably even any ordinary physician. Perhaps under the glare of a public courtroom hearing, DeBakey might have been reluctant to assert that privilege. The instances are numerous where persons who have said in private that they would claim such a privilege have been unwilling to do so when faced with the necessity of requesting it publicly. What is more, a judge has the prerogative to order a witness to testify. If he exercises this right, in contradistinction to Judge Singleton's leniency, he imposes a powerful constraint upon a reluctant or resistant witness, who would be in contempt if he refused to give testimony.

The interplay of factors that led Judge Singleton to make the decision he did could well constitute a study in itself. Irrespective of its origins, one of the most serious consequences of the ruling was that it created great difficulties for Mrs. Karp and her counsel in effectively arguing their case. These difficulties in gaining access to critical evidence were increased because the judge also impounded the Baylor records that bore on the case. As the data presented earlier in the chapter indicate, those records were unusually probing and revelatory, since in addition to the medical data they contained they also included al the materials pertinent to the Karp case gathered by the two Baylor committees that conducted investigations into the ethical issues associated with it.

In these various respects, Judge Singleton's decision seems to have served more as a deterrent than as an aid to the truth's being fully known about the case of the artificial heart. It runs counter to one of the fundamental premises of the legal system: the assumption that unless there can be redress in the courts, some rights cannot be adequately protected. Rights as basic as the minimization of physical injury and the preservation of human life were involved here. The way they were dealt with by the court leads one to profoundly question whether persons like Haskell Karp, on whom therapeutic innovations are tried, are adequately protected by the present legal process.

This lawsuit constitutes the strongest action taken in the case of the artificial heart. Apart from Mrs. Karp's initiative, the formal and informal sanctions that have been brought to bear upon the defendants have been mild. Cooley's and Liotta's professional activities have been restricted only in relatively minor or short-term ways. The professional norms of privacy, autonomy and self-regulation, decorum, and disinterestedness have converged more to protect than to penalize the many individuals who were involved in the events that culminated in the implantation of a mechanical heart in Haskell Karp. Their relative immunity has also been fostered by the mass communication system. The media paid far more attention to the fact that for the first time in medical history an artificial heart was implanted in a man, and to the process by which a cadaver heart donor was flown to Houston, than to the serious moral issues the case raised, or to the events following Mr. Karp's death that were concerned with these questions.[30]

In our view, this case and its outcome show that the medical and law professions, and the larger society to which they belong, have not satisfactorily dealt with the social, moral, and legal issues involved in therapeutic innovation with human subjects.

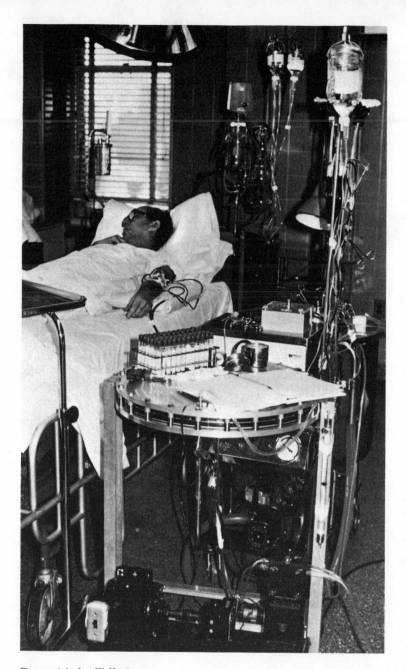

Photograph by Lee W. Henderson

3

*Patterns in Therapeutic
Innovation: Dialysis*

7

"To Give Life": A Study of Seattle's Hemodialysis Program

In the early 1940s Dr. Willem J. Kolff, an internist associated with the Municipal Hospital in Kampen, Holland, built the first artificial kidney that could be used on human beings.[1] He constructed it out of an old bathtub and spare parts from an automobile foundry, partly because he was working under wartime conditions during the Nazi occupation of Holland. Kolff subsequently migrated to the United States and joined the Cleveland Clinic Foundation.

By 1950, inspired by Kolff's prototype, several American medical centers, including Georgetown University, Mount Sinai Hospital, and, most notably, the Peter Bent Brigham Hospital, had assembled their own artificial kidney machines. These variants of the Kolff model were still highly experimental and were only capable of providing short-term, intermittent treatments for persons suffering from acute, temporary, and life-threatening loss of kidney function. Patients generally could not be maintained on this machine for more than a few weeks. The physicians who used it hoped that the detoxification effected by the artificial kidney, along with the "rest" it afforded the patient's own kidneys, would help him regain adequate renal function. But all too often this did not happen. As late as 1960, Dr. George E. Schreiner and his colleagues exulted because they had succeeded in dialyzing a patient for 181 days, the "longest reported maintenance of life in true oliguria [decrease in urine excretion]" (Schreiner 1966, p. 126).

From 1950 to 1960, sustained treatment on the artificial kidney was restricted by the fact that each time a patient was dialyzed he had to undergo surgery to insert cannulas (tubes) into an artery and a vein. Because each artery or vein could be used only once, the number of cannulations, and thus the number of possible runs on the machine, was limited. For this reason, in the early stage of its development and use the artificial kidney was not able to prolong the life of patients in the terminal renal failure stage of chronic kidney disease. Perhaps its most effective role at that time was to remove from the bloodstream specific, dialyzable poisons that cause acute renal shutdown.

In 1960 long-term hemodialysis became possible, making feasible the continuing treatment of patients with chronic, irreversible kidney failure. This was largely because Dr. Belding Scribner and his colleagues at the University of Washington School of Medicine in Seattle solved the problem of the cannula sites by developing a semipermanent apparatus.

The impetus for Scribner's innovation was the death of one of his patients, Mr. Joe Saunders. Saunders was referred to the University Hospital in January 1960 for dialysis treatment of what was thought to be acute reversible kidney failure. "I cannot recall ever having seen a sicker patient survive on the artificial kidney than Joe Saunders," Scribner has written.

When he entered the hospital, he was in coma, and his heart failure was so bad that foam was oozing out of his lungs and mouth. Yet one week [after dialysis began] Joe was up and about, feeling amazingly well as a result of several treatments on the artificial kidney . . . and yet despite this amazing result all was not right. Mr. Saunders had not passed any urine in a week, a fact that made the original diagnosis suspect. A biopsy of his kidney revealed the tragic answer. The original diagnosis was wrong. Mr. Saunders had a disease which had totally and irreversibly destroyed his kidneys. They would never function again.
What to do? . . . We did the only thing we could do. We had an agonizing conversation with Mrs. Saunders and told her to take her husband back home to Spokane where he would die, hopefully without much suffering. . . . He died quietly [at home] about two weeks later. . . . The emotional impact of this case was enormous on all of us, and I could not stop thinking about it.
Then one morning about 4:00 a.m. I woke up and groped for a piece of paper and pencil to jot down the basic idea of the shunted cannulas which would make it possible to treat people like Joe Saunders again and again with the artificial kidney without destroying two blood vessels each time. And, indeed, basically it was such a simple idea—just connect the tube (cannula) in the artery to the cannula in the vein by means of a connecting tube or *shunt*, and the blood would rush through without clotting and

maintain the cannulas in functional condition indefinitely. Then when an artificial kidney treatment was needed, we could simply replace the shunt temporarily with the blood circuit of the artificial kidney.

The most amazing thing about this idea was that unlike most such ideas it worked right from the start. [Scribner 1972]

The advent of chronic hemodialysis as an alternative or adjunct to the then fledgling procedure of renal transplantation created a penumbra of complex and often painful issues. These included questions concerning the prolongation of life, available and appropriate ways of supporting such an important and costly therapeutic innovation, the allocation of scarce medical resources, the respective roles of the local community and the federal government, and the part the mass media could and should play.

As one physician from the Seattle dialysis program reflected, "Doctors now find themselves able from time to time to enter a gray, limbo-like area where they are able to prolong life without, however, being able to cure the disease or heal the injury. . . . The first great anxiety, then, that one faces in approaching the question of hemodialysis is whether from the patient's point of view the whole procedure will turn out to be a blessing or merely a labored and painful hanging on to life" (Norton 1967, p. 1267). Given evidence that maintenance dialysis could indeed rehabilitate many patients so they could work and otherwise lead a relatively normal life, a second core problem immediately loomed. In the face of a large patient population but a limited number of dialysis facilities—including machines, hospital beds, and medical personnel—and the great expense of long-term treatment, who gets on the artificial kidney, who makes the decision, and what criteria should be used? Dr. H. E. de Wardener of the Charing Cross Hospital Medical School in London provides a succinct and pointed statement of what he regards as the "ethical problems" with which "this form of treatment bristles":

(1) Is it justifiable to prolong life in this way?
(2) Who should be chosen?
(3) What are the financial consequences?
(4) Who ought to pay?
(5) Ought the large sums involved be directed to this purpose?
(6) Ought the large numbers of skilled persons involved be directed to this work?
(7) Should home dialysis be encouraged?
(8) What ought to be the relation between intermittent haemo-

dialysis and renal transplantation? (de Wardener 1966, pp. 105–6).

A perspective on these issues, which we will examine in the next three chapters, is provided by data on the prevalence of kidney disease and its social and economic costs. In 1964, major urinary diseases ranked as the nation's fourth largest killer, after cardiovascular diseases, cancer, and pneumonia.

In considering the impact of kidney diseases we find that between July 1964 and June 1965 there were 58,788 deaths, a prevalence of 7,847,000 cases, 139,939,000 days of restricted activity, 63,494,000 days of bed disability, and 16,729,000 days of work loss in the United States. Likewise, in 1964 the total economic cost of kidney disease was $3,635,000,000. The indirect costs of morbidity and mortality accounted for $2,000,412,000 of the total cost with the larger portion due to morbidity loss. This is in contrast to economic costs in the other leading disease categories in which the mortality proportion is higher and reflects the earlier age of death of many patients with kidney disease. [Goodman 1968, p. 1]

In response to the magnitude of the problems posed by renal disorders and the coexistence of hemodialysis and transplantation as "by no means optimally developed [but] sufficiently well advanced" forms of therapy to treat them, the United States government appointed a Committee on Chronic Kidney Disease. In September 1967 the committee, led by Dr. Carl W. Gottschalk from the University of North Carolina School of Medicine, issued what has come to be known as the Gottschalk report. They found that:

Approximately 5,000 patients with chronic uremia died in fiscal year 1967 because of lack of adequate treatment facilities, and by 1973, when treatment capabilities may meet demand, a minimum of 24,000 additional medically suitable patients will have died without the opportunity for treatment by chronic dialysis or transplantation. Until capability meets demand, agonizing decisions concerning patient selection are inevitable at both the local and national level, creating psychological, ethical, and political problems. [*Report of the Committee on Chronic Kidney Disease* 1967, p. 5]

Although the Gottschalk report brought the supply and demand problem in the treatment of chronic renal failure before the public eye, its expensive proposals [$800 million to $1 billion for the first six years] for a national treatment program were not carried out. During the years since the report was issued, the annual number of patients receiving dialysis and transplantation has risen and the costs of these procedures have decreased. Treatment capabilities, however, still fall far short of demand. At the end of 1970, approximately 3,100 persons in the United States were being maintained on chronic hemodialysis, about double the 1968 figures, and some 1,000 other patients received kidney transplants (Schmeck 1970). Given a median estimate of 7,500 medically suitable dialysis or transplantation candidates per year, over 3,000 persons died in 1970 who might have lived had treatment facilities been available.[2]

The painful economic and moral problems involved here have been vividly summarized by H. E. de Wardener. He views them both from the perspective of the total medical system and from the vantage point of the individual patient and his family.

The cost of maintaining life with intermittent haemodialysis is such that few can afford it from their own pockets. This throws into very sharp relief the differences in socio-political thought amongst various people in various countries and of course their enormous economic differences. In some countries I am told there are establishments for chronic haemodialysis in which are treated only those patients who can pay. There are other countries in which intermittent haemodialysis is provided by the State. And there are those countries where intermittent haemodialysis does not exist.

Even when patients can pay there are not many for whom the expense will not severely lower their standard of living. . . . More often I think the patient who has to pay to survive can only find the money if he sacrifices so much that his family's standard of living is involved. His children's future may even be jeopardized. In this situation the patient may then be forced to choose between altering his family's way of life or dying. . . .

Unfortunately a patient with chronic renal failure may be faced with these tormenting alternatives when his judgment is obscured by his disease. He may therefore, without realizing the full implications of his decision, decide that he wishes to pay for his life to be prolonged. Later, when he is being treated and feels well, he is trapped. Now if he decides that he wishes to save his family further financial embarrassment he has to stop his treatment, a much more deliberate and obvious step. [de Wardener 1966, pp. 110–12]

In this and the following chapter we will focus on how the pioneering Seattle Artificial Kidney Center has tried to respond to these questions. Our central interest will be how a given group of physicians, patients and their families, and a particular community have dealt with the medical-ethical and socioeconomic issues posed by chronic hemodialysis. It will quickly become apparent that a considerable amount of trial-and-error experimentation has been involved as this center has attempted to reach practical and humane solutions to problems whose scope and significance extend far beyond the particularities of investigating and treating kidney disease.

March 1970 marked the tenth anniversary of chronic hemodialysis. It was "celebrated" in Seattle in a special way by three patients. Clyde Shields, Harvey Gentry, and Rolin Hemming, the first terminally ill renal patients in the world to participate in clinical trials of long-term dialysis, were guests of honor at a reception held for them and for Dr. Belding Scribner, whose cannula-shunt device had made their ten-year survival possible. At the reception, Shields, Gentry, and Hemming presented a scroll of formal tribute to Scribner, the physician who had cared for them and experimented on them.

In 1960, the first year of the chronic dialysis program in Seattle, Scribner and his associates had worked intensively with these three patient-subjects and subsequently a fourth one. Scribner describes the crisis of success he and his colleagues unexpectedly faced with these first chronic dialysis recipients, a crisis which led to the creation of Seattle's Artificial Kidney Center.

Late in March 1960, just 3 weeks after Mr. Shields began treatment, we started our second patient on chronic dialysis without thinking much about the implications since at that point we really did not expect the patients to live more than a few weeks or months. This patient was taken simply because he was in clinic and would have died shortly thereafter. Then in May we took a third patient, and in July a fourth. Then suddenly the hospital administration blew the whistle and ordered us not to accept any new patients. They had good reason— for suddenly it became apparent that the treatment was working but was going to cost tens of thousands of dollars per patient per year. Furthermore, we were taking up valuable hospital beds, since the concept of an artificial kidney center for chronic care had not even occurred to us at that point. . . .
For the next year we took the advice of the administration and shut out of our thinking the idea of accepting any more new patients. Then in the summer of 1961 we felt we had made enough progress with the technique of chronic dialysis to attempt

to set up a feasibility study to determine whether a community artificial kidney center could function as a service oriented treatment center outside a hospital. [Scribner 1972, p. 4; see also Scribner et al. 1960, and Hegstrom et al. 1961]

Scribner's group worked from August through December 1961 planning the establishment of an outpatient artificial kidney center, to which patients would come from their homes twice or more each week to undergo dialysis. Their feasibility study was made possible by a $250,000, three-year grant from the John A. Hartford Foundation to plan, build, and begin operating a three-bed treatment center.[3]

As its innovators realized, this venture would make chronic dialysis a social as well as a medical experiment, in part because it would have to function without the organizational and financial support of the University Hospital and its research grants.

In a sense, fortune intervened or the time was ripe in the Seattle area for just this type of experiment. The relationship between the relatively young medical school and the county medical society was good. The county medical society, in the face of its premonition of impending change in the medical-social area, was experiencing one of those recurrent upsurges of new and progressive leadership. This leadership was community-oriented, experimental in mood, and progressive in its outlook. It took seriously its view that insofar as possible the medical community should take a leadership role in the area of medical-social change. [Norton 1967, p. 1271]

The location and organization of the center, the mode of patient selection, and funding were the three major problems worked out during the planning phase (Murray et al. 1962). The choice of a community hospital in which to house the center was entrusted to a lay-dominated committee appointed by the King County Medical Society and the Seattle Hospital Council. From among the several institutions that vied for the center, the committee selected the Swedish Hospital. Space for the center was located in a separate building a block from the main hospital. The process of appointing key personnel, preparing the patient treatment area, laboratories, and other facilities, and acquiring equipment was begun. The center was opened on 1 January 1962 and was scheduled to move into full operation, with a seven-patient capacity, by the beginning of 1963.

An estimate of the potential number of patients the center might serve was based on an analysis of responses to a memorandum sent to members of the county medical society, telling them about the program and inviting them to refer candidates for dialysis. On the basis of this survey and actuarial data from the Metropolitan Life Insurance Company, five to twenty "ideal candidates" per million population per year were expected to be eligible for dialysis. From the outset, therefore, it was clear that the center could not accommodate all those seeking treatment, and that some type of selection procedure would be necessary. A Medical Advisory Committee, composed of physicians interested in renal diseases and a psychiatrist, was appointed by the King County Medical Society to choose candidates who met the medical criteria for treatment. Since the number of these candidates still exceeded the center's treatment capabilities, the medical society also established an Admissions and Policy Committee. This group, made up of laymen and physicians, was charged with formulating and applying nonmedical criteria to select which medically qualified candidates would receive treatment. In the next chapter, when we examine the history and workings of the center's patient selection committee in greater detail, we shall see why it soon became a subject of national attention as it executed its arduous task of allocating a scarce new medical resource among persons who would soon die without it.

Money has always been one of the most important scarce commodities involved in allocating medical care. With chronic, intermittent dialysis the expenses continue, month in and month out, as long as the patient's life is maintained. Since the early 1960s, however, the cost of dialysis has been somewhat reduced by a number of technological advances. Chief among these is the development of a portable dialysis unit for home use. In its initial years of operation, in-center dialysis twice a week averaged approximately $20,000 per patient per year. By 1970 this figure had been reduced to as low as $12,000, but costs still ran as high as $66,000 a year in some cases. The cost of home dialysis, though far less, was still a formidable obstacle to meeting the goal of treating all qualified candidates. Initial in-center training, plus purchase of home dialysis equipment, ran from $9,000 to $13,000, with an annual cost thereafter of $3,000 to $5,000 for supplies, physician care, and backup dialysis at the Seattle Center (Blagg et al. 1970).

The program proved that it could function effectively as a medical enterprise, but in 1963 it came close to financial collapse. Federal funds like those from the National Institutes of Health that financed dialysis research at the University Hospital were not available for continuing treatment programs, and the Hartford grant, which had been given with the understanding that the center would become self-supporting, was expiring. "We were so busy making the Center run well technically," Scribner recalled, "that we never even thought about money. We just assumed the Hartford Foundation would renew their grant, and suddenly we found out they weren't going to. They had done their job by providing research money to demonstrate the feasibility of a dialysis center" (Scribner, personal interview).

The center's 1963 financial dilemma was resolved by foundation, community, and federal government support of the fledgling dialysis program. The Hartford Foundation offered $60,000, as Scribner said, "to bail us out for one more year." Community and government assistance, Scribner feels, was triggered in large part "by the most dramatic part of the crisis: the Seattle *Times* ran pictures of the center's nine dialysis patients across the top of page one, headlined, 'Will These People Have to Die?'" In response to this appeal, the employees of Seattle's major industry, the Boeing Corporation, gave the center a grant from their Good Neighbor Fund, the first major sign that community sources might help underwrite a dialysis program. Following the *Times* story, Scribner continued, he and his colleagues "had a noon meeting at the Ranier Club with a representative from the U.S. Public Health Service" (Scribner, personal interview). As a result of that meeting, the Public Health Service's Kidney Disease Control Program initiated its grant support of dialysis centers with a three-year demonstration grant of $350,000 to the Seattle center (Goodman 1968).

During the same period, from early 1963 to late 1966, Scribner's group at the University Hospital also received financial support from the NIH for their program of laboratory and clinical research. A separate NIH subsidy was given to cover costs of inpatient care for six chronic hemodialysis research patients in the hospital's Clinical Research Center (Norton 1967, p. 1296).

Both the Hartford Foundation and the Public Health Service grants to the center stipulated that it should take steps to establish sound business management and a program that would make it largely self-sustaining. In an effort to remedy its management problems, the center was made an independent, nonprofit corporation in December 1963, a board of trustees was organized, and an experienced administrator was added to the staff. Within the next year, through improved administrative practices, more vigorous and effective public relations efforts, and the development of new sources of funds, the center became essentially self-supporting.

Continuing state aid had been obtained, and work with unions and insurance companies and a thorough review of existing medical insurance revealed hitherto untapped medical insurance resources. A successful fund drive had been accomplished as a precedent for future annual drives. Useful and friendly liaison had been established with the local mass media so that the Center emerged as a significant factor in the public eye. With an annual budget in its third year of operation amounting to $350,000, this attainment of financial independence represented no small social accomplishment. It demonstrated, among other things, that chronic dialysis as a very tangible and concrete lifesaving accomplishment had the ability . . . to attract considerable public attention and support. [Norton 1967, p. 1272][4]

Despite its now sound management and improved finances, the problem of meeting the high costs of dialysis continued to beset the center. Scribner and his colleagues at the University Hospital had foreseen the economic problems with dialysis conducted by a professional team in a medical institution. When plans for the center were still being formulated, they had already begun to think about reducing costs and widening the availability of treatment by developing a portable home dialysis unit that could be operated by the patient and members of his family. In 1963 the Hartford Foundation agreed to underwrite the development of a home dialysis program in Seattle.[5] The University Hospital dialysis research program and the university's department of engineering joined in an intensive effort to design and build a safe, effective dialysis system for home use. Other portions of the Hartford grant were paid out in salaries to the physician hired to supervise the home program and to nurses and technicians who trained patients to operate the dialysis equipment. The Hartford money was also spent to supply a room for training and to cover the costs of home dialysis for a small trial group of patients over a period of three years. The foundation stipulated that any patient accepted for the home program during this period must be assured of continued financial support once the grant terminated. Because the University Hospital could not assume such long-term financial responsibility, the Artificial Kidney Center agreed to cover the costs of home dialysis for these patients after 1966.

The first clinical trial of home dialysis in Seattle grew out of the medical team's desperate desire to save a terminally ill patient who could not be placed in the Kidney Center.

> In 1964 an intelligent 16-year old high school girl was dying in Seattle with terminal renal failure. There was no space available in our dialysis program. Because she was highly motivated and her parents were intelligent and devoted to her, the decision was made to train the patient and her parents to operate an artificial kidney in their basement. Hemodialysis was begun April 5, 1964, and by August her parents were able to dialyze her in their home without medical supervision. [Eschbach et al. 1967, p. 1149][6]

By 1967, the University Hospital had trained twenty-three patients for home dialysis, sixteen of whom lived in areas remote from Seattle and its treatment facilities. Over 2,500 home dialyses had been performed, and only four times had it been necessary to summon a physician to the patient's home during dialysis. Twenty-one of the twenty-three patients were alive, and all of them were judged to be "fully rehabilitated, the majority without any complications of uremia other than anemia" (Eschbach et al. 1967, p. 1161). With these results, the Seattle group felt they could characterize their program as one that was "initially a cumbersome experimental endeavor but has evolved rapidly into a practical and successful means of treating end-stage kidney disease" (Eschbach et al. 1967, p. 1149).

During these first three years, the home training unit gradually worked out the most successful procedures, both medically and psychologically, for the patient and his family to follow. The ideal-typical home training program that emerged is still followed. It consists of a two-month period in the University Hospital's outpatient facility, a motel room remodeled to simulate the home environment. A nurse, technician, and physician are in attendance, each with a distinctive function. Although the doctor is in charge, the technician and especially the nurse have more continuing and extensive responsibility for training the patient and the relative who will assist him with the dialysis. In this setting the patient is dialyzed regularly to correct his uremia and other symptoms of chronic renal failure.

Beginning with the first run, the nurse teaches the patient to perform his own dialysis. She also instructs him in cannula care and the technique of cannula declotting. Subsequently, the technician shows the patient and a family member how to clean and assemble the dialyzer and maintain the dialysate delivery system. The technician also helps the patient order equipment and supplies that will be needed at home. From the beginning of the two-month period, the patient is trained to keep the log book he will be required to maintain. Data such as the length of each treatment, blood pressure, pre- and postdialysis weights, and weekly hematocrits are recorded in this book. The dialysis physician's chief tasks are helping the patient adjust to unattended overnight dialysis; preparing him to respond to medical or equipment emergencies; discussing details of his medical management, such as the strict dietary control that is essential to successful maintenance dialysis; and, finally, giving instructions to the patient's own physician. The training group considers the involvement of the patient's local physician to be very important to the program; for even though he may know little about dialysis, he must be able to oversee the patient's posttraining medical care (Fenton et al. 1968, p. 1098).

In the training procedure itself, the nurse plays a primary role, one that is very different from her usual function in an inpatient center. It is she who must cope most directly with the implications of transferring responsibility for managing a complex, risky treatment from medical professionals to a terminally ill patient and close relative.

Instead of doing everything for the patient in a rapid and efficient manner, the training nurse must watch patiently as the trainee fumbles and blunders while he learns to dialyze himself. She must stifle her natural tendency to take over when the patient falters and learn to reinstruct and stand by while the patient laboriously tries again. [Fenton et al. 1968, p. 1099]

By trial and error the Seattle group evolved these new relationships within the dialysis team, and between the team and the patients and their families. In addition they had to grope their way toward a home dialysis schedule that would be biochemically effective without unduly disrupting the patient's family and work life. The two weekly dialysis periods of twelve to sixteen hours each that were customary at the center proved unsatisfactory at home. If dialysis was conducted during the day, it interfered with the patient's job and other waking activities. If it was carried out at night, a family member had to stay up and supervise the treatment. A schedule of three dialyses a week, each for six to eight hours, was tried next. This proved biochemically equivalent to the two longer treatments, but three of the first four patients soon developed neuropathy, and hypertension proved hard to control. To provide longer periods of dialysis without overtaxing the patient and his family, the Seattle research group developed monitoring devices and other techniques permitting unattended, overnight dialysis. Patients were subsequently trained to sleep during their treatment periods, for eight to ten hours, three nights a week (Eschbach et al. 1967, p. 1150).

One of the most crucial and delicate problems that the Seattle home program had to resolve concerned the division of labor between the patient and the family member running the dialysis unit with him. To begin with, home dialysis confers an unusual amount of "responsibility for operating a complex life-support system" on lay persons (Daly and Hassall 1970, p. 509). It also runs counter to the tendency in modern urban American society for serious illness to be cared for outside the kinship system and the family's residence. Furthermore, the majority of patients receiving hemodialysis treatment for chronic renal failure in Seattle, as in the United States at large, are middle-aged married men.[7] Given the structure and dynamics of the American family, this means that in most cases the relative most eligible and appropriate to assist the patient with home dialysis would be his wife. The Seattle group had no difficulty in reaching this conclusion. What they did not foresee were the social and psychological difficulties that would arise when the patient's wife was put in charge of the dialysis process. That kind of superordinate responsibility proved to be a severe emotional burden for the wife. It tended to make the husband, already dependent on a machine for his life, even move passive and subject. And because it entailed a certain degree of role reversal in the usual male–female relations, it disturbed the equilibrium of the entire family.

Beyond these stresses associated with family dynamics, sex roles, and the unusual amount of medical responsibility assigned to lay persons, home dialysis involves a gift-exchange relationship that also imposes strains on its participants. In a way that is analogous to donating and receiving a live kidney transplant, home dialysis requires a family member to make an extraordinary gift of herself (or himself) so that a close relative may survive.

Although dialysis does not entail donating a part of oneself in the same literal sense that an organ transplant does, its life-giving implications are as momentous. In home dialysis, life is exchanged for death not through a single act of giving as in transplantation, but rather by a continuous donation of time, energy, skill, and concern. This recurrent gift confronts those undergoing chronic dialysis with the same problem of reciprocation that transplant recipients face.

It took time for the Seattle team to become aware of some of these strains and their consequences and to restructure the home training procedure accordingly.

Initially, the spouse or another family member was instructed to be responsible for the dialysis procedure. This approach proved unsatisfactory because in two immature male patients it fostered excessive dependence upon their wives. Eventually, the stress on these wives increased to such an extent that, when combined with the insecurity of the patient, it seriously threatened family stability. On the basis of this unfortunate experience patients are now taught to dialyze themselves and assume primary responsibility for their own treatment. Therefore, whenever possible, cannulas are inserted initially into the leg so that both hands are free to accomplish self-dialysis. . . . This approach has resulted in better patient adjustment to [the] disease and its treatment and has minimized the dependent attitudes that are prone to develop in any particular patient on maintenance dialysis. In addition, by making the patient himself primarily responsible the amount of stress felt by other family members has been eased considerably. [Eschbach et al. 1967, pp. 1149–50]

By 1968 the Seattle physicians felt that these and other problems had been sufficiently remedied to deem the home training program a success. In turn, this recognition led to a major re-orientation in the University Hospital and Artificial Kidney Center programs, both of which were now training patients for home dialysis. Those who had been engaged since 1960 in developing maintenance dialysis now believed that "home dialysis must be made to work for all types of patients, and center dialysis must be abandoned, or dialysis programs will continue to flounder in terms of meeting the needs of the thousands who die for lack of this life-saving treatment" (Fenton et al. 1968, p. 1097). A simple calculus lay behind this judgment: the resources (money, facilities, and health and administrative manpower) necessary to provide one patient-year of treatment at the center could train six new patients a year for home dialysis. Thus, committed to offering treatment to as many qualified candidates as possible, the Seattle program adopted a new policy.

Being able to accept several patients for home dialysis in lieu of one patient for center dialysis means that it is morally wrong to take on any more patients for center dialysis until all candidates for dialysis in the home are given a chance. Because of these considerations, accepting new patients for center dialysis has been discontinued in Seattle for the foreseeable future. [Fenton et al. 1968, p. 1097]

In the spring of 1970 the Seattle Artificial Kidney Center was officially renamed the Northwest Kidney Center (NKC). The change was adopted to signify a twofold expansion that had already taken place in the treatment program that the center, in conjunction with the University Hospital, offered to patients with terminal renal disease. Geographically, "Northwest" replaced "Seattle" because less than one-third of the center's patients now came specifically from the Seattle area. This regionalization of the program had begun with the advent of home dialysis seven years earlier. The word "artificial" was deleted to reflect an enlargement of the center's treatment modalities. The Seattle group was now willing to use renal transplantation as well as chronic hemodialysis, rather than devoting themselves exclusively to the latter.

The Seattle renal transplantation program is a relative latecomer; it has been accepted slowly; and in terms of size and scope it is very much a junior partner to the home dialysis program. The University Hospital began kidney transplants in 1967 when Dr. Thomas Marchioro, a surgeon, was invited to join its staff. He came to Seattle after spending five years in Denver as a member of Dr. Thomas Starzl's team of renal and hepatic transplant specialists. In comparison with Denver, Dr. Marchioro felt in 1970, "Seattle's medical community is still rather conservative about transplants. They are very slowly reaching the point of committing themselves to renal transplants, and are not yet ready to consider the transplantation of other vital organs. At this time, I'm the only surgeon in the area engaged in organ transplantation work of any kind." Marchioro attributes the Seattle group's "conservatism" regarding transplantation to their social and emotional, as well as medical, involvement in hemodialysis:

Through the very worthwhile efforts of Dr. Scribner and his
associates, Seattle became the Mecca of chronic hemodialysis.
There has been a tremendous drive for dialysis here; the public's
sentiments and support have been mobilized, and dialysis has
received a great deal of constructive publicity. One byproduct
of this community-wide commitment to dialysis has been slowness
in considering and accepting organ transplantation. [Marchioro,
personal interview]

Scribner would not deny that his center's involvement in chronic
hemodialysis retarded the initiation of a transplant program in
Seattle. In fact, he feels that this kind of fervor has been essential
to the relatively favorable results he has obtained with this mode
of treatment:

It's a historical fact that out of the first round of dialysis that
was started in 1960–61, only Seattle patients survived; no other
patients in the world survived. In my view the major reason
was that other people who started dialysis in the early days were
all associated with transplant centers. And their motivation was to
use dialysis as a means to an end and get a transplant. They
did the least they could instead of the most they could to make
dialysis work, and the results were disastrous. It wasn't anybody's
fault. . . . We were not better than anybody else. It was just a
question of attitude and motivation. . . .
Now again, speaking historically, after we succeeded in Seattle
and got things going, the next successful programs started around
the world were all started de novo, away from transplant
centers. . . .
I don't know what to do to guarantee the quality of dialysis in
the future. It's so intimately tied to the motivation and the
personality of the people running it. I think dialysis could
deteriorate very badly in the next ten years because of this
problem. It takes devotion of the highest order to make this thing
work. . . . I guess my message to the transplanters is, "For God's
sake, don't downgrade dialysis, because it's your backstop, it's
the thing the patient goes back to if he ever gets in trouble."
[Scribner, personal interview]

But these attitudes were not the only deterrent to launching
transplantation in Seattle. In Scribner's words, "We [the University Hospital group] wanted to start renal transplants in 1964,
but we had enormous obstacles to overcome." These obstacles,
he explained, began with the task of finding a well-trained transplant surgeon like Marchioro to begin Seattle's program. "We
didn't want someone starting transplants de novo. Thus we blocked
some local surgeons, because we felt they weren't properly
trained."

Marchioro, Scribner went on, came to Seattle under "strange" and "frustrating" financial circumstances. In contrast to Denver's well-funded research and clinical transplantation program, "Seattle had no funds for transplanters, and none to go for. It took from 1967 to 1970 to convince laymen in the community to back transplantation. Businessmen, for example, argued against cadaveric transplants on the grounds that the procedure would cost around $10,000, and half of the transplants would fail" (Scribner, personal interview). In part, these difficulties were a consequence of the Seattle community's deep commitment to the value of chronic dialysis, and of the time it took to sufficiently "deconvert" them from this allegience so that they were willing to help support transplantation.

Community support for the center depends to a considerable extent on business management and public relations. The center has established an unusual set of collaborative relationships between the medical and lay persons who govern and operate it. It recognizes that fund-raising and community promotion considerations intersect with the medical and moral issues involved in selecting and maintaining patients.

At the May 1970 meeting of the executive committee, for example, these interrelations were apparent in the items that made up the agenda and in the exchanges that took place between medical and lay persons. The meeting began with the center and the University Hospital reporting the following breakdown for the 187 persons in their treatment programs:

> Renal transplantation 36
> Home hemodialysis 111
> Home peritoneal dialysis[8] 9
> Home dialysis training at the
>   NKC's outpatient facility 14
> Home dialysis training at the
>   University Hospital's facility . . . 9
> In-hospital dialysis prior to
>   home training program 8

The ceaseless financial problems underlying this patient treatment report quickly surfaced at the meeting, both in various business reports and in related discussions among those present. This was particularly clear in some of the remarks made by the center's medical personnel, who often expressed frustration because economic considerations must bear so heavily upon their professional decisions, and in the comments of the lay members of the committee, who repeatedly referred to the necessity of maintaining a responsible fiscal policy.

When the chairman of the Patient Admissions Committee stated that seven patients had been accepted for treatment and home training during the previous month, the businessmen on the executive committee voiced concern over "stepping up the rate of patient acceptance to the point where it will be more than the center can handle by the end of the year." In response, the medical director admitted that "the medical team is not sure of where we're going in terms of new patient numbers." He explained that the center had been adding about sixty patients a year, as had been projected on the basis of the approximately two and one-half million people in the geographical area it serves. But this year, he admitted, the figure would probably run closer to seventy new patients. Another physician hastened to add that, "medically, the center has not fallen behind. We have no stack-up problems, and the number of patients we can accept is being expanded with added income and with the addition of transplantation and peritoneal dialysis." The executive committee was also assured that the admissions committee checks the center's latest financial statement at each of its meetings, "in order not to overcommit our resources."

One of the meeting's longest discussions dealt with whether the center should begin accepting children under sixteen for treatment by hemodialysis, peritoneal dialysis, or transplantation. In this matter too financial considerations were aired along with the complex medical and psychological aspects of chronic dialysis and transplantation of children. On the basis of some recent indications that children could be dialyzed or transplanted without deleterious effects upon growth and development, the Medical Advisory Committee had proposed in March 1970 that the executive committee reconsider its policy of not accepting children. A pediatrician from Seattle's Children's Hospital spoke favorably about a policy change at the meeting and estimated that three to five children a year might be candidates for treatment. In the ensuing discussion, a physician-member of the board of trustees reported that the center's lawyers had found no legal barriers to accepting minors. He felt that potential for rehabilitation was not as appropriate a primary selection criterion as it was for an adult. The Special Committee on the Acceptance of Children had suggested that the major consideration should be the "family atmosphere and the determination of the parent that the child get well."

Various medical, economic, and legal arguments for and against accepting children were then advanced by both physicians and laymen. Strong emotional and moral sentiments underlay the businesslike reports. One could sense the tragic image of a sick and dying child. Finally, a lay member of the executive committee put the implicit feeling of the group into words: "I think this is something we *have* to do." Only the Protestant minister-chairman of the admissions committee voiced doubts about the medical and psychological problems that might be encountered. With little further discussion, the executive committee voted unanimously that the center adopt a policy of accepting children, using its regular selection criteria "with additional inquiry into its impact on the family unit."

The executive committee moved on to consider the creation of a "corporate image" for the center and its larger import. One of the center's trustees, president of an advertising agency, had been authorized to engage a commercial artist to design an insignia that could be used for letterheads, posters, and other sorts of publicity. The artist sketched some of the symbols associated with other voluntary health organizations, such as the heart and torch of the American Heart Association, the sword of the National Cancer Society, and the Red Cross. The symbol that would be most suitable for the NKC's image, he suggested, was the familiar bean-shaped kidney itself, a symbol that would transcend any future changes in the center's name or its range of services.

Two of the most enthusiastic reports given were those by the chairman of the center's finance committee and by its auditor. They declared that the center now presented a very different picture from its early years, when uncertain funding and inadequate management nearly caused its demise. In 1970, the finance committee chairman proudly announced, "We finally have financial records we can rely on, so that we know what is really going on. The center is now putting out monthly statements, and the patients know exactly what they are being charged, and what they owe." The audit report focused on a particular form of the center's income, donations given for the treatment of designated patients. The center had found that this money was often not fully expended for the particular person for whom it was given. Some of these patients could partly meet their own expenses; others had died before the funds were used up. When the center sought legal advice on what should be done with the residual funds, it was told that a designated donation is legally defined as a "true gift" for which a tax deduction may be taken, and the center was therefore not obligated to return any unspent money to the donor. It had decided to put these sums in a reserve fund. This now rather large fund, and the "very generous" funding of new patients by the Division of Vocational Rehabilitation, had meant that thus far in 1970 the center had not been forced to reject any candidates for financial reasons. It had even been able to surpass its original patient quota. At this juncture, the center's president reaffirmed its currently sound financial status but warned that:

As nice as it has been to have state funds, the Committee should not assume that they will always be available, for the political picture might shift very rapidly, as it has in the past. As long as we can get tax dollars, we're in good shape. But we must not forget that we're committed to a certain number of patients, and if the legislative situation should change, this will not alter our obligation to these patients. If we ever get to the point where the Division of Vocational Rehabilitation doesn't pick up new patients, we'll have a real problem.

As the various reports presented to the executive committee suggest, the operation of the NKC is dependent upon continuing and diverse fund-raising and public relations efforts. To meet the costs of operating the center, continuing treatment of those patients already on home dialysis, and adding an expected fifty-five new patients to the program, the NKC's projected budget for 1970 was $1,268,294.[9] It was anticipated that 61 percent, or $767,294, of this sum would be met by the patients' own resources, including their health-insurance coverage. Another 21 percent ($271,000) of the funds was expected to come from federal and state governments. The goal of the center's 1969–70 fund drive was to raise the remaining 18 percent ($230,000) of the budget as undesignated funds to finance treatment for those patients unable to meet expenses on their own or from government sources.

The 1970 fund drive, operating under the center's motto "To Give Life," was initially scheduled to run for ninety days ending

7 February. During that period, community auxiliaries of the NKC and various civic and fraternal organizations engaged in specific fund-raising activities, while another network of more than one hundred volunteers from the Seattle community solicited other public contributions. At the same time, parallel fund drives were undertaken by county chapters of the center. These chapters, organized in 1968, are representative of the regional area the center has come to serve. Each chapter that has a delegate on the board of trustees is given an annual "dollar goal" to cover the treatment costs of old and new patients living in the territory it covers.

As in most well-organized fund-raising drives, solicitors for the NKC were provided with an "information sheet" and other literature about the operation and needs of the center's program. The material emphasized the life-or-death situation of the patients involved and the "normal lives as productive working members of society" that "in most instances" could be theirs if they were maintained on an artificial kidney.

A second set of themes on which the fund-raising appeals dwell is the high cost of treatment and the necessity for the community's help in meeting these expenses through contributions to the NKC.

Since its origination, costs of NKC treatment have been reduced through advances in technology . . . from $21,000 per year to $13,401 for the first year . . . and $3,432 (supplies) thereafter.

Insurance, personal and government funds are not sufficient to fully fund hemodialysis patients. Hence, approximately 50% of all existing and new patients need additional funds to continue treatment—and to continue living.

Artificial kidney treatment is *not* financed by the United Good Neighbor Fund, as UGN . . . does not support on-going medical care. Therefore, the continued success of NKC's life-giving care rests largely on public contributions. . . .

On a dollar basis, donated funds buy life for an otherwise doomed victim of renal disease. One dollar buys two hours of life for a present patient being treated at home. . . . Or $1.00 buys nearly 45 minutes of life for a patient new to NKC's "life-continuing" program. . . .

The Need: To stop the needless loss of life.

The Challenge: To eliminate finance as a selection criterion.

Third, and perhaps most important to ongoing public support of the NKC, the fund-raising literature stresses that the donor's money will be used within the community to treat his less fortunate fellow citizens and appeals to pride in helping to maintain a pioneering, world-famous local program. It is not reluctant to invoke negative as well as positive xenophobic sentiments, particularly in the form of allusions to regional distrust of East Coast domination.

All money donated to NKC for patient care is spent right here . . . the money is not sent East to maintain a national organization or fund drive. Locally donated dollars are locally spent to assist in the care of your fellow Washingtonians. . . .

NKC is a non-profit organization operated by a board of responsible community leaders—both doctors and laymen—in the Swedish Hospital Medical Center complex. . . .

The Seattle Artificial Kidney Center is the largest dialysis treatment center in the world. . . .

Seattle is the world focal point for improving treatment techniques, modernizing equipment, developing training programs, and pioneering cost-reduction methods.

The 1970 fund drive was extended to 15 April 1970, with additional special fund drives scheduled to run through the summer. For at the close of the regular campaign in February the drive was nearly $80,000 short of its $230,000 goal. This shortage was all the more acute, the fund drive chairman reported, because the number of new candidates accepted in the first quarter of the year indicated that seventy to seventy-five new patients, rather than the anticipated fifty-five, would go on home dialysis by the end of the year. Those at the May 1970 executive committee meeting were told that at the end of the 15 April extension period, approximately $168,000 had been collected in undesignated funds (still $42,000 less than the original goal), $96,800 in designated funds, and $14,000 for capital expenditures.

In his report in the center's newsletter, "To Give Life," the drive chairman attributed the shortage of contributions to Seattle's "momentarily depressed economy." The city then had one of the nation's highest unemployment rates, owing in large part to cutbacks by its major employer, the Boeing Corporation. At the same time, the chairman observed, public contributions thus far in 1970 were 64 percent greater than in 1968–69, when the drive's goal was $200,000 in undesignated funds.

The fund drive is only one of the activities conducted by the center's public relations and fund-raising office to maintain and broaden its treatment program. Philanthropic support is sought all year. The various forms this type of donation may take, and income-tax benefits and legal procedures, are explained in a 1968 booklet entitled "Your Gift of Life to the Seattle Artificial Kidney Center: A Summary of Methods of Philanthropic Support."

Diverse groups in the communities served by the center also are engaged in different enterprises to publicize, promote, and raise funds for home dialysis. The range of these activities is revealed by a sampling of the stories appearing in the center's quarterly publication, "To Give Life." The November 1968 issue, for example, reported on four "Helping Hands." Individuals, clubs, or corporations were invited to again support the center through its Christmas card program. A second item noted that the Seattle Junior Chamber of Commerce had begun its third year of sponsoring a speaker's bureau, which arranges talks on the center's history and activities for clubs and other organizations in the greater Seattle area. One of the center's major "helping hands," the Employees Good Neighbor Fund of the Boeing Corporation, made a grant for construction of a home-training area. A smaller but no less important contribution received the most prominent coverage in this issue of "To Give Life": a winning crew in Seattle's annual Dinghy Derby sold their prize, "a very old cow," for $104.50 and donated their proceeds to the center.

Our content analysis of the center's publication identifies the main forms of community support for the center. There are episodic gifts, such as that by the derby winners. Second, the employees of many businesses and industries in Seattle, as well as other Northwest areas, regularly support the center. The names of employee groups, along with those of individual benefactors, are listed on a plaque at the center—the "Major Donor Honor Roll" of supporters who contribute $500 or more to the NKC. The spring 1970 issue of "To Give Life" listed sixty-seven additions to the honor roll. In some instances, employee groups will "adopt" a specific patient and conduct fund-raising activities for his or her treatment. A third important source of funds, as well as volunteer service work, comes from the many women's auxiliaries that have been organized on behalf of the NKC.

A profile of some of Seattle's major enterprises, voluntary associations, and groups of citizens, as well as of traditions, social attitudes, and value commitments characteristic of the city and region, emerges from this glimpse of the Northwest Kidney Center's public relations and fund-raising activities. The degree to which supporting the center through "gifts of life" has become institutionalized in this community is nowhere more apparent than in the way it responded to the 1971 fund drive during a year of deepening economic recession. "Seattle, as you may know, is hit very hard by the current sagging economy with unemployment running about 14 percent," the director of fund raising and public relations for the center has written.

The obvious reaction to this situation would be, "This is not the time to try to raise money." But amazingly enough, we are running about 20 percent over 1970's fund drive . . . public contributions are running 2–1 over last year. There is a tendency, I believe, on the part of the people to give to charity when times are rough, but they are working. For example, United Good Neighbors (UGN) was off in their fund drive because contributions are tied to payroll deductions. But individual contributions of those working were up over the previous years. [R. C. Howard, personal communication]

Furthermore, despite their massive economic reverses, corporations in the area matched the donations they had made in previous years.

Because they realized that "things [were] tough," those in charge of fund raising "tried harder" and attempted to be "more professional in [their] approach." In addition, a "relative deprivation" phenomenon may have worked in favor of the drive. Comparing themselves with the many residents of Seattle who had lost their jobs, those who were employed seem to have experienced a quickened appreciation of their own good fortune. A sense of privileged abundance may have increased their generosity to those in acute need whom the Kidney Center tries to help. Quasi-magical sentiments could also have been involved: in the face of generalized adversity, a donation to the NKC functions as a symbolic petition to destiny to continue to smile upon one because of one's charity and good works in which one has been engaged. But underlying the specific reasons for the 1971 fund drive's success are the more general and enduring social structural conditions that the Northwest Kidney Center has helped to create and mobilize—conditions that have "allowed and encouraged sentiments of altruism, reciprocity, and social duty to express themselves" (Titmuss 1971, p. 225). In his analysis of the commitment of the British people to a voluntary blood donor program, Richard M. Titmuss has suggested that "the ways in which society organizes and structures its social institutions—and particularly its health and welfare systems—can encourage or discourage the altruistic in man; such systems can foster integration or alienation; they can allow the 'theme of the gift' . . . of generosity towards strangers—to spread among and between social groups and generations" (Titmuss 1971, p. 225). The Northwest Kidney Center of Seattle has become a community-oriented social institution that, to quote Titmuss once more, provides "opportunities for ordinary people to articulate giving in morally practical terms outside their own network of family and personal relationships" (Titmuss 1971, p. 226).

8

Patient Selection and the Right to Die: Problems Facing Seattle's Kidney Center

From its inception in 1961–62, the most controversial and publicized feature of Seattle's chronic dialysis program quickly became its Admissions and Policy Committee. This board of laymen and physicians was appointed to formulate and use nonmedical criteria for deciding who among the medically qualified candidates approved by the center's Medical Advisory Committee would receive one of the limited number of kidney machines available. The decision to form the admissions committee was also prompted by a desire to "protect those in charge of the Center from pressure to take a given patient" (Murray et al. 1967, p. 316). A third function, more difficult to fulfill since the committee members wished to remain anonymous, was to have the committee "represent the Center in the community." "The future of the Center," its founders wrote in 1962, "rests, in large part, on assessment of its acceptability as a community service by this group" (Murray et al. 1967, p. 316).

National attention was drawn to the Seattle center's program, particularly to the workings of the admissions committee, through an article by Shana Alexander that appeared in *Life* magazine in November 1962. Colorfully but accurately entitled "They Decide Who Lives, Who Dies: Medical Miracle Puts Moral Burden on a Small Committee," the story captured the inherently dramatic nature of the artificial kidney program: the frankly experimental nature of chronic dialysis; the dependence of the patient upon the workings of a machine—the fact that for the rest of his life he must "surrender his life's blood to a medical laundromat twice a week"; and, above all, the radically unorthodox step of involving laymen in making life-or-death decisions about a candidate's acceptability for this medical procedure.

"As I recall that period," Belding Scribner wrote in 1972, all of us who were involved felt that we had found a fairly reasonable and simple solution to an impossibly difficult problem by letting a committee of responsible members of the community choose which patients [would receive treatment] among several who were medically ideal . . . through pre-screening by the Medical Selection Committee. In retrospect, of course, we were terribly naive. We did not realize even then the full impact that the existence of this committee would have on the world. [We] simply could not understand why everyone was much more interested in the existence and operation of the lay selection committee than in the fact that in two years we had taken a disease, end-stage kidney disease, and converted it from a one hundred percent fatal prognosis to a ninety-five percent two year survival. Nor were any of us prepared for the very severe criticism that was to be forthcoming both at the annual medical meetings and in the scholarly literature. [Scribner 1972, p. 5]

Although patient selection has been the most visible and therefore most discussed issue posed by the limited availability of chronic dialysis, it is by no means the only socially and ethically troublesome matter that this procedure has paradigmatically raised. In his 1964 presidential address to the American Society for Artificial Internal Organs, for example, Dr. Scribner dealt with four of the most ethically difficult problems that he and his colleagues had encountered in their experience with chronic dialysis. These problems, he believed, are all the more acute because they will "recur again and again as other new, complicated, expensive, life-saving techniques are developed" (Scribner 1964, p. 209). The first problem Scribner discussed was patient selection, for to him it was "in many ways the easiest [one] to talk about," in part because "there are those in this audience who maintain that there is no problem with respect to selection because there is no need to select." To Scribner, simple figures tellingly rebutted this viewpoint:

All I can say is that at the present time in the United States there are not more than 50 to 100 patients on transplants plus chronic dialysis—yet in the last four years, since these techniques have become available, 10,000 or more ideal candidates have died in this country for lack of the treatment, so obviously rigid selection of one sort or another must have taken place.

The other three interrelated problems Scribner raised, which we shall explore, are overt termination of dialysis by the physician, termination by the patient himself, and "death with dignity." As he had expected and still recalls with some pride, Scribner was roundly "criticized from the floor for discussing such things," for as he knew firsthand, these subjects are "tough, uncomfortable, unpleasant" ones which most physicians would prefer not to dwell upon, much less to air publically (Scribner 1964, p. 209).

These "uncomfortable" subjects, of course, are not peculiar to the dialysis program in Seattle; they confront all dialysis centers. In 1967, A. H. Katz and D. M. Proctor conducted the first comprehensive study of dialysis centers and patients in the United States, collecting extensive questionnaire data from 93 of an estimated 120 centers and from 689 (81 percent) of the estimated dialysis patients. As they point out in their section on "Patient Selection Criteria and Process," patient selection is an important and prominent aspect of dialysis because "basic issues of social policy, the limits of medical responsibility, major ethical and legal considerations are encapsulated in the decision to choose or reject patients for dialysis" (Katz and Proctor 1969, p. 22). A summary of their findings about patient selection documents the nonuniform and uncertain nature of this decision-making process at all dialysis centers. It also provides a comparative frame of reference for the in-depth look at Seattle's admissions committee that follows.

Katz and Proctor found that the "prevailing pattern of selection" in the eighty-seven centers responding to their survey begins with an evaluation of the candidate's medical suitability for treatment, using information collected by the center staff and by the referring physician. The medical "problems of uncertainty" in dialysis are akin to those we have discussed with reference to transplantation, as is made evident by the finding that only half the centers "reported that they had explicit medical criteria for accepting or rejecting a hemodialysis patient" (Katz and Proctor 1969, p. 22).

Candidates judged medically suitable are then evaluated by the "patient selection decision-makers" in terms of the criteria employed by the particular center. Only eight centers reported that they utilized a lay or community advisory selection committee, and, Katz and Proctor found, "the actual role of such committees was unclear, for in no case were they reported to participate by *voting* in the final selection of patients" (Katz and Proctor 1969, p. 26). (At the time of this study, as we shall explain more fully, the Seattle admissions committee's role was being reformulated because of changes in their dialysis program.) Thus in the vast majority of centers the final screening and selection process is primarily a function of the physician.

The predominant role in voting on patient selection was played by physicians (facility directors voted in 73 centers, staff physicians voted in 64 centers and referring physicians in 11 centers). Ancillary personnel such as staff nurses, social workers, psychiatrists and psychologists voted on the selection of patients in only a small minority of centers (20 or fewer centers). [Katz and Proctor 1969, p. 27]

The type of information about a dialysis candidate, and how it is gathered for a selection committee, also varies widely.

Data preparation for the selection committee was done by: the referring physician (46 centers), social workers (45 centers), center director (40 centers), psychiatrist (33 centers), and staff physicians (32 centers). A minority of centers (23) administer intelligence, personality or vocational aptitude tests to prospective patients.
Eighty centers reported that they routinely interviewed a prospective patient's spouse. . . . Other sources interviewed were: the patient's children (22 centers); parents of minor or unmarried patients (53 centers); employers (28 centers); local social agencies to whom the patient is known (19 centers); family or referring physician (10 centers); and social groups of which the patient is a member (16 centers).
Sixty-seven percent (62) of centers informed prospective patients and their families of the selection criteria employed, while one-third (23) gave little or no information. [Katz and Proctor 1969, p. 23]

To further assess selection methods, Katz and Proctor asked dialysis center directors what criteria their centers employed. One point these investigators were interested in was what conditions would definitely *exclude* a candidate's selection. Centers were given a checklist of seven items and permitted to check as many as were applicable (see table 5).

A second list of seventeen criteria were to be rated according to the following degrees of importance in the selection process: "not used; minor importance (occasionally used); important (but occasionally not considered); or highly important (always used)."

Table 5.   Conditions Which Definitely Exclude Selection of a Patient

100 Percent = 87 Centers

Criterion	Percentage of Centers
Mental deficiency	68
Poor family environment	29
Criminal record	25
Indigency	21
Poor employment record	20
Lack of transportation	17
Lack of state residency	17

SOURCE: Katz and Proctor 1969, table III–4, p. 25.

The eight most frequently employed criteria, "i.e., highly important criteria which were reported by centers to be always used," were as follows: "willingness to cooperate in treatment regimen (86 percent of eighty-seven centers); medical suitability (good prognosis with dialysis) (79 percent); absence of other disabling disease (69 percent); intelligence (as related to understanding treatment) (34 percent); likelihood of vocational rehabilitation (32 percent); age (29 percent); primacy of application for available vacancy (26 percent); psychiatric evaluation (25 percent)."

The members of the Seattle Artificial Kidney Center's Admissions and Policy Committee were appointed jointly by the board of trustees of the King County Medical Society and the Seattle Hospital Council. The committee convened in the summer of 1961 to begin drawing up guidelines for the nonmedical screening and selection of dialysis candidates. It was envisaged as representing a broad socioeconomic spectrum of the Seattle community, in hope that this would mitigate any bias in favor of candidates with certain social backgrounds or occupations. The committee's first seven members consisted of a lawyer, minister, housewife, labor leader, state government official, banker, and surgeon, plus two physician-advisors. Thus the center's ideological position notwithstanding, the admissions committee it chose was relatively homogeneous, largely upper middle class in education, occupation, income, and general social background. This was to result in certain biases in the selection criteria the committee evolved, biases which helped to trigger a lasting and sometimes strident debate about the ethical propriety of such a triage process.

The admissions committee requested and was granted the right to work anonymously. They did so to protect themselves from direct pressures to select particular candidates, to mitigate the strains of their task, and to reduce their involvement in argument about its overall merits or demerits. Apart from deciding not to reveal candidates' names to the committee, the center gave them the freedom to investigate applicants in any way that seemed appropriate. In its early days, the group relied primarily upon data gathered by the center's physicians and on reports from referring physicians. At least one member of the panel soon expressed his discomfort at depending only upon these sources of information plus his own intuitive judgment about a candidate and urged that the committee be given an investigative staff including a social worker, psychiatrist, and vocational guidance counselor (Alexander 1962, p. 118).

In their first deliberations, the committee decided to accept only candidates from the State of Washington, and also to exclude from consideration children or adults over age forty-five. The adoption of these first two nonmedical criteria reduced the initial number of candidates to three, the number of places that were available when the center opened. Space soon became available for another patient, and when four candidates met the residency and age requirements, the committee had to begin formulating additional selection criteria. In her *Life* magazine story, one of the first accounts of the Seattle program, Shana Alexander reported that the committee members weighed factors such as "sex of patient; marital status and number of dependents; income; net worth; emotional stability, with particular regard to the patient's capacity to accept the treatment; educational background; nature of occupation, past performance and future potential; and names of people who could serve as references" (Alexander 1962, p. 106). Using these guidelines to evaluate the four candidates for the center's one vacancy, the group selected "a 33 year-old electrician whose 7 dependents almost certainly would become dependent upon state aid if he were unable to continue to work" (Murray et al. 1962, p. 316).

As applications for dialysis mounted, the committee members were increasingly forced into this type of decision-making, able to choose at most one or two out of a number of candidates.

"The choices were hard," Mr. N, a lay member of the committee told us, "and I wasn't happy about some of the decisions I made. For example, I remember voting against a young woman who was a known prostitute. I found I couldn't vote for her, rather than another candidate, a young wife and mother who had proved her responsibility and worth. I also voted against a young man who had been a ne'er-do-well, a real playboy, until he learned he had renal failure. He promised he would reform his character, go back to school, and so on, if only he were selected for treatment. But I felt I'd lived long enough to know that a person like that won't really do what he was promising at the time."

The reasons for which Mr. N rejected these two candidates illustrate the "social worth" criteria that entered into the committee's selection process. The patient's "marital status," "net worth," "occupation," and "past performance and future potential" were the types of social worth criteria that the committee members avowedly considered. Within these very general criteria, the specific, often unarticulated indicators that were used reflected the middle-class American value system shared by the selection panel. A person "worthy" of having his life preserved by a scarce, expensive treatment like chronic dialysis was one judged to have qualities such as decency and responsibility. Any history of social deviance, such as a prison record, any suggestion that a person's married life was not intact and scandal-free, were strong contraindications to selection. The preferred candidate was a person who had demonstrated achievement through hard work and success at his job, who went to church, joined groups, and was actively involved in community affairs.

Since these values do predominate in American society, it is interesting that their explicit, overt use in a life-or-death patient selection process has evoked great indignation. In discussing whether any group has the "ability or right" to impose arbitrary selection criteria, for example, Dr. George E. Schreiner pointed out that:

If you really believe in the right of society to make decisions on medical availability on these criteria you should be logical and say that when a man stops going to church or is divorced or loses his job, he ought to be removed from the programme and somebody else who fulfils these criteria substituted. Obviously no-one faces up to this logical consequence. [Schreiner 1966, p. 128]

One of the sharpest criticisms of the Seattle selection process has come from David Sanders and Jesse Dukeminier, a psychiatrist and a lawyer, in a 1968 paper on transplantation and dialysis:

> The ethical muddle of selection committees comparing human worth is well illustrated by the operations of the selection committee at the Seattle Artificial Kidney Center. The descriptions of how this committee makes its decisions . . . are numbing accounts of how close to the surface lie the prejudices and mindless clichés that pollute the committee's deliberations. . . . What is meant by "public service," a phrase so difficult to define in a pluralistic society? Were the persons who got themselves jailed in the South while working for civil rights doing a "public service"? What about working for the Antivivisection League? Why should a Sunday-school teacher be saved rather than Madalyn Murray? The magazines paint a disturbing picture of the bourgeoisie sparing the bourgeoisie, of the Seattle committee measuring persons in accordance with its own middle-class suburban value system: scouts, Sunday school, Red Cross. This rules out creative nonconformists, who rub the bourgeoisie the wrong way but who historically have contributed so much to the making of America. The Pacific Northwest is no place for a Henry David Thoreau with bad kidneys.
> The Seattle selection system was begun when chronic hemodialysis for renal failure was truly an experimental program. If a project is experimental, the use of broad discretion in selecting candidates who can demonstrate the validity of the project is not objectionable. Once a procedure proves its merit and passes from the experimental to the standard, however, as has happened with chronic hemodialysis, justice requires that selection be made by a fairer method than the unbridled consciences, the built-in biases, and the fantasies of omnipotence of a secret committee. [Sanders and Dukeminier 1968, pp. 377–78]

It is difficult to grasp the emotional strains that the burden of patient selection placed upon the members of the admissions committee, for few nonphysicians are ever cast in such a life-or-death decision-making role. One member of the original selection panel, a Lutheran minister who has continued to work with the center and currently serves as chairman of the admissions committee, spoke to us about how "we all came out of those meetings with empty feelings." When he received a letter inviting him to become a member of the committee in 1961, he recalled, he felt himself "shying away from such a task, because I didn't want to play the God role." He discussed his doubts with a physician friend, the president of the King County Medical Society, "who probably nominated me because of my broad interests in theology and medicine and my willingness to explore and express ideas." The Reverend Mr. X learned of the many "agonizing appeals" that Scribner and his associates had been receiving from private physicians and their patients, and recognized that the decision to form the committee had been prompted because "the doctors didn't want face-to-face confrontations with these patients," as well as by the belief that the community served by the program should "share some of the responsibility for these selection decisions." The Reverend Mr. X agreed to join the admissions committee, with the proviso that he would be free to resign if, after attending the first meeting, he "felt in good conscience he could not serve." Two factors, he said, helped persuade him to remain on the committee. "First, I felt that as a citizen I had no right to shove this responsibility on to someone else just because there were some unpleasant things associated with it." The second reason was his perception of the role he and his colleagues were playing in the allocation of treatment:

I would not be deciding who was to die, but rather I would be deciding who would have a greater chance for life. . . . . Those with renal failure, I realized, are going to die anyway, and making no decision means that all will die.

The other members of the committee justified their selection role to themselves and others in ways similar to the Reverend Mr. X's formulation. For example, when he was interviewed by *Life* reporter Shana Alexander, the banker on the panel voiced his worries about the "morality of choosing A versus B," and said: "I finally came to the conclusion that we are not making a moral choice here—we are picking guinea pigs for experimental purposes. This happens to be true; it also happens to be the way I rationalize my presence on this team." The lawyer expressed a comparable viewpoint: "We are dealing in this work with life that is being artificially sustained for experimental purposes. The so-called 'rejected' patients would have died with or without the Committee. . . . I cannot honestly say I am overwrought by the plight of the patients we do not choose—the ones we *do* choose have an awfully rugged life to look forward to" (Alexander 1962, pp. 115, 117).

In the decade since its inauguration, the Admissions and Policy Committee has undergone several shifts in its functions and modes of patient selection, corresponding with changes in the center's facilities and patient load, its move into home dialysis, and its financial resources. When the center's treatment facilities were enlarged in 1964–65, for a time there was enough space to accept all medically qualified candidates. During this period, with some forty-five patients receiving in-center dialysis, the admissions committee was gradually phased out. In the words of a member of the Medical Advisory Committee, "they were hardly ever called upon to make a decision about a patient's eligibility." At this juncture, a new group, composed of the center's administrative and medical directors and a social worker, was formed to act as a review board for the Medical Advisory Committee.

The center had only a brief respite from the pressures of too many applicants for its facilities and funds to handle. Increasing numbers of candidates, and dwindling grants from government, foundation, and other private sources, were powerful incentives behind the decision for the center and the University Hospital to launch a home dialysis program in 1965. The availability of home treatment eased many of the allocation problems caused by the limited facilities and high costs of center dialysis. Out of these changes, a staff physician on the Medical Advisory Committee recalled, "came the philosophy that if there are funds and no major medical problems, you give the patient a chance even if he has social or psychological problems." However, he continued, the new review board did occasionally reject a candidate, and "the Medical Advisory Committee was unhappy, feeling that no one medically qualified should be turned down for home dialysis. We physicians got upset, because we felt there should be no restrictions . . . we sort of revolted."

The revolt of the center's medical staff resulted in the re-institution of the center's Admissions and Policy Committee. It was reduced from seven to five persons: two physicians—the center's medical director and chairman of the Medical Advisory Committee; and three laymen—the center's administrative director, and two members from the board of trustees. In contrast to the lay members of the original admissions committee, who served for the duration of the group's existence, the medical director of the center now appoints the lay members to serve for rotating one-year terms.

The present screening and selection process at the center begins when a patient is referred for treatment by a formal letter from his private physician. One physician affiliated with the program estimates that:

We see about 80 percent of all patients in the state who need dialysis, and accept 90 to 95 percent of these. We see fewer out of state candidates than we used to, because of the greater acceptance of and growth in number of dialysis facilities. The 20 percent of patients in Washington who need treatment but do not come for evaluation are not seen for several reasons. These include the hesitancy of doctors who do not believe in keeping people alive in an artificial way, the patient's own reluctance about dialysis, and the fact that many private physicians, and the community at large, are not aware of our loosening selection criteria.

After his referral, the home dialysis candidate goes through a series of evaluative procedures administered by the center's staff. These include medical and psychological tests, interviews with the patient and his family by a psychiatrist and social worker, and a financial assessment. As many members of the original selection committee had urged, the center began to use psychological and psychiatric assessments of candidates in 1963. These evaluations, along with studies of patients already on dialysis, sought to identify in advance the characteristics relating to "superior," "good," or "poor" adjustment to chronic dialysis. The "psychological team's" first published paper, in 1966, reported that they had evaluated forty-two candidates for the Medical Advisory Committee from 1963 through 1965, three of whom were subsequently rejected "primarily for psychiatric and social reasons." Another study sample of eighteen patients receiving dialysis were rated for their adjustment to treatment to assess the "predictive accuracy of pretreatment evaluation" (Sands, Livingston, and Wright 1966, p. 604).

On an a priori basis, from knowledge of "the stresses and demands placed on all chronic hemodialysis patients," the center's psychiatrist and clinical psychologist evaluated candidates and patients in terms of three sets of factors concerned with "psychological suitability" for dialysis. The first were characteristics related to self-care, the patient's ability to "take an active role in maintaining his own physical well-being." The team predicted that patients "unlikely to show adequate self-care" would include persons with self-destructive wishes, those with special difficulties in relating to authority figures, those whose self-concept and defenses are seriously compromised by medical requirements, individuals with a life history marked by impulsive, irresponsible behavior, and persons with a low intelligence.

The second factor evaluated was potential for rehabilitation: whether the patient can live a "satisfactory, useful life," either by "his own standards or those of the community." Individuals "particularly likely to show inadequate rehabilitation" were expected to include "persons showing low self-esteem and lacking firm identifications with family, friends, or occupation," and "the patient who has in the past demonstrated strong tendencies to use his symptoms for secondary gain." The team also observed that:

Whether it is necessary that the chronic renal patient assume near-normal social and economic responsibilities is, of course, an ethical question rather than a psychological one. Assuming however that this is a goal, the patient's performance as regards employment and motivations to function up to the limits of his physical capacity . . . deserves close attention. This should give some impression of forces either within the patient himself (such as obsessive anxiety or hypochondriasis), or within his environment (such as an overprotective spouse . . .) which might compromise rehabilitation.

Finally, candidates and patients were assessed with respect to their ability to tolerate the "frequent and recurring stressful situations" that accompany dialysis. These include "uncertainty about life expectancy, stresses individual to each patient and his family," and "the extremely immediate stresses of medical complications and emergencies."

On the basis of their three-year pilot study, the psychological team and the center's medical treatment staff judged that the "great majority" of dialysis patients were "making an at least adequate adaptation" to dialysis. Preliminary psychological and psychiatric assessment was felt to be a valid and useful selection tool, for it led to "predictions about the patient's potential level of adjustment which agrees at quite respectable levels with staff judgments of actual adjustment to treatment." Finally, as they had theorized, the patients in their treatment study sample who were deemed to be adjusting most successfully to dialysis "appear to be differentiated from the less adaptive patients in showing (1) higher intelligence, (2) a less defensive attitude about admitting to anxiety or emotional difficulty, (3) less reliance on emotional defenses that involve the use of physical symptoms, (4) more satisfactory emotional support from family members" (Sands, Livingston, and Wright 1966, pp. 608–9).

The third step in the Northwest Kidney Center's selection process occurs when the Admissions and Policy Committee meets to discuss and vote on the candidate, reviewing together the material in his application file and, whenever possible, hearing about the patient's case from his private physician. The committee then votes on whether to accept, reject, or defer the dialysis candidate. The option of deferral is a relatively new one employed by the selection committee, and, its members feel, "has done a considerable amount of good, because it has forced us to secure more information, or to think through our decisions more fully." In our observation of transplant teams, we found that they also frequently choose to defer a patient, a move that serves not only to give them additional time to judge his case, but also one that at least temporarily relieves them of the burden of flatly rejecting a candidate.

Although the former policy of not revealing the candidate's name to the selection committee is no longer followed, the committee still adheres to the practice of not meeting the applicant personally. The Reverend Mr. X, chairman of the admissions committee when we visited Seattle, vividly illustrated some of the pros and cons of not seeing candidates in person by recalling "one of the most painful things I've ever had to endure."

Six or seven years ago, the committee suddenly found themselves confronted by a patient, Mr. J, and his attorney. Mr. J was a very fine, upright, and worthy gentleman, but he was beyond the age limit we had established. With the patient, as well as his lawyer, in the room, we could not be objective in our discussion of his candidacy. The whole situation was absolutely intolerable. When you're dealing with a fine man, pleading before you for his life, let me tell you, it's rough. We were so uncomfortable and shaken when faced with Mr. J that we bent the rules and accepted him. Mr. J later spoke at a dinner held in connection with the center, and described the meaning to him of the chance he had been given for extending his life and how he intended to use that life purposively. At the end of his speech, he received the longest standing ovation I've ever heard.

We saw how in error we would have been to reject Mr. J just because of his age. It proves that our batting average is not 100 percent. But I've learned to live with the fact that we make some mistakes in our judgments. If I couldn't accept that fact, I'd have to get off the committee.

In contrast to some phases of the first admissions committee's activities, The Reverend Mr. X feels that the present group "now has other than rubber-stamp powers vis-à-vis the medical people. The philosophy about the selection process has changed since the mid–1960s, to the belief that if you have financial responsibility, then you must have some power to decide about the process by which patients are selected." The Reverend Mr. X, however, realized why the physicians were inclined to accept any medically qualified candidates, and sympathized with their tendency to do so. "They know these patients so well. They're often in the same situation the committee was when Mr. J came to plead his case before us. The doctors do a lot of agonizing with and pleading for patients. I sometimes wonder how they can still smile in the face of all the anguish they see."

The physician members of the committee also acknowledge their patient advocate role. Said one of them:

The doctor ends up identifying with his patient, and wants to get him treated. That's why we have built a safeguard into the selection procedure: if a doctor-member of the committee presents his own patient, he's not allowed to vote on that patient's acceptance. It's also why we have a businessman on the committee; he can be more objective than the physician, and look at a patient's candidacy more like a balance sheet. On the other hand, he doesn't have to see the patient in his office, and he isn't faced with the responsibility of telling the patient and his family, "I'm sorry, but there isn't anything more we can do."

The Admissions and Policy Committee, informally known as the "Patient Processing Committee," meets twice monthly at 7:30 A.M. in a small conference room at the Northwest Kidney Center. We attended one of these meetings in May 1970, observing and recording the committee's deliberations about three dialysis candidates. Present at the meeting were the five members of the committee, another physician from the center's staff, a private physician there to present his patient's case, and the member of the center's social service staff responsible for the financial evaluation of dialysis candidates.

In presenting the cases acted upon that day, we will first cite representative material from the application files that are compiled for the selection committee. The files typically contain a summary of the patient's medical history and prognosis, a financial statement, a psychiatric evaluation, and an extensive social service report. We will also recapitulate the committee's discussions of each candidate, examining as we do so the dynamics of their decision-making process, particularly with respect to the selection criteria explicitly and implicitly employed.

Case 1

Mr. Edward A, age twenty-two; "married"; education—tenth grade; occupation—unemployed long-haul truck driver.

Medical History. Proteinuria noted five years ago on pre-induction physical. Renal disease evaluated two years ago; said to have 30 percent renal function. . . . Now has advanced renal failure, normal size kidneys, twelve grams proteinuria per day. Biopsy shows end-stage renal disease. Hypertension present since 1969.

Psychiatric Summary. Mr. and Mrs. A are plain, ordinary folk, pleasant enough, and stable appearing. Their marriage relationship appears to be a happy one. So far as I can see they ought to be able to manage home dialysis satisfactorily.

Social History.

Referral: Mr. A is being followed at University Hospital and is referred by that agency. He stated that he has had kidney problems for about three years, and "possibly before then". . . . He has been off work since fall 1969, and understands now that his kidneys are "totally destroyed". . . .

Identifying Information: The As are not legally married. Although Mrs. A is still apparently legally married to her second husband, the couple presents themselves as "married" since summer 1968. Mrs. A's two young daughters, ages four and six, live with them. The A's are renting at _____. They have no telephone number. Mr. A last worked for a domestic employment office. He terminated his employment there last fall and has not worked since. Presently, the family receives welfare payments, approximately totalling $200 monthly. Mrs. A is not employed. Neither the patient nor his wife has completed high school. . . . The patient is not religious, and states that his wife is a Catholic but inactive.

History: Mr. A was born in _____ and "grew up everywhere in the United States." During the years he was in school, he was mostly in New Mexico.

Family: . . . The marriage of the patient's father and mother to each other was the second for each of them. They were divorced in 1961 and the father remarried a few months later. Mrs. A was remarried, to her third husband, in 1970. The patient lost contact with her for many years after 1963. He told me that she "drinks excessively," and I got the impression that she had drifted around the country. . . . According to Mr. A, his father "drank and gambled," which his mother "tolerated but hated." While the patient was growing up, there were many financial problems,

family instability, and fighting, both verbal and physical. . . .
Mr. A remembers his father as "strict, but a good father."
According to the patient, for reasons still unknown to him, his
father "threw me out when I was seventeen." Mr. A has forgiven
him for this now, but they are still not close. His mother he
regards as a "pal." . . .

Education: Mr. A completed one-half of his junior year. He
made grades of B and C without "ever cracking a book." At that
time, he had no desire to study, and as I understand him,
associated with a semidelinquent group. He felt that he could have
made straight As had he applied himself. He felt that he got
along well with his peers, and told me that he had been manager
for several of the sports teams while he was in high school. I felt
that Mr. A was considerably above average in intelligence. He
demonstrated this through a vocabulary far beyond the amount
of formal school he has had, as well as in insightful thinking.

Military Service: None

Working History: . . . .

Marriage: The As met in a bar in _____ and were "married"
the following month. . . . The patient's wife weighed 150 pounds
when he met her, and now weighs 257 pounds. When I interviewed her, she was quite adamant in insisting she is hypothyroid
and that her weight problems are "glandular." She also
mentioned that several physicians had "given me diets and other
useless information," which had greatly annoyed her, as they had
not paid attention to the "true nature of my problem." The As
seem to be happy and satisfied with each other. Mrs. A referred
several times to her husband as "my little baby" during the joint
interview I held with them. She is subject to wide mood swings . . .
she appears to become quite excited, angry, and unduly depressed
or elated very quickly. Many of her comments struck me as
being considerably hostile, especially toward the medical
profession. . . .

Home Visit: The As are presently renting a one-bedroom,
frame house. . . . From their description of it, installation of a
dialysis machine does not sound difficult. They wish to move into
a sixty-foot trailer, if he can become employed and they can
afford it. Storage of supplies would prove somewhat of a difficulty
at their present location. They have been offered a small house
behind a gas station where Mr. A is dickering for a job.

Interview Data: Mr. A is a slight, wispy-looking man who
related to me in a very casual and informal but likeable manner.
His wife is an obese woman who appears and acts angry. I felt
that a psychiatric examination might reveal her to be an oral-
hostile personality. She relates to Mr. A in a smothering and
domineering manner, which he appears to appreciate. His inter-
actions with her are mainly compliant and self-subordinating.
Neither of the As impressed me as having any real understanding

of the severity of his illness, or the demands of the treatment regime that would be made upon them. They seemed quite blithe, and almost unconcerned. (However, I did feel that part of this is a defense against, and an attempt to minimize how upset they are.)

Summary: Overall, the *present circumstances* of this family offer little to recommend them. Their financial prospects are poor, the legal situation is murky, and the family history indicates much instability and acting out of problems. However, in spite of all this I was struck by the fact that neither of the As appeared at this moment to be overwhelmed by these problems, and that both of them are still striving fairly energetically to overcome them. . . . In summary, this family will present many problems in training. Mrs. A mentioned to me in passing that she is "afraid of the dark," and asked me if it would be possible for her to stay with her husband every night while he is in the home training unit. In spite of the drawbacks, they struck me as having enough energy to make a go of the program, and I believe there is some rehabilitation potential here. Overall, I would rate the situation as fair to good.

Financial: No assets, no insurance, and no income other than public assistance.

Admissions Committee Discussion of Mr. A

Dr. F (the private physician presenting Mr. A's case): I really don't know much about his job history. But medically, I think he's a good candidate.

Rev. X (chairman of the admissions committee): Mr. A is not precisely married; he has a common-law marriage because the woman he is living with is not divorced from her previous husband.

Miss S (the financial evaluator): Mrs. A would be the greatest management problem if Mr. A went on home dialysis, because she seems to be a defensive, manipulative, and overreactive person.

Various persons then commented on the As seemingly unstable home condition, and on Mr. A's unhappy childhood history and emotional problems.

Mr. W (the businessman member of the committee): Given their unstable home condition and the physical setup of the home, I wonder if a home dialysis unit and the necessary supplies can be accommodated.

Dr. F: If you really try, you can get a unit in about anywhere.

Rev. X: The As have a visionary hope of moving into a trailer, which would solve the equipment-storage problem.

Miss S: The move is at best a long way off, since now they can't even afford for Mrs. A to get a divorce from her legal husband.

Dr. F: It would be an important but hard goal to get Mr. A to work by himself on home dialysis, because he's a cooperative but dependent and passive person.

Several persons then questioned Dr. F about whether he truly thought Mr. A could ever act independently given Mrs. A's character, and whether Mrs. A's possible hostility toward the medical profession might not also be a problem regarding her "husband's" medical management.

Dr. F: I don't think Mrs. A has greatly resented my management of Mr. A while he's been in the hospital, though I don't know if this would hold true in the home situation as well. Mrs. A does think she is full of medical problems that I should treat, but I've simply avoided getting into that kind of relationship with her.

Mr. Y (the center's administrative member on the committee): Mrs. A is now twenty-five years old, and on her third husband. What happens when she gets her fourth? Who will be around to help Mr. A with dialysis?

Dr. F: In all probability, Mr. A will need treatment within the next couple of months, because he has little or no reserve renal function left, although his condition is fairly stable now. The As do seem to know quite a bit about dialysis. I think they had a relative on the artificial kidney, who died in the course of treatment. There are plenty of potential problems, such as the fact that Mrs. A thinks she has to be here the whole time he's in home training, her domineering relationship with Mr. A, and financing.

Dr. G (a physician-member of the committee): It will take lots of care to hold things together in this case, but that's part of our job. There are lots of problems, but nothing to rule him out.

Dr. F: Mr. A has been a cooperative patient. He wouldn't follow his salt-free diet, so his blood pressure has been out of control again. But I think he now understands the necessity for a strict diet.

Mr. W: How could they live, economically, if Mr. A went on home dialysis?

Miss S: They receive $240 monthly from welfare. Funding for his dialysis could come from the center, and there's a possibility that the State Division of Vocational Rehabilitation might help.

Dr. H (a physician-member of the committee): I think the greatest thing going for this kid is the fact that he's tried to work even when he's known he is sick.

Mr. W: Is Mr. A a transplant candidate? I would think that a transplant would be a much better long-range solution for him than home dialysis.

Dr. F: He has a brother, but we haven't even considered using him as a donor, because he and Mr. A don't get along well.

Dr. H: Even if a cadaver transplant were possible, it would probably be six to twelve months before a kidney was available, so Mr. A would have to go on dialysis in any case.

Mr. W: I still think that at his age and in his condition a transplant would make a lot of sense.

Rev. X: If there are no other comments or questions about Mr. A, let's move on to the next candidate.

Case 2

Miss Isabelle C, age fifty-two; single; education—high school; occupation—bookkeeper.

Medical History. A single lady with known polycystic kidney disease and known infection, at least dating back some twenty-five years, with a long history of hypertension, who has at least a year or two history of anemia, easy fatigability, malaise, nausea, and pruritis of one year's duration. Of further significance is the fact that she did have tuberculosis of the pulmonary tract, treated from 1940 through 1944. . . . She has a strong family history of polycystic kidney disease. . . . She also has a history of detached retinas on three occasions. The reason for this is unclear to me.

Psychiatric Summary. . . . Over the last year Miss C has had nausea and vomiting, but she is still able to function on her job and has had no recent acute increase in symptoms. Miss C is the eighth of nine children. Her father was a farmer who died when she was nine. She graduated from high school and went halfway through nurse's training. She took some college night courses in business administration. She has supported herself working in an office as a bookkeeper. She has worked at her present job for the last three years. Miss C has been active in the Methodist church and some of its groups and organizations. Until a year ago she maintained her own home in _____. During the last year she has lived in an apartment, by herself. . . . She has a sixty-five-year–old divorced sister who . . . has discovered within the last year that she has polycystic kidney disease. Miss C also has a widowed sister in _____. She thinks she may be able to work something out with one of these sisters so far as having someone available to assist her with home dialysis. On the whole, Miss C appears to be an intelligent, rather tough and independent sort of person who ought to be able to manage home dialysis satisfactorily.

Social History.

Identifying Information: . . . Miss C belongs to the Working Woman's Guild, a fraternal organization. She has no car, feels that she is unable to afford owning one, and does not feel that she should drive.

Education: . . . Miss C impressed me as being of somewhat average intelligence.

Home Visit: No home visit is planned. . . . In a general discussion, the prospect of moving into the duplex her sister owns, and enlisting her sister's support in assisting in dialysis sounded like the best possible present plan. Miss C was not very enthusiastic about this, and remarked vaguely that she was "afraid of going up the outdoor stairway."

Interview Data: Miss C presents herself as a small, quiet, reserved and polite woman. She tended to be vague and tentative during my interview with her and was not especially optimistic or enthusiastic about becoming a dialysis patient. At the same time, she was not openly restive or hostile toward the prospect. She appears to have a better than average knowledge about her problem, and the treatment program.

Summary: Overall, Miss C strikes me as being a fair to good prospect for our program. At this time she impresses me as having somewhat weak motivations; however, this may be attributed to her present physical status. Information that she gave me about her hobbies indicates that she is a fairly active person. The main problems here appear to be mechanical in nature—transportation difficulties in getting here, lack of adequate living situation, and, most importantly, lack of someone who could assist her in her treatment regime. If she is accepted, I think that it would be wise for me to initiate a family conference between herself, her sister, and her brother to attempt to clarify what living circumstances might be arranged for her in which they could assist her in dialysis. I think the patient will also require some emotional support and encouragement during the initial training phase and we should help her build up motivation.

Financial. Annual income of $5,100. Has invested $20,000. Has a basic medical insurance policy that will not pay for equipment and supplies.

Admissions Committee Discussion of Miss C

Dr. H (a physician-member of the committee, who presented Miss C's case because her private physician could not attend the meeting): At the present, Miss C's hypertension is well controlled and she has no kidney infection. Medically speaking, she has no other real problems at this time except her polycystic kidney disease. I would classify her as a cooperative patient.

Rev. X: I've checked into her job situation, and there seems to be no reason she couldn't continue working if she goes onto home dialysis.

Dr. G (a physician-member of the committee): I'd like a clearer statement about her medical prognosis, and about how she could manage home dialysis.

Miss S (the financial evaluator): Her main problems are transportation to the center, her inadequate housing situation, and no one to help her with dialysis. She doesn't seem keen on going to live with her sister. I don't think the sister has even been consulted about the possibility.

Dr. G: Is there a possibility that she could go on peritoneal dialysis?

Dr. H: Given her large kidneys and her small stature, she might have a complicated course on peritoneal dialysis.

Mr. W (the businessman member of the committee): She doesn't seem too motivated about going on dialysis.

Dr. G: I think her work history and her substantial savings account are pretty good indicators of her motivation.

Miss S: Miss C doesn't have insurance for dialysis, so the costs of her treatment would have to come out of her savings.

Mr. W: Does she need treatment immediately?

Dr. H: It sounds to me like it's pretty close; a matter of one to three months.

Mr. W: It seems to me that very little thought has been given to how her home treatment could be handled.

Dr. H: I think it's a little premature to raise that issue. The appropriate time to do so might be after we've decided whether or not to accept her.

Mr. W: But we did reject another patient because he had no one at home to help him with dialysis.

Rev. X: That patient was borderline in other ways. We didn't reject him just because he had no one to help him.

Mr. W: What about Miss C's age? She's fifty-two. The fellow we turned down, who lived alone, was much younger. We don't have anyone on the home program who manages alone, do we?

Dr. G: Yes, we do have one person running dialysis alone, because he was divorced after going on the program.

Dr. H: Where there's a will, you can do it. But it is an increased risk, and we don't like it. Someone will have to sit down and discuss all these things with Miss C, and on that basis decide whether hemodialysis or peritoneal dialysis will be the best treatment.

Rev. X: Are there any other questions or comments?

Dr. I (a physician from the center attending the meeting): The center's general funds are getting hit pretty hard this morning; two out of the three patients you're considering might have to be subsidized that way. I think there should be a review of the funds available and the funds that are already committed before final decisions about today's candidates are made.

Case 3

Mr. Ernest B, age forty-eight; married; education—high school; occupation—claims adjuster.

Medical History. Mr. B had a tubercular kidney removed twenty-two years ago. At that time it was noted that his remaining kidney was small and undeveloped. At the time his kidney was removed he was treated with high doses of streptomycin and developed a marked nerve deafness. Mr. B has had high blood pressure for some time. In the last three to four months he has had symptoms of kidney failure, and a tentative diagnosis of TB in the remaining kidney has been made. He is currently on an anti-TB program. Apparently he has been able to function on his job until recently. He is in the hospital now because of what is thought to be a reaction to the anti-TB drugs he is taking. He is receiving peritoneal dialysis.

Psychiatric Summary. I was unable to interview Mr. B personally because of his deafness and because he was quite drowsy from medication when I saw him in the hospital. Therefore I had to depend on Mrs. B for information about him. Mr. B has been married twenty-seven years and has two children, one of whom is married. He belongs to a number of lodges but is not active in any of them. According to Mrs. B his interests are mainly bookish. He is currently writing a book about his life. He is not much for doing things around the house. Mr. B has a history of migraine headaches many years ago which went away

after he talked to a psychiatrist. Following that he developed an
ulcer, which apparently cleared up and has not bothered him
again. Mrs. B appears to be a rather nervous and insecure person.
She first went to see a psychiatrist when she was thirty-five and
continued in treatment for six years. She has a tendency to get
anxious around people and has difficulty relaxing. She tried some
hypnotherapy and is currently taking meprobamate. The family
would appear to be fairly stable and middle class. Mr. B is
apparently fairly successful occupationally despite his deafness.
Mrs. B is not the sort of person who is able to offer her husband
strong psychological support in times of crisis. Psychologically I
would guess that Mr. B would be required to go it pretty much
on his own, and it would be he who was required to support
his wife. My guess would be that this family could probably
handle home dialysis satisfactorily. However, the family psychological situation reminds me somewhat of that of Mr. Z
[a patient who committed suicide by pulling out his shunt while
on home dialysis training] and it wouldn't surprise me if Mr. B
decided it wasn't worth the effort of carrying on. This, however,
is speculation on rather small amounts of information.

Social History.

Identifying Information: . . . Mrs. B is not employed. . . .
The Bs are not particularly religious, although they do attend
church occasionally. Both have completed high school, and Mr. B
has also completed a study course making him a "Certified
Claims Adjuster."

Family: It was my impression that Mr. and Mrs. B must have
talked together many times about his early life, in a somewhat
therapeutic manner—she remarked that "when we got married, he
wouldn't even talk about it at all, but now he can accept his
feelings better." According to Mrs. B, the family was very poor,
and ate "what they could raise and catch fishing." The father
farmed, did odd jobs, and worked as a casual laborer. According
to Mrs. B, the father must have carried on many extramarital
affairs, and finally deserted the family when the patient was
eleven. When Mr. B was about nine, he apparently found out
something about his father's activities. This knowledge resulted in
a confrontation, wherein his father threatened to "drown him,
or something," if he revealed his knowledge. The patient's mother
came across as a nonentity. Mr. B felt his mother did not take an
interest in him, and once remarked that she "wished he were
not around."

Military History: Mr. B served in the Coast Guard from 1939
until 1944, when he was discharged on medical grounds.

Health History: Mrs. B told me that her husband had been
"nervous" for many years, and finally told me that he had
consulted a psychiatrist in Seattle, whom he had seen about four
times before entering the hospital because of his kidney condition.
Mrs. B also has been "very nervous." She told me she had

benefited from the psychiatric treatment she received, and "learned much about myself." In spite of this, she has a phobia about meeting strangers, and frequently refuses social invitations, preferring to stay at home, rather than go into public and experience the subsequent anxiety.

Marriage: When I asked Mrs. B to describe their marital adjustment, she said "we're just like two peas in a pod—we were born on the same day in different years, and we're so much alike." Specifically, they are both "shy, quiet, reserved, stay-at-homes". . . .

Interview Data: In general, I assume Mrs. B to be a relatively passive, retiring person. She did not experience any of the psychiatric or emotional difficulties she complained about in relating to me, and commented upon this herself. When we discussed the training period, she did not feel it would upset her to participate in this. Overall, I feel that her difficulties in relating to others would not be a detriment in the training situation at the center.

Summary: The picture I get of Mr. B is that of a retiring man, who is a good worker, and mostly a family man. He and his wife appear to me to have reached a good adjustment with each other. Overall, I think Mrs. B an asset to her husband in his training and treatment. I see this as being a suitable case for us, and would rate Mr. B without interviewing him personally, as ranging from a fair to good patient.

Financial. . . . The applicant's government insurance plan, which pays up to $50,000, is the most likely source of funding resources.

Admissions Committee Discussion of Mr. B

Dr. G (a physician-member of the committee): Overall, Mr. B's renal failure just took off faster than anyone else's I've ever seen, perhaps due to his tubercular condition. Mrs. B is definitely a nervous individual who needs to be given a lot of explanations. I was on the phone with her about five times over the weekend, telling her things about her husband's condition. But I don't see that this is an insurmountable problem. I'm not sure I agree with the psychiatrist's view of similarities between Mr. B and Mr. Z. I don't think his various medical complications would bar his being a home dialysis patient. I do admit he's going to take more support than the usual patients, but he does want to get well and go back to work. I'm worried now about deciding whether his tubercular kidney should be taken out, or if he should be kept on these very potent anti-TB drugs. I put him in the hospital last Friday because of his reaction to the drugs, discharged him on

Monday, and he was back in on Tuesday and had to go on peritoneal dialysis, because his condition went downhill so fast.

Mr. W (the businessman member of the committee): Could Mr. B be transplanted?

Dr. G: He would be at best a marginal transplant candidate. For example, he's likely to have tubercular sites elsewhere in his body, and they would go wild with steroids.

Mr. W: I'd like to know more about his financial situation.

Mr. Y (the center's administrative member on the committee): The condition that led to his being reviewed today developed so rapidly there wasn't enough time to assemble all the information on him before the meeting.

Mr. W: It seems to me that Mr. B has a lot going for him. He's married, with a family, a good job, and insurance.

Dr. G: He won't be an easy patient to take care of. I'm not saying we shouldn't treat him, because I feel that we should. But his medical and psychological problems are complicated. I think he will make it, but it will be touch and go all the way. His psychological problems can be handled by a good physician talking things out with him. Therefore I don't consider them serious. It's harder to know how deep Mrs. B's emotional problems are.

Rev. X: If there's no more discussion for now about Mr. B, let's look at the financial sheet before we vote on the candidates.

A brief review of the center's current financial status followed, ending rather abruptly when Dr. H said, "I move that all three patients be accepted." Dr. G promptly seconded the motion.

Mr. W: Hold it. That's a very broad motion. I want to discuss each patient individually, because I think they're too different to vote on together.

Rev. X opened the quasi-parliamentary voting procedure to a discussion of each candidate, beginning with Mr. Edward A.

Mr. W: I'm dubious about him, given the social worker's report. His financial position is poor, his legal situation is murky, and his psychological situation is unstable. I wonder if he clearly understands his medical situation?

Dr. G: I think it's often better if patients don't know their situation too clearly in a case like this. Some ambiguity keeps young people like Mr. A going.

Mr. W: I still think, especially because he is young, that he'd be a good transplant candidate.

Dr. G: He probably might be, but he'd still need dialysis until we could get him a kidney. I'd give him anywhere from a week to two months until he's going to need dialysis.

Mr. W: Do you think he could be trained for dialysis before his living situation changes?

Dr. H: In marginal situations like this, we have to get into the nitty-gritty of what is the best form of therapy for the patient: hemodialysis, peritoneal dialysis, or a transplant. That's something for the doctor to work out with his patient.

Rev. X: Mr. A would have to move to different living quarters for home dialysis? Who assumes responsibility for getting this done?

Miss S: That can be done through social service agencies here and in his home town.

Dr. G: I think the physicians at the center are a lot more capable now of handling this kind of patient, with all his problems, than we were a year ago.

Mr. W: I move we accept Mr. A with the understanding that we will need to look further into his finances, home facilities, and the possibility of a transplant.

Mr. A was accepted unconditionally by the committee, with the understanding that Mr. W's suggestions would be taken into account by the physician handling Mr. A's case.

Rev. X: What about Mr. B?

It was moved and seconded that Mr. B be accepted as a home dialysis training patient.

Mr. W: Can we add to the motion that no center funds be used for him?

Various persons immediately protested this suggestion, pointing out that such a proviso "makes it very final for Mr. B, because if his personal financial situation changed in the future and he needed center funds, he would be cut off from them."

Mr. W withdrew his motion, and Mr. B was unanimously accepted.

Rev. X: I've just remembered that Miss C was presented once before to the committee, but at the time it was felt she was not sick enough to warrant acceptance.

Mr. W: I think she should be rejected until we can find out whether she could handle the home dialysis situation.

Dr. I: That's no problem. We can work everything out.

Miss S: Do you want to defer her?

Mr. W, who did not comment on the possibility of deferral: She's a fifty-two-year-old single gal who doesn't seem very enthusiastic about treatment.

Dr. G: I do think we have to make it very clear to her that she has to handle it in the home. We just don't do in-center dialysis any more on a continuing basis. I share your concern that she might suddenly come in here and say, "I can't do it, take care of me." I don't know if we've been strong enough in the past to say to a patient, "It's home dialysis or nothing."

Dr. H: We will have to emphasize to her that she will have to handle home dialysis and not expect to be taken into the hospital for chronic treatment. She's too old for a transplant. Her private doctor has presented her twice, and he's not even a kidney-type physician. So either he's very aggressive, or he is very convinced of her desire to live. Maybe we should defer her and talk to her doctors about things like her motivation and her vision problem. But I really don't want to defer her case until the next meeting because her condition might necessitate moving very quickly. I'd really like the decision left to Dr. G's and my discretion after we've talked to her doctors by telephone.

Dr. G: I move that Miss C be accepted, pending the decision of our medical director about the feasibility of home dialysis.

With one dissenting vote, Miss C was accepted.

Rev. X then opened the meeting to a discussion of some other patients: those on a deferred status, those "approved pending processing," and "old patient status changes," primarily concerned with the mounting problem of hepatitis. He also reported that the "Division of Vocational Rehabilitation, after some pressure, has finally authorized the center to use some of its funding to cover the costs of cadaver transplants."

Rev. X then announced that "the next meeting of the class will be held on June 4 at 7:30."

Dr. I: These meetings are held at an awfully depressing hour.

Dr. H, as the meeting adjourned: Maybe if we could only talk of something cheery for a change, the early hour wouldn't matter.

The patterns that emerged in the course of this bimonthly meeting of the Admissions and Policy Committee are not idiosyncratic. Rather, they exemplify significant aspects of the patient selection process as it currently takes place at the Kidney Center.

Although the committee members are reluctant to base their decisions on economic factors and somewhat abashed about invoking them in their deliberations, the "financial balance sheet" of the center looms over their decision-making. The fact that resources for hemodialysis, even though they are more ample in Seattle than in other communities, are inherently limited is one of the major reasons the committee exists. The committee members are aware of this and they are determined to be fiscally responsible. But as the proceedings of this meeting indicate, except for episodic moments when budgetary matters surface, members prefer to keep them latent.

These economic restrictions notwithstanding, it is striking that there are very few, if any, medical, psychological or social factors that easily disqualify a candidate. At the meeting recorded here, for example, a medical diagnosis of tuberculosis along with terminal kidney disease, advanced age, the lack of appropriate physical facilities at home for the installation of a kidney machine, the unavailability of a family member to assist with dialysis, the presence of psychopathology in the patient or his spouse, unemployment, the total absence of personal funds, a "murky" legal situation, an irregular marriage—none of these, singly or combined, were sufficient to render Mr. A, Mr. B, or Miss C ineligible for the program. This openness contrasts sharply with the two prior eras in the history of the committee when "social worth" and subsequently "psychological suitability" criteria of choice predominated. At present, the committee tries to give all patients who apply the benefit of the doubt and to provide them with dialysis facilities. To a remarkable extent it succeeds in doing so, because of the reduced costs of home dialysis and the community support the center enjoys, as well as the shift in its philosophy and policy of selection.

The dynamic interplay between physicians, social workers, businessmen, and the clergyman-chairman at the meetings of the committee is significant. Although they are all oriented toward selecting rather than refusing the patients whose cases come before them, each plays a somewhat different role in the process. The social workers present the most richly detailed psychological, sociological, and economic background data on each case. The physicians generally act as patient advocates. The businessmen raise a series of "Yes, but . . ." qualifications regarding the advisability of accepting a patient, with special emphasis on the state of the center's finances. The pastor-chairman remains as judiciously neutral as he can.

The great involvement of the committee in hemodialysis and their lesser zeal about transplantation is apparent in the committee's discussions. Finally, as their meeting adjourns with a touch of gallows humor and some last admissions about the "awfully depressing" nature of their deliberations, it becomes clear how stressful the work of the Admissions and Policy Committee continues to be for those who most actively participate in it. "If I have to play God," a physician on the committee said to us shortly after the meeting adjourned, "it's a lot more reassuring to only play one-fifth God; to share these decisions with other people."

Many physicians, social scientists, ethicists, theologians, and lawyers have grappled with the difficult question of how to decide "Who shall live when not all can live?" (Childress 1970). There is not, and perhaps can never be, any wide accord about what standards and criteria should be used to choose recipients of a scarce medical resource such as chronic hemodialysis, or about who should make this decision. As its members are the first to acknowledge, Seattle's selection committees are only one imperfect and uneasy attempt to deal with these issues.

The changes in the criteria employed by the admissions committee during the past decade reflect more than the increased availability and lower cost of dialysis through the development of home treatment. The committee's shift away from "social worth" criteria to professionally evaluated indexes of "psychological suitability" and its reluctance today to reject a candidate on *any* nonmedical grounds are evidence of its members' profound disquiet at having to "play God." The moral burden of such a task has been eloquently stated by Paul Freund:

The more nearly total is the estimate to be made of an individual, and the more nearly the consequences determine life and death, the more unfit the judgment becomes for human reckoning. [Freund 1970, p. xvii]

According to Katz and Proctor's study, Seattle is one of only eight dialysis programs to employ a lay or community advisory selection committee. Their data, however, show that the physician committees which make the final selection of patients in most centers have found themselves utilizing similar screening processes. Such factors as the congeniality of the patient as an individual, economic burdens of dependents if the patient is not selected, "demonstrated social worth," and "future social contribution," which have overtones of moral judgment and middle-class bias, were considered of minor importance by the majority of centers, although from one-fifth to one-third of the centers rated them important (Katz and Proctor 1969, p. 24).

Given the uncertainties about both medical and nonmedical indicators of how well or poorly a patient will do on dialysis, selection committees also find it difficult to evaluate every candidate uniformly, by whatever criteria they employ. Thus, Katz and Proctor felt that "one of the most impressive features of [their] data" was the finding that "57 percent of Centers said the 'criteria varied in their application from patient to patient' " (Katz and Proctor 1969, p. 25).

Critics of Seattle's selection process have objected less to the involvement of laymen in the decision-making process than to the use of standards that are influenced by the value system of the selectors. Sanders and Dukeminier, for example, assert that:

If selection of patients by *ad hoc* comparisons of social worth is objectionable, comparisons by a committee composed of physicians, hospital personnel, and social workers rather than by a lay committee is no less objectionable. Medical men are no more qualified to play God—to look at two persons and say one is worth more than the other—than ordinary mortals. [Sanders and Dukeminier 1968, pp. 378–79]

However, as Sanders and Dukeminier recognize, "one can know what is a bad method without knowing what is the best method" (Sanders and Dukeminier 1968, p. 380). Dialysis programs have experimented with a number of other selection procedures in an attempt to avoid the ambiguities and ethical problems inherent in the use of psychological and social criteria. These include ability to pay as the sole nonmedical factor; a first-come, first-served policy; and lottery or random selection. Each such stratagem, as their proponents themselves acknowledge, has its defects; none are perfectly equitable, impartial methods for allocating chronic dialysis. Ability to pay, for example, obviously discriminates against the poor. And unconscious selection biases or overt pressures to accept a given patient may work their way into the operation of such seemingly neutral systems as first-come, first-served or random selection.

In a paper titled "Psychological Dilemmas of Medical Progress," psychiatrist Harry Abram also points out that medical screening precedes a random or first-come method. That this medical screening often includes appraisal of psychological elements such as the patient's "willingness and ability to cooperate" in the treatment regime and his "stability and maturity" means that "preselection" is occurring. "In considering the problem of [preselection or] selection on psychological grounds," Abram writes, "one can then inquire 'should they be included with medical criteria?' " Abram, one of the most thoughtful and judicious authorities on the psychological aspects of dialysis, tends to say no, while still affirming the importance of psychiatric study of the dialysis candidate and recipient:

the issues concerning selection are vague and complex. Terms, such as first-come, first-served, cooperativeness, and emotional maturity, need further definition. In view of the ethical questions which have been raised in selecting one man over another for life-sustaining procedures and the lack of specific evidence that psychiatric screening can prevent behavioral disturbances (such as repeated dietary indiscretions and suicides) after a patient is placed on dialysis, I seriously question whether patients should be refused this treatment solely for psychological reasons except clearly defined and validated instances of severe psychosis and mental deficiency making dialysis unfeasible. This is not to say that all patients should not be studied psychiatrically. (Indeed greater knowledge and research is desperately needed in this area.) And certainly psychiatric treatment remains an essential element in the overall care and rehabilitation of the dialysis patient. [Abram 1972, p. 56]

Finally, one can raise the question of whether the use of methods such as first-come, first-served and random selection represent an abdication of the decision-making responsibilities that are an inherent part of the physician's role.

As Abram indicates, the gatekeeping role of dialysis physicians is not abolished by the involvement of laymen in the patient selection process. In Seattle, indeed, the necessity for physicians to exercise their gatekeeping role led to the creation of a third patient review board, the University Hospital's Dialysis Utilization Committee, composed of five physicians appointed by the dean of the medical school. Scribner, a member of the committee, explained that its formation was generated by two problems. "The University Hospital gets undiagnosed renal cases from all over the state, and virtually all of them turn out to be chronic cases. In part because most of these patients don't have their own doctor-advocates, many people here at the hospital get very emotionally involved with individual patients. This committee sprang from a need to attenuate the degree to which this emotional involvement was affecting the decision about a chronic patient's acceptance for dialysis treatment. The immediate stimulus was the case of Ernie Crowfeather" (see chapter 10). The Dialysis Utilization Committee, Scribner went on to say, was also "formed out of desperation, to try and help patients the service arm of our program, the Kidney Center, could not accept." In 1968–69, coincident with the Crowfeather case, Dr. Henry Tenckhoff had obtained clinical research funds to place patients on home peritoneal dialysis. At that time, Scribner said, "peritoneal dialysis was not an accepted form of treatment by the Kidney Center. The formation of the Dialysis Utilization Committee enabled us to successfully buck the center's policy by getting the peritoneal dialysis patients treated via the University Hospital" (Scribner, personal interview).

The Dialysis Utilization Committee, like the center's admissions committee and the transplant "gatekeepers" discussed in chapter 1, must make difficult decisions about a candidate's eligibility for treatment. Even though there are clinical research funds that enable the Dialysis Utilization Committee to admit indigent candidates for long-term, in-hospital dialysis as research patients, the committee still must consider cost-effectiveness factors such as the probable total investment in a patient's care, especially if he has unusual medical complications and his prognosis is dubious, and weigh this cost against the number of other patients who might be treated by these same funds and manpower. "Our problem," a member of the Dialysis Utilization Committee said to us, "is not one of supply and demand in the usual sense, but of how much emotional energy as well as money, bed space, etc., you're going to invest in any one person." He illustrated his point by referring to a patient discharged from the renal service that day. "This woman probably never should have been admitted to the renal service in the first place. She has a poor prognosis because of her terrible medical problems. Her bill was easily

$40,000, and we can't afford to spend that much money just to get a patient back to the point where she or he can be dialyzed. The community can't afford it. . . . One bad patient can wreck you financially."

Even were there a utopian state of unlimited treatment resources, the physician-gatekeepers would still be confronted by existential decisions about whether there are strong indications that a candidate's life on chronic dialysis would be so dismal that it would be more humane to deny him treatment. Dr. W, a member of the Dialysis Utilization Committee, told us about a recent meeting in which the physicians had been confronted with this type of decision.

We had to consider the case of Mr. H, a man in his forties, who was turned down by the center as a home dialysis patient for various reasons, including a lack of finances. Mr. H has a low IQ, around 70, and therefore has never been able to hold a job, except for occasional part-time work with agencies like Goodwill Industries. He's always lived with his family, and has no money of his own. For the past twenty years he's been sleeping on a cot in his older brother's one-room apartment. In terms of financing, his home living situation, and his mentality, Mr. H simply could not do home dialysis, and we don't do in-center dialysis any more. For a number of medical reasons, he's not a good transplant candidate. I guess Mr. H's biggest problem is that he's stupid. He's a happy idiot whom everybody loves. We have money to treat indigent patients, so finances weren't the reason that we too rejected Mr. H at our Monday meeting. He has so many other problems. For instance, he'd be in the hospital constantly, because with his mentality he'd keep mucking up his dialysis treatment. We had a long, agonizing discussion about Mr. H, and in the end we decided to stick to the center's judgment that he was not a good dialysis prospect. So now the guy is going to die. The real dilemma is that we can never say with that much accuracy that a person won't do well if we give him a chance, despite factors such as a low IQ. We often consider the question of whether it might be more merciful to let a dialysis candidate die. But it's a lot harder to make such a decision when a guy is walking around than when, for example, you decide to pull an I.V. tube out of the arm of a terminal cancer patient lying in bed.

One could hear the Seattle group's discomfiture over their emergency meeting decision not to admit Mr. H into the home dialysis program. "The doctor at this stage of the game should not walk around with a guilt complex all the time because he can't save every uraemic individual in the free world or even in

the under-developed countries of the world," Dr. George Schreiner
of Georgetown University Hospital has written (Schreiner 1966,
p. 130). Their selection policy notwithstanding, the physicians
associated with the University Hospital and the Northwest Kidney
Center are still highly prone to this kind of guilt.

At the same time, even though the Seattle program has abandoned its social worth criteria of selection, there is a covert sense
in which the medical staff considers being chosen for dialysis (or
a transplant, or both) a privilege which should transmute a person's whole outlook and existence. They tend to feel this way not
only because these treatments are potentially life-saving, but also
because given their relative scarcity, and the technical, physical,
and psychological demands that they make upon those who are
gravely ill with renal disease and their families, there are patients
like Mr. H to whom the medical team regretfully feels it must
deny such therapy. This expectation becomes most visible when
a patient has been far from a "pillar of the community." One
such case which various members of the Seattle team independently told us about was that of Ernie Crowfeather (see chap.
10). "How would you like to go over to the county jail and see
one of our successful outcomes?" was the rueful way in which a
physician began his description of the case. Ernie had been put
on chronic hemodialysis and subsequently had been given a renal
transplant. His "habitual occupation," they said, had been that
of "robber," for which he had several times been sentenced and
jailed. After dialysis and a transplant, provided by the University
Hospital, Ernie resumed his previous activities, and at the time
we visited Seattle he was back in the local penitentiary. "We
really didn't expect him to be converted," another physician
maintained, "but we didn't think he'd go back to his former occupation!" "One must simply accept the fact that some people are
not going to change," the Reverend Mr. X commented. "But,"
he admitted, "having to give what help you can knowing this is
one of the rough things I've had to learn to accept."

Although the members of the Seattle group are inclined to
react to such a case in a naive, moralistic fashion, they have a
wry perspective on their tendency to do so. What might be termed
their metaphysical outlook was expressed in the statement about
suicidal behavior in chronic dialysis patients that Belding Scribner made in his 1964 presidential address before the American
Society for Artificial Internal Organs:

I want to bring to your attention . . . the problem of the patient
himself overtly terminating treatment, in other words, a form of
suicide. . . . So far, [this has] not been a problem in chronic
dialysis, despite the ease with which it could be accomplished by
a patient wearing an arteriovenous shunt. To my knowledge, there
have been only two suicide attempts in the entire world experience to date. Actually, this fact should come as no surprise, for if
one examines the psychology of suicide, one would have predicted that the suicide rate among patients on chronic dialysis
would be extremely low. Studies of suicide have demonstrated
repeatedly that among persons whose lives are threatened by
external factors, such as disease, famine or war, the suicide rate is
extremely low and the greater the threat, the lower the rate. If
these conclusions are correct, then we should expect that as the
quality, security and safety of chronic hemodialysis improves and
the threat to life from treatment failure becomes less and less,
the suicide rate among the patients may gradually increase—a
paradox indeed! [Scribner 1964, p. 210]

In a courageous and continually self-searching way, the Seattle
team has faced up to the many ramifications of the question
whether, for some of their patients, in the words of the Reverend
Canon G. B. Bentley, "dying would be a lesser evil than the
treatment proposed" (Wolstenholme and O'Connor 1966, p.
119). Although, as we have seen, the center and hospital do
everything they can to give life-saving treatment to renal patients,
the physicians on their staffs do not automatically succumb to
what Paul Ramsey has termed the "triumphalist temptation to
slash and suture our way to eternal life" (Ramsey 1970, p. 238).
By and large, they share the point of view that "some patients
should be permitted to die," and that "there are worse things
than death. . . . It's not an absolute evil."

Like other renal units in the country, the Seattle group has had
to make hard decisions about what they ought to do when a
patient in need of dialysis and accepted into the program does
not want to begin treatment on the kidney machine. "We have
had personal experience with intelligent people who have decided,
not for financial reasons, but for purely intellectual and artistic
reasons, not to have this treatment," Schreiner has stated. "One
man said this was not the image he wanted his children to carry
around" (Schreiner 1966, pp. 119–20). We were also told of a
clergyman who had moral and religious scruples about starting
chronic dialysis because he believed that it was "not right" for

the center and his family to spend "thousands of dollars . . . to artificially prolong his life" when the same amount of money could be used to feed hundreds of impoverished, hungry, but essentially healthy persons. The Seattle group feels that the individual has the right to refuse such expensive, extraordinary treatment, providing his "decision is made in lucidity" and that it is not his "uremia talking." What is difficult for the medical team to ascertain is whether the nondialyzed patient in terminal renal failure is in a biochemical and psychological state that permits such clear-mindedness.

Scribner has publicly spoken out in favor of allowing the patient confronted with the prospect of dialysis to opt for "death with dignity" in still another way, by preventing uremic poisoning with limited treatment. "Death from uremia can be one of the most horrible known. . . . How much more humane and less expensive it would be to offer such a dying patient a weekly hemodialysis for a limited period. Then he could live a normal life right up to the end and die quickly without prolonged suffering" (Scribner 1964, p. 210). Scribner and his colleagues have never put these convictions into action, on the grounds that "under existing moral, ethical and religious guidelines . . . such a maneuver" would be "utterly impossible," because it would constitute active euthanasia (Scribner 1964, p. 210).

As a growing number of psychological and psychiatric studies have documented, chronic dialysis patients and their families are subject to stresses, frequently acute, associated with the patient's medical problems, the rigors of his treatment, consequent changes in the family's way of life, and financial worries (see, for example, Kaplan de Nour et al. 1968; Menzies and Stewart 1968; Sands, Livingstone, and Wright 1966). The major problems of patients on dialysis are "being able to adhere to the dietary restrictions and to tolerate the dependency imposed by the treatment, as well as the recurrent physical complications associated with dialysis" (Abram 1972). In addition, hemodialysis often significantly changes intrafamily dynamics and compounds the other physical and emotional stresses the patient must tolerate. Faced with such stresses, patients and their spouses commonly exhibit defense mechanisms such as denial, displacement, isolation, reaction formation, and projection. These defenses generally have a positive, adaptive function, enabling the patient and his family to function adequately, both emotionally and socially. But in some instances the dialysis patient finds his life so uncomfortable, unsatisfying, and stressful that he no longer wishes to continue treatment.

The most common ways in which patients on dialysis signal to a renal team that they wish to forego life are requesting their physicians to allow them to discontinue treatment and engaging in behavior that consciously or unconsciously is intended to be self-destructive. As Harry Abram's inquiries have shown, these phenomena take place "with uncomfortable frequency among dialysis patients" throughout the United States. For example, Abram found that "suicidal behavior" occurred in approximately 5 percent of the dialysis population in the sample of 127 dialysis centers that replied to the 201 questionnaires he mailed out. (The returned questionnaires comprised a total sample of 3,847 living and dead patients.) Exsanguination, overdosage, and food or drink binges ("ingestion of large amounts of fluids and foods forbidden by the dialysis regimen") are the most common means of suicide (Abram, Moore, and Westervelt 1971).

One of the most striking of Abram's findings was "the increased incidence of suicidal behavior in center as compared to home patients (significant at the .001 level)." This is borne out by Seattle's home dialysis program, for the rate of suicide that the hospital and center physicians have experienced is considerably lower than the 5 percent reported by Abram. In 1970, the University Hospital's dialysis research team reviewed their six-year experience with home dialysis, involving fifty-two patients followed for six to sixty-four months (Blagg et al. 1970). The mortality rate in this group of patients was 31 percent, predominantly caused by infections and cardiac problems. No suicides are listed among the causes of sixteen patient deaths. In the judgment of the physicians, by indexes such as "rehabilitation" and "psychological response," the majority of the home dialysis patients showed satisfactory physical and psychosocial adjustment to their condition.

Rehabilitation at present or before death, as judged by return to predialysis occupation, school or household duties, was considered good in 43 patients (83 per cent), and partial in four but only poor in five, who were incapacitated by medical complications. . . .

. . . Continued severe stress with maladjustment to dialysis was present in 10 patients (19 per cent), and the majority had occasional stressful episodes due to medical, technical or cannula problems. The ability to adjust to such problems depends on emotional stability, their frequency of occurrence and the emotional support provided by family, friends and physician. In general, older patients adjust readily to the rigid schedule and time loss entailed by dialysis, whereas teenagers and young adults usually find this more difficult.

Another indicator of stress is insomnia. Although all but one patient were trained to sleep during dialysis, 16 (31 per cent) are sleeping poorly. Eight of these are among the 10 patients with continued stress and poor adjustment to dialysis. [Blagg et al. 1970, pp. 1127–28]

Another study of the social and family functioning of twenty-three Northwest Kidney Center patients similarly indicates that although psychological, social, and economic stresses are common, most patients and their families make at least functionally adequate adjustment to home dialysis.

After an average of 2 years of living with a home maintenance hemodialysis regime, 23 couples report work, friendship, and the companionship aspects of family as high areas of satisfaction in their lives. In relation to finances, they live more comfortably after 2 years of treatment: i.e., after the initial crisis subsides and the patient is medically stabilized. Significantly more patients feel financially secure than do their spouses and significantly more spouses feel vaguely insecure. This may reflect the use of denial as an emotional defense by the patient group. If so, it is a selective use of denial only in relation to feelings of insecurity. Another explanation for this difference is that spouses face more uncertainties in their future.

The common concerns of the patient group are related to their health, with slightly over 40% also reporting feelings of depression and frustration. The spouse group report feelings of depression, frustration, and vague insecurity as their common area of discomfort.

About one-third of the patients wish, or perhaps have wished, they were dead. This ambivalence about their existence is associated with feeling circumstances are against them, feeling extremely depressed at times, and not achieving their ambitions in life. The spouse group presents a different picture in relation to depression. For spouses, feeling extremely depressed at times is associated with feeling vaguely insecure, feeling circumstances are against them, and feeling that people are unappreciative of their efforts. [Holcomb and MacDonald 1973]

Such findings enhance the Seattle physicians' belief that chronic dialysis can be a viable, worthwhile treatment for many of their patients. At the same time, through observation of their patients and discussions with them, they have become keenly aware that the many rigors to which the dialysis patient is subject can make his existence on the kidney machine "too long a life" or "a living death" (Abram 1972). The strains associated with chronic dialysis have become more evident to the Seattle team since they have begun their still very limited transplantation venture. As members of the Seattle group told us, physicians are now discovering how many of their patients "do not seem to have reservations about transplantation because the biggest thing for them is getting rid of the machine." Patients consider transplantation more desirable and "more natural" than dialysis because "they're not tied to a machine, they don't have cannulas, they have a kidney, they pass urine, and they can eat what they want."

With combined amusement and chagrin, a physician at the Northwest Kidney Center described to us the unexpected content of a speech about what it feels like to be on the artificial kidney machine that one of his "prize patients" made to a group of visiting doctors: "I've seen a lot of transplant patients," the patient said, "and I've talked to a lot of doctors. I'm not totally convinced by what I see. But while I'm on the kidney at home, all those patients Dr. Marchioro has transplanted are getting better and better. And some day, I will have a transplant, too."

Such sentiments on the part of their patients may help to deepen and expand the Seattle group's commitment to a transplantation program. In turn, this extra option may reduce still further the number of patients who choose to withdraw from an extraordinary method of treatment for their otherwise fatal illness. But at present the Seattle doctors periodically must try to respond in a rational, humane way to those of their patients "who do not find dialysis a solution for the treatment of their terminal kidney disease." These physicians have the impression that there are two groups of patients who are especially determined to discontinue dialysis:

The first of these groups are persons in their late teens or early twenties. . . . Usually, these are young people who have had prolonged kidney disease, and who haven't really lived what they consider life. . . . They are willing to take any chance, accept anything but life on the machine which for them is death. . . . The second category of patient who does not adjust well to dialysis are certain people in the older age group. Some of those

who are older do remarkably. . . . But older persons who have led full, independent lives, and who are more intellectual, often find this particular form of treatment difficult. Some such patients have tried dialysis, and then, after having experienced it, have turned it down flat. Or, they have tried it, and then simply stopped. . . . They feel they have met many of their responsibilities, that a good deal of their work is done, that their children are grown up, that their wives have been taken care of. And perhaps their intellectual proclivities make them more reflective about the kind of future that awaits them if they are kept alive.
[H. Tenckhoff, personal interview]

The policy of the Seattle group is to listen with empathy and respect to those of their patients who affirm that they want to end their dialysis and who appeal to their doctors not to stand in their way through disapproving attitudes, psychiatric intervention, or enforced hospitalization. Physicians try to test whether the patient's motivation for wishing to stop dialysis is both reasoned and resolute. If they are persuaded it is, then they accede to the patient's wishes.

In so doing, have these doctors legitimized suicide? Have they performed euthanasia? Have they acted in an ethically responsible way? These are haunting moral and metaphysical questions that physicians involved with chronic hemodialysis debate with their consciences, with each other, and more than occasionally with theologians, philosophers, lawyers, and social scientists. They discuss them with the dawning conviction that they are dealing not only with matters specific to present-day techniques such as dialysis, but with issues that will be even more central to the medicine of tomorrow.

9

Ernie Crowfeather

Artificial Kidney Use Poses Awesome Questions
by Lawrence K. Altman

SEATTLE, Oct. 23 [1971]—Ernie Crowfeather, a bright, charming part American Indian with a history of personal instability and brushes with the law, died recently at the age of 29 after he refused further life-supporting therapy.

By what was regarded as a suicide, Ernie averted the frightening possibility that his doctors would have had to purposely turn off, for lack of funds and because of his irresponsibility, the artificial kidney that for two years had kept him alive on public money totaling $100,000.

Ernie Crowfeather and the problems associated with chronic dialysis and transplantation that he experienced and personified were introduced to a national public through these lead paragraphs of a front-page story in the *New York Times*. We had first heard of Ernie from his physicians at the University Hospital, Seattle, when we were conducting field research there in 1969. We were struck with how intensely the doctors of the dialysis and transplant teams were preoccupied with his case. Although we never met Ernie, he came to exemplify for us all the medical dilemmas and the human and moral anguish that these modes of treatment can entail.

Our study of the Seattle dialysis program, which included some facets of Ernie's case, had been completed and was being reviewed by Dr. Belding Scribner and his associates when we learned of Ernie's death in June 1971. Later that summer, Scribner urged us to include an extensive account of Ernie's story in our book. For to Scribner, still haunted by the implications of Ernie's life and death, this was a "classic case," "the epitome of all the problems," "the personification of everything at once." We expressed our interest, but indicated that we would not be able to return to Seattle to interview those who had been closely involved with Ernie. Scribner offered to make available the necessary data, including extensive interviews that Dr. Lawrence K. Altman of the *New York Times* was conducting with the principals in the case. We then consulted Dr. Altman, who felt it was appropriate that we use the materials he was collecting, and he subsequently made them available to us, with the consent of those interviewed.

Ernie Crowfeather can no longer speak for himself. But his experiences and their import live on in the testimony of the medical professionals who cared for him, his family, members of the community who rallied around him, and the journalists who wrote about him. This chapter is based on what they felt, said, and did.

Ernie Crowfeather was first admitted to the University Hospital with a renal disease of unknown origin on 23 January 1969. Thirty months later, on 29 July 1971, he died in the emergency room of the Ellensburg, Washington, hospital. For Ernie, those thirty months were a constant struggle for eligibility to receive treatment by dialysis and transplantation, the only means that offered him a chance of survival. He was also faced with painful "quality of life" problems, which finally confronted him with a classically tragic dilemma. In the words of his primary physician, "Ernie felt so miserable that he really didn't want to live . . . but he couldn't face death either. He couldn't summon up the courage, as some of our patients have, to say 'I want to stop.' "

Ernie's response to his medical situation was conditioned by his social background and his personality traits. These same factors contributed to the ways physicians and the local community became involved in his case. For everyone concerned, Ernie and his situation evoked the life and death issues, the sense of obligation to actively intervene, the problems of meaning, the uncertainties, and the feelings of guilt and failure that terminal kidney disease, chronic hemodialysis, and transplantation can trigger.

I. Personal Vignettes

To understand Ernie Crowfeather's last thirty months of life, it is necessary to know something about his personal history. What we have learned about Ernie indicates that his attitudes and behavior patterns, independent of his illness, were strongly influenced by three factors: his half-Indian ancestry, his home life as a child, and his loss of a kidney during early adolescence. Similarly, it seems clear that the feelings and actions of the medical personnel and laymen who were involved with Ernie after the onset of his terminal renal disease were due as much to his "Indianness," his personality, his economic situation, and his social record as to his medical condition.

Ernie Crowfeather, the son of a full-blooded Sioux father and a German-American mother, was born at Fort Yates, North Dakota, in 1942. Although Mr. Crowfeather was the only member of his family who had attained a college education, according to Ernie's mother, he had "worked on a ranch for a white guy" before joining the army in 1941. A year after Ernie's birth, his parents had their sixth child. Soon after, Mrs. Crowfeather moved her five daughters and her son to Yakima, Washington, where her own mother was living. As one of Ernie's sisters explained, "Mother didn't want to be in Fort Yates, as a white woman among Indians, while our father was in the service." Although Yakima is a predominantly white town, it is adjacent to a reservation. Thus Ernie's family lived in close proximity to an Indian community. In 1946, Mr. Crowfeather left the army and rejoined his family in Yakima. Within a year he died of a coronary thrombosis, leaving his wife with little money and six young children to raise.

When her husband died, Mrs. Crowfeather related, she "shipped his body back to the Indian reservation in North Dakota because that's where he'd always wanted to be buried." Subsequently, she had little contact with her husband's relatives, and so "the kids grew up without knowing much about their father's family and the Indian way of life. I didn't know much about this either."

Of the Crowfeather children, Ernie alone seems to have been in conflict about his Indian inheritance. His feelings about his background, as we shall see, were strikingly manifested during the fund drive that made his dialysis treatment pohsible. Ernie's Indianness was made the focal point of this effort to "save" his life, and it was the Indian community who responded most strongly to the fund appeal.

A psychiatrist who worked with Ernie at the University Hospital was struck by the fact that "Ernie simply didn't identify with Indians. Whenever I tried to involve him at all with the Indians, he cooled off completely. . . . I think it was partly a denial of this part of his ancestry, and also a certain sense of uneasiness about being identified with a group which on the whole has not been held in very high esteem."

Ernie's mother and an older sister to whom he was very close both remember vividly how from early childhood Ernie had reacted to his Indian heritage. They imply that he may have been more troubled about his ethnicity than the other children in the family because, as the only son, he felt more closely and indelibly identified with what he viewed as the largely negative status of Indian. His mother said that he "was always ashamed and resentful because 'Crowfeather' was his last name. He always felt rejected in school because he was an Indian. I know I probably spoiled him by letting him have things like the good clothes he always asked for. He always wanted to dress and look nice, because he thought that would hide the Indian part of him and make him be more like white people. I know that being Indian hurt him a lot. But near the end, after the fund drive, he used to say to me, 'If it weren't for the Indians, I wouldn't be here.'"

His sister, too, knew how sensitive Ernie was about his lineage. Although he was very close to many of his doctors at University Hospital, she noted, "Ernie still felt that some of them were rejecting him and picking on him because he was an Indian. Dr. N [a young physician with Indian origins who helped launch the fund drive] was the only one who could call Ernie 'the chief' and get away with it." "Ernie," his sister continued, "always used to say he envied me because I could get married and change my name. I never experienced the rejection he felt he got from white people, maybe because I was never looking for it."

At the same time that he resented his half-Sioux background, Ernie's sister felt, he sought from Indians an acceptance he felt denied by the white community in which he was raised. "Ernie used to search Indians out all the time because he felt rejected by whites. He'd tell me he only felt accepted by other minority groups, like Indians and Mexicans and Negroes. Ernie just couldn't accept things. I suggested that he shorten or change his name, but he didn't feel that would help him."

Ernie, his sister believes, was also strongly affected by two features of his childhood environment: the female-dominated home and the German-Catholic religious atmosphere in which he was raised. "It was hard for him to grow up in a household of women. Ernie didn't like or see much of my mother's relatives; he felt they disliked him because he was part Indian. So he never had any strong male influence. He was just around women. And he was brought up, at home and in school, under a strong Catholic influence." "Ernie never could conform to the strict rules of Catholicism," his sister added, "but he had religious beliefs, and his family was very important to him."

When Ernie's mother and sister were asked what he was like as a child, they described a charming, handsome boy, who loved sports and reading and showed a marked artistic ability. Even as a little boy, they acknowledged, Ernie was often "hard to manage"; Catholicism was one of the many types of authority he found hard to accept. And, they remembered, Ernie often "got his own way," for he always showed a great ability to manipulate people and situations for his own ends. They also depicted an often lonely, withdrawn, and insecure boy, bothered by many things besides the name Crowfeather.

The course of his life from midteens on, they believe, was strongly influenced by two events: his mother's brief second marriage and the loss of his kidney. After these incidents, Ernie became an increasingly troubled youth, rebellious against a society he felt would not accept him, and at the same time seeking out a guidance and discipline he was unable to provide for himself. He also seems to have been deeply affected when an older sister, Bernice, died from a kidney disease in 1960. These aspects of Ernie's life, before the onset of his own kidney disorder in 1969, are captured by the following vignettes from our case materials.

University Hospital. Social Service Report
Crowfeather, Ernie. 1/28/69

Background Information:

At age 14 Ernie was hurt in a fall from his bicycle injuring his kidney. His mother described his kidney as pulverized and added that the organ was removed by a Yakima physician.
The patient's mother had been married a year to a Mr. _____ at the time of the patient's bicycle injury. The step-father was angered by the patient's need for care and so vindictive that the mother took her children and left him. . . .
Ernie apparently recovered satisfactorily from his kidney surgery and resumed his interest and participation in football, basketball, etc. His doctor, however, refused to sanction his playing. In his last year of high school the patient was much interested in a white girl, whose parents restricted her from seeing the patient because he was an Indian. His mother feels that the patient had

social problems from this point on and a difficult time adjusting. . . .

[Ernie's mother] spent many years working to support her children. Though she is a small person, she did much heavy work. For years she picked and packed apples.

> *University Hospital. Vocational Counseling Report.*
> Crowfeather, Ernest. 4/4/69

Educational and Work History: In 1956 (9th grade) Ernie dropped out of high school. He worked at an uncle's hop ranch for something over a year. After a six month abortive attempt to stay in and finish his schooling, he was caught in an effort to rob a store (bar?). He spent 22 months in the Monroe reform school. There he worked as a kitchen worker, orderly, and library helper. On a parole violation, according to the client, he returned for another 21 months. He spent three more periods, 9 months and 6 months and 90 days, for similar violations. The reformatory also provided him with training in a clerical and supervisory capacity in a warehouse and as a barber. He completed his high school equivalency (GED) also. Prior to his hospitalization he was waiting on a Job Corps placement with the Bureau of Indian Affairs.

Ernie's Mother: Ernie was always a good kid, until he lost that kidney. He had loved sports, especially running—he was like a little deer. Then the doctors told him he couldn't run and play ball. I think he'd have had a different life if that hadn't happened.

Ernie's Sister: After he lost his kidney, Ernie got more and more quiet and reserved. He never complained about pain, unless he was really suffering. The day he hurt himself in the bicycle accident, he lay in bed bleeding all day. He wouldn't tell anyone, until I came home from school and he told me.

Mother: Ernie read a lot. He liked medical things, and stories about what people do when they get desperate—like those books by Thomas Wolfe. He did a lot of art work, too. And he liked animals, and loved children.

Sister: As a young boy, Ernie loved poetry. He used to write me little notes and poems and put them in my school lunch pail. He read a lot. He was always quiet within himself. He was capable of learning, but it was hard for him to stay in school, or keep a job, because he couldn't conform to everyday things.

Ernie wasn't malicious. He was a quiet boy, and did the little, everyday things he was told to do. But he couldn't cope when it was time for him to grow up and strike out on his own. He functioned best when he had someone to tell him what to do, and help him.

I think a lot of Ernie's problems about accepting responsibility came when Mother divorced her second husband, after

Ernie lost his kidney. Then, Ernie wanted to be his own boss, and that's when he started getting into trouble. Mother never could handle him, although I usually could, maybe because I'm forceful.

Ernie was a terribly lonely, frightened person. He was scared to do anything on his own. But he was a con artist from the day he was born. He could make you believe he had blue eyes, when you were looking right at him and could see they were brown. When he first got into trouble, the police tried to help him, and he conned them—he talked his way right out of it.

· · · · · · · · · · · · · · · · · ·

Mother: Every time he did something wrong, he was sorry. He'd say he didn't know why he acted that way. He just would get to a point where he had to do something, because he felt rejected all the time. He used to do things, even like robbery, to get attention because he was so desperate to be rescued. He'd always feel bad afterward. I'd hear him cry.
Sister: In the last few years, after he started feeling sick, he'd be out of Monroe Reformatory a while, doing fine, and then he'd get into trouble. He admitted to me he was lonely, and wanted help and supervision. He used to write beautiful letters home from the Reformatory. He was always happy in prison.
Mother: When my oldest daughter, Bernice, got pregnant, she discovered her kidney trouble. I don't know its origin; her husband wouldn't let them do an autopsy. She was treated at the University Hospital, too. I think her dialysis was paid for by the hospital because the treatment was so new then, and they experimented with her. She just lasted two weeks. She died in 1960, at 26, with complete kidney failure.
Sister: As a little boy, Ernie talked a lot about religion. He was brought up in a religious atmosphere, where he thought a lot about the meaning of life and death. Later, after Bernice died [when Ernie was 17] and Ernie knew he only had one kidney left, he focused a lot of his worries on getting a kidney infection. He often said he'd never live to be an old man.

II. December 1968–April 1969

Soon after Ernie was paroled from the Monroe Reformatory in October 1968, his health began to decline. Around Christmastime, when he began to cough up yellow sputum and blood, Ernie became frightened enough to go to his family's physician in Yakima. He was given antibiotics, and his condition seemed to improve. On 2 January, following "some heavy New Year's drinking," his face swelled markedly for twenty-four hours. Ernie then noticed that he was having difficult and painful urinations (dysuria), and that traces of blood were appearing in his urine (hematuria). He was hospitalized briefly for his condition, and told he had anemia and a urinary tract infection. Tests indicated that his remaining left kidney had no obstructive disorder, and Ernie was discharged, with medication for the infection. His course from this episode through his referral to the University Hospital on 23 January 1969 is recorded in his medical chart as follows:

Since that time he has felt weak, fatigued and nauseated, drinking around a case of beer every other night. Two weeks prior to admission he noted the onset of frontal headaches and over the past 10 days, he has had swelling of the face, hands, and feet, gaining around 5 to 10 pounds. He then developed intractable vomiting and was hospitalized on January 19. His BUN [blood-urea-nitrogen level in the blood—an index of kidney function] was then discovered to be greater than 100 and his urine output around 150 ml/24 hours. Consequently he was transferred here for further diagnosis and treatment.

The day after his admission to the University Hospital, Ernie was started on peritoneal dialysis to alleviate his uremia, and his doctors began an exhaustive series of tests to determine the nature and cause of his renal problems. The physicians soon discovered, to their dismay, that attempts to treat Ernie by either peritoneal or hemodialysis would be fraught with difficulties. Ernie himself began to suffer a round of new and serious complications, related both to his disease and to the efforts to treat it. The extensive problems of uncertainty, both diagnostic and therapeutic, that he presented during his first two months of hospitalization are graphically documented in the following excerpts from his clinical record.

On admission the patient was felt to have evidence of hypertensive encephalopathy [brain damage] with recent renal failure, possibly secondary to hypertension. He was initially treated with hydrazine in an effort to lower his blood pressure, which was successful. . . .
A peritoneal catheter was inserted [on 1/24/69] and the patient was begun on peritoneal dialysis. Initially this procedure went smoothly with good dialysis, but the patient soon developed fever, abdominal pain, and bleeding around the site of the cannula. . . .
The patient was started on steroids and intravenous heparinization. However, the patient then began to lose blood into the peritoneal fluid during peritoneal dialysis, and heparinization had to be discontinued. . . .

Because of further difficulties with peritoneal dialysis, the patient was placed on hemodialysis [on 2/7/69]. There were marked difficulties with this procedure because of problems with cannula clotting [recannulations were required on 2/14, 3/3, and 3/4/69] and [artificial] kidney clotting. The patient developed a pericardial effusion on Feb. 17 and underwent a pericardiocentesis. . . . On Feb. 21 the patient was taken to surgery and had open drainage of the pericardial effusion and creation of a pericardial window, with drainage into the left pleural space. After a few days of production of large amounts of bloody drainage from the left chest tube, the patient stabilized and the chest tube was removed. . . .

Soon thereafter the patient developed signs and symptoms of cardiac failure and because the pericardial tamponade could not be ruled out, he underwent cardiac catheterization. . . . Because of further difficulties with cannula clotting the patient was placed on peritoneal dialysis on March 5. Thereafter he has been maintained on peritoneal dialysis with no complications and having good dialyses with maintenance of adequate control of his creatinine and BUN. On March 7 a renal biopsy was performed. . . . [The biopsy showed] changes compatible with both intervascular coagulation and hypertensive nephropathy.

One week after the renal biopsy the patient passed a small amount of blood in his urine and complained of left flank pain. . . . On March 12 he developed a supraventricular tachycardia with potassium elevated to 7.4 and was treated with intravenous calcium, with lowering of his potassium to 6.0. . . . After the patient had been stabilized on peritoneal dialysis, further hematologic evaluation was carried out which showed that he had a markedly abnormal platelet half-time of 2½ days and marked elevation of fibrinogen turnover time. This was felt to be evidence for continuing intravascular coagulation and hypothesis was raised that the patient's remaining kidney was responsible for continuation of this process.

The hospital record describes what Ernie's physicians called a "medical disaster." From a social service report, the physicians also learned that their new patient might provide nonmedical management problems, and that financing the costly treatment of his life-threatening illness would be difficult and probably impossible for his family.

Social Service Report: 1/28/69

Impression: It appears that the patient, his mother and sister are all very much aware of the gravity of the patient's problems. They all recall vividly the demise of the eldest daughter and are saddened and frightened.

This patient is on parole. . . . He is described as being fond of women and has been involved in two common-law marriages. When the first wife became pregnant, the patient left. She and her child are supported by the Welfare Department. The patient then became involved in the second relationship.

The Parole Officer describes the patient as immature, irresponsible and impulsive, adding that he has always been over-protected by his mother. The mother has had "nervous breakdowns." The Parole Officer states all the other children are responsible citizens and that the step-father is a hardworking laborer who pays his bills and conducts himself very well. The Parole Officer verifies that the patient is talented artistically.

The patient has a pleasant and winning manner but has evaded discussing himself.

In checking with the Hospital Business Office, his sister made a $300 down payment on his admission and his mother and sister have signed an agreement to pay up to $2,000 at $30 per month. The patient has not lived on an Indian Reservation since he was 2 years old. . . . [The] Director of the Indian Health Office at U.S.P.H. Hospital . . . was positive that since the patient had not lived on the reservation since age 2, he had no benefits coming.

By the end of March 1969, Ernie's condition under peritoneal dialysis appeared to have stabilized. For his family and his physicians at the University Hospital, the source of funds for long-term treatment now became a central concern. The costs of any one of the three treatment options available to Ernie—transplantation, hemodialysis, or peritoneal dialysis—seemed to be beyond the limited resources of his family or of the hospital.

"We had no way to pay for his treatment," Ernie's mother stated. "We barely lived from paycheck to paycheck, and had no insurance. And Ernie couldn't get any insurance because he only had the one kidney. By the time he died, Ernie's doctor bills were over $280,000. For a family, that's an impossible cost. Unless you have a silver spoon, no one can raise that kind of money."

After his death, Ernie's mother and sister recalled their emotions during his first months of treatment. In their voices, one could still hear the anguish they felt at the pain and suffering they saw him endure, and at the financial barriers that seemed to block any alleviation of his plight. The cost of a transplant, they knew, was beyond their means. And, as they understood Ernie's case, money rather than the problems he had encountered with dialysis was preventing the implantation of a permanent dialysis catheter for long-term treatment. In their words and tone, however, there seemed to be no bitterness against the University Hospital physicians, but rather a profound sorrow and amazement that a situation such as Ernie's could exist in the United States.

"You hear Apollo this and Apollo that," Ernie's sister declared, "and you suddenly realize that people are dying because they haven't any money for treatment. . . . I appreciated the efforts of the hospital, and the doctors' kindnesses to Ernie. But to have the doctors keep puncturing his stomach with those peritoneal catheters, over and over again, and say they can't implant a permanent catheter because they need $5,000–6,000 first or to say they won't transplant him until they know the $20,000 cost will be paid—that's pretty hard to take. How do you weigh a life against $20,000, even though that's a lot of money?"

Ernie's mother, who had moved to Seattle after his admission to the University Hospital, also talked with distress about "how the doctors said they had no funds, so they couldn't put in a permanent dialysis catheter. I remember how he lay there and just took it. Each time they put another catheter in, the pain got a little worse, and he got more and more upset. We were all there with him as much as we could be. He and I would talk sometimes, and it was heartbreaking. I think it was the worst thing possible, next to death—to sit there and see him suffer, because you haven't got the money to take care of your child."

In early April Ernie's physicians sought to resolve his financial problems by applying for home dialysis treatment through the Northwest Kidney Center. For several reasons, neither they nor Ernie and his family were optimistic about his candidacy. His case was complex medically, especially in view of the shunt and kidney clotting problems he had experienced with hemodialysis. Dr. Henry Tenckhoff, one of Ernie's primary physicians at the University Hospital, felt that Ernie might do well on home peritoneal dialysis. But Dr. Tenckhoff had only recently developed techniques to permit long-term home peritoneal dialysis, and (in a colleague's words) he was "battling" to have the Kidney Center accept it as a mode of home treatment. In addition, the center's selection committee would consider other nonmedical facets of Ernie's case in deciding his eligibility for home dialysis treatment. "The doctors [at the University Hospital] told Mother and me," Ernie's sister recalled, "that the center would weigh Ernie's financial status and the fact that he hadn't been a very 'productive' citizen."

Ernie's application was rejected by the Kidney Center's Medical Advisory Committee. Ernie's lack of financial resources and his personal history, including an "unstable home situation with a common-law wife," entered into their deliberations. Ernie's unconventional life-style evoked a certain amount of moral disapproval from committee members. But they were also more neutrally concerned with the difficulties that his domestic situation might create for a safe and effective home dialysis regimen.

Ernie's prison record was also considered by the committee. "We knew he'd been in the Monroe Reformatory for breaking and entering, or something." However, in the words of one committee member, "it didn't sound like a major crime so it wasn't in itself a strike against him."

The committee's final judgment was stated purely in medical terms. In their opinion, Ernie's shunt-clotting problems, coagulopathy (blood clotting in the artificial kidney) and other medical factors indicated that he would not do well on home dialysis.

At least in front of his family, Ernie reacted calmly to the news of his rejection by the Kidney Center. "All he said to me," his sister recalled, was 'Well, they told me they wouldn't accept me. Maybe I won't be around as long as I thought I would be.' Ernie even joked about it some. He had a good sense of humor about his situation until the end, when he just lost his will to live."

Ernie's family then began a desperate effort to find money for continuing his treatment. "I told him there were ways to get money, and we would," his sister related. "We first tried to get money from Welfare, asking if funds were available from the Indian Agency in North Dakota. The agency didn't even reply for a long time, and then we finally got a short note saying there were no funds. Then we wrote to a state senator, but he told us no funds had been appropriated for a case like Ernie's."

III. The Clinical Research Center, April–September 1969

Ernie's physicians at the University Hospital shared his family's distress over his rejection by the Kidney Center and were determined to find a means for continuing his treatment. They realized that certain unusual and puzzling aspects of his renal disease might make Ernie eligible for admission to the hospital's Clinical Research Center (CRC), where he could be treated and his case studied through research grant funds. A "historical review" of

Ernie's case, prepared for us by his primary physician, recognizes that his transfer to the CRC was not solely impelled by his challenging medical problems.

Because of the rather unusual features of his renal disease, a "unique opportunity study" was formulated, applying to the Clinical Research Center for six months of dialysis support including initial nephrectomy and final renal transplantation in an effort to demonstrate whether the coagulopathy that was involved in his renal disease would abate after nephrectomy and whether transplantation could be successfully performed thereafter without recurrent disease. This became necessary because the patient was turned down for dialysis support by the Northwest Kidney Center on account of his medical history, his background including the lack of a stable home, and lack of financial support.

Ernie's rejection by the NKC, as we indicated earlier, was the primary stimulus for the formation of the University Hospital's Dialysis Utilization Committee, which has enabled a limited number of dialysis patients to receive in-hospital dialysis treatments and home training by means of research funds. When members of the Kidney Center staff were asked how they felt about the hospital treating a patient like Ernie, whom the center had rejected, they responded as follows. Dr. A: "They've got the right as long as they don't expect us to fund them. I guess that's what it comes down to. Any private physician could do it if he wanted to, as long as he's expending funds from somewhere else." Dr. C: "This has been the problem historically. In the earlier days a number of the patients that were rejected here were then accepted at the University Hospital on a research grant basis. When the grant money runs out, what happens to these patients? They're on dialysis, we feel a community commitment to treat all patients with chronic renal disease, and therefore, we are obligated to take these people on and assume their financial burden."

The commitment Ernie's physicians felt to him was not unique. The bond between Ernie and his physicians in many ways typified the close, intense, at once personal and collegial relationship that often develops between clinical investigators and the patients they care for and study. As Belding Scribner said to us, using Ernie as an example of his own and his colleagues' involvement with their patients: "You get locked into these things and can't quit. At some point in time we become committed to these patients. We don't know exactly when that is, but once it happens, then we find it impossible to let them die."

The response of Ernie's physicians to his rejection by the Kidney Center, then, was in many ways prototypic. But at the same time, their relationship with Ernie had some special nuances and was increasingly stressful. The fact that Ernie was half-Indian, and thus belonged to a minority group whose history and present socioeconomic conditions disturb many more advantaged persons in this country, was one element in the physicians' reactions to Ernie and their relationship with him. As one physician put it, "There was a special sense of injustice about his having so many problems."

Second, and perhaps more important, were Ernie's own personal qualities. His physicians knew that he had many nonmedical problems, as evidenced by his prison record. He was often labeled by psychiatrists, social workers, and others as a sociopath.[1] The hospital staff found him "difficult" in many ways. But they all liked Ernie Crowfeather.

Dr. Scribner: Ernie wasn't that clever, but in his own uneducated way he was a very intelligent type of guy, intuitively. He was a con man in certain ways. The way he manipulated people was unbelievable. . . . I liked Ernie, but I tried to stay clear of his case because of the terrible complexities. Dr. Tenckhoff seemed willing to take the brunt of our side of it, so he was the guy who sort of carried it all.

Dr. Tenckhoff: Despite all the problems and headaches he gave us, Ernie was very much liked by his doctors, which is strange. His inability to get along with his medical regimens was extremely frustrating to us. He had many appealing qualities. He was artistic, and very verbal about his feelings. He was honest, except for self-deceptions—and then he'd deceive others, too. Ernie was always pleasant, and very apologetic about his failures. He had the appeal of a child who needed help.

Dr. G (a psychiatrist): When I first met Ernie, I could see very quickly that he represented a chronic challenge. The nurses didn't quite know how to handle him. He would be rather uncooperative about his dialysis; moody, demanding, difficult.

Ernie's knowledge of himself was that he was a man doomed. I'm reminded of a few other young patients I have known, who knew that they were facing a life-threatening illness with a probably fatal outcome. Without a prior history of what we might call sociopathy, they, too, decided "as long as I have to die anyway, I might as well try to get all I can out of life." Ernie really didn't seem to appreciate all the special things that were done for him; he took it all for granted. And, like every person whom one might diagnostically call sociopathic, there was really no awareness of one's death and obligations. . . . Ernie, like sociopaths generally, was very impulsive, and the immediate gratification of his wishes was a predominant concern of his. . . .

One of the unfortunate things about Ernie is that he stereotyped the prejudices or images that people have about the American Indian—unreliable, shiftless, demanding, alcoholic, somewhat potentially or actually criminal, unable to form long, intimate relationships. . . . But I was aware of the fact that I really liked Ernie in spite of it all.

On 27 April 1969 Ernie was admitted to the Clinical Research Center "for his nephrectomy, then repeat studies, and subsequently for renal transplantation." Ernie was to receive a cadaver kidney, when one became available, for "a search for a living donor was made, but no compatible donor was found."

Ernie's physicians had cause to be pleased with the outcome of their "unique opportunity study" strategem. For the next six months, Ernie's treatment, including the cost of a transplant, would be borne by the CRC. Then, *if* the new kidney functioned well and was not rejected, the major part of Ernie's financial problems would be over. Ernie and his family, too, were relieved of a major worry. But his transfer to the CRC did create some apprehensions. "I was frightened when the doctors told me he could be treated by a research grant," Ernie's sister remembered. "I didn't want them to try things on him. One day, he called me and said 'the doctors want to put an artificial kidney in me. Maybe it will work.' I said, 'Ernie, you're kidding. You're on the top of the transplant list. Just wait.'"

The day after his admission to the CRC, Ernie's single kidney was removed, and he started peritoneal dialysis three times a week. After recovering from his nephrectomy, Ernie was allowed to leave the CRC between most dialysis sessions. In addition to receiving treatment and undergoing various studies, Ernie also was taught home peritoneal techniques, "and learned them rapidly." The CRC staff, however, like the Kidney Center, found that Ernie did not have a home situation that would be favorable to a successful home treatment program until his transplant occurred. Ernie's mother could not stay in Seattle indefinitely to help him with dialysis and manage his strict diet because she had a husband and a teen-age daughter in Yakima. Ernie's girl friend was initiating divorce proceedings against her husband and planned to marry Ernie when the divorce was final, in about three months. In the interim, she could not provide Ernie with the type of home assistance he would need. And, even assuming that Ernie could manage his own care, he had no income to provide himself with housing. Thus, "due to lack of a home," Ernie's physicians "elected to keep the patient [on dialysis] at the CRC."

Ernie's six-month course of treatment and study at the CRC was not a smooth one. "Largely due to inconsistencies in sterile techniques, he contracted a total of three peritoneal infections." Never an ideal patient, Ernie became increasingly "moody, demanding, and difficult," and uncooperative about following his medical regimen. "On one occasion," his record notes, "when he got mad at the nurses, he disconnected his dialysis cathether with his bare hands and left the hospital."

The problems that CRC personnel encountered with Ernie also involved their plans to have him train for a job that he could assume after his transplant. The week he was admitted to the CRC, Ernie was interviewed by a vocational counselor and given various intelligence and aptitude tests. His report read in part as follows:

Counselor's Impression:
The patient was most cooperative, congenial, and verbal in the interview. He appeared relaxed and confident and spoke frankly of his reform school experiences. At the same time he greatly oversimplified and "played down" the reasons for his several stays there. His smooth interaction with the counselor and others, his history of trouble with society's standards, his embellishment of his experiences impressed this counselor as being rather typical of the sociopath (another conjecture!).
Summary and Recommendations:
Ernie's present condition might be expected to demand 3–7 nights per week on dialysis. He appears to be mildly anxious and compulsive in his behavior, and might have some difficulty adjusting to social demands made of him. . . .
The following recommendations seem to be tenable:
1) that, in spite of his social history, medical condition, and prognosis, Ernie should be considered a candidate for vocational rehabilitation,
2) that such rehabilitation, limited in scope, be sponsored and undertaken by the Division of Vocational Rehabilitation, if possible,
3) that the patient's training be directed toward a vocation allowing him considerable autonomy, and which also enables him to perform certain minimal administrative functions, e.g., warehouse dispatcher, stock clerk, sales clerk, office clerk, or worker, etc.

Ernie had some training as a barber, and following the vocational counselor's findings, his physicians "went through many procedures and problems to get him enrolled in barber school, and get special hours for him." "Multiple and persistent efforts" were made to motivate Ernie to utilize this opportunity about which he expressed enthusiasm, but "he completely fell down on this; he barely followed through, going only to a few training sessions."

Ernie's sister was familiar with the behavior patterns he showed on the CRC —his moods, failure to accept responsibility and act on his own initiative, his difficulties in adhering to regimentation, and his "charming con man" approach to most people and situations. She had seen all these patterns in Ernie since he was a young child, but she also attributed many of his attitudes and actions while at the CRC to an increasing fear of the endless studies and dialyses. "At first, Ernie truly was a very good patient. He'd let the doctors do anything to him without complaining. But after a while, he got so frightened of pain he couldn't bear the thought of anything else being done."

To his psychiatrist, in turn, Ernie's reactions to his medical regimen represented a familiar pattern of denial, a reaction to his illness that was exacerbated by Ernie's "sociopathic personality."

As is frequently the case with men who are sick, their illness, to them, is identified with weakness and weakness is identified with lack of masculinity. I think I would explain Ernie's almost desperate attempt to deny to himself over and over again the fact that he needed treatment two or three times a week, and just had to lie there and take it, partly on that basis. . . . I think it's likely that the sociopathy he displayed was present without his illness, and then was tremendously accentuated.

Near the end of Ernie's allotted six months on the CRC, his fiancée obtained her divorce, and they were married. With public assistance funds the couple were able to rent an apartment in Seattle. Subsequently, because Ernie's time on the CRC was running out, he was started on home peritoneal dialysis.

IV. Transplantation and Rejection: October 1969– November 1970

Ernie's physicians were not optimistic about his prognosis on home dialysis. They felt it was fortunate that on 14 October

1969, just a few days after he started home treatments, a cadaver kidney was obtained and Ernie received his transplant. Ernie's new kidney, from a twenty-year-old woman, was a "C" match. The implantation went smoothly, and his postoperative course was "essentially uncomplicated." Ernie was discharged from the CRC on 29 October on an immunosuppressive therapy of prednisone, Imuran, and ALG. He was scheduled to report at regular intervals to the hospital's Renal Transplantation Clinic for post-transplant checkups.

On 5 November, through a laboratory error that yielded a falsely high creatinine level, his physicians diagnosed an acute rejection crisis. Ernie had a renal biopsy, received intravenous prednisone and a radiation treatment at the graft site, and had his oral prednisone dosage increased. The following day, when his creatinine test was within normal limits, the laboratory error was discovered. Ernie's prednisone dosage was reduced to its former level, and he was discharged.

After this episode, Ernie's transplant appeared to be functioning satisfactorily, and his prednisone dosage was further reduced. There were indications, however, that Ernie would again be a management problem for his physicians. His chart, for example, notes that on 18 December, Ernie "was admitted for a planned platelet survival study. However, patient leaves hospital the same evening without giving reason."

From late December through February, Ernie spent much of his time in the hospital, fighting off a rejection episode and the infections that are a constant hazard for patients on immuno-suppressive therapy. When he was discharged on 5 March, "essentially improved," Ernie boarded a train for his mother's home in Yakima. By now his life was further complicated by a failing marriage, and he and his wife had separated. "I know Ernie really loved his wife," his sister related. "We tried to tell her how ill he was, but she married him anyway. Ernie was very hurt when his marriage didn't work. He had hurt her a lot, but he still expected her to stand behind him."

En route to Yakima on 5 March, Ernie felt a sudden pain in his chest and shoulder. The pain increased over the next few days, and he entered a hospital in Yakima with a fever and chest and shoulder pains. On 27 March, Ernie was transferred back to the University Hospital. A presumptive diagnosis of splenic in-farcts was made, but his physicians decided not to remove his spleen because he still had an infected wound in his abdominal wall. Ernie was discharged "improved" on 31 March to be followed weekly at the Renal Transplantation Clinic.

In the first six months after his transplant, as we have seen, Ernie experienced a series of complications—rejection reactions and infections—common to many organ recipients. These problems, as we read in the following extract from his case history, continued over the next eight months, culminating in the removal of his transplanted kidney on 23 November 1970. During this period Ernie again struck out against society, or as many feel, again appealed for help and the institutional guidance he seemed to need and desire. Ernie committed an armed robbery, immediately surrendered to the police, and then attempted suicide in his jail cell.

Although in good physical health on the whole, the patient did not try to find employment and most of the time hung out with friends. About the middle of May, after ample alcohol ingestion, he was involved in an armed robbery in a local motel, following which he gave himself up to the police in a nearby bar. He was taken to the local jail, where he attempted suicide and was transferred to Western State [psychiatric] Hospital on 5/20/70. From there he would come to his clinic appointments under guard. . . . During this time at Western State Hospital it was noticed that his renal function was declining, and on 10/8/70 he was readmitted to the University Hospital for renal biopsy because of more rapid deterioration of renal function and duodenal ulcer.
There has been some question about the consistency of his taking the prescribed immunosuppressive therapy. By 10/27/70 his renal function had deteriorated to the point at which it no longer sustained well-being and he was transferred to the medical service. He was restarted on peritoneal dialysis on 11/6/70 with the intention to retrain him for home dialysis with the possibility of a future second transplant. On 11/23/70 his renal graft was removed.

The loss of Ernie's transplant was not the only rejection he underwent in the fall of 1970. At the end of October, when it was evident that his kidney function was irreversibly failing, Ernie faced the same plight he had when first admitted to the University Hospital: how to pay for dialysis treatments. Once again, his physicians turned to the Northwest Kidney Center. On 5 November, the center's patient admissions committee met to review Ernie's candidacy. The record of that session states:

Ernie Crowfeather presented by Dr. _____ is a 28 year old
separated male who had been previously rejected by the Medical
Advisory Committee in April 1969. He subsequently received a
transplant . . . and is being re-presented for dialysis at this time
because the transplanted kidney is failing. Careful evaluation of
the medical, psychiatric, social, and rehabilitation reports revealed
a long history of recidivism, and that he was again in custody
for a felony at the time of his present University Hospital
admission. Mr. Crowfeather has been historically uncooperative
in his medical management both before and after his transplant.
Medical, psychiatric, and social worker opinions reveal little
hope for successful reform and indicated a highly probable
inability to manage home dialysis. The consensus of the Committee was that Mr. Crowfeather would be an unsuccessful
dialysis patient due to medical and emotional instability. It was
moved and seconded that Mr. Crowfeather be denied treatment.
Motion passed unanimously. Rejected.

A year after Ernie's second rejection by the Kidney Center, in
the course of interviews conducted by Dr. Lawrence K. Altman
of the *New York Times*, several staff members discussed why
Ernie was twice refused treatment by the center, and the pros and
cons of those decisions. They also considered whether the center's
policy had changed sufficiently in the interim that if Ernie were a
candidate today he would have a better chance of acceptance.

Dr. E: I think at the present time the situation with respect to
selection is a little bit different from Ernie's day. . . . at the
moment, I think it's fair to say that people are only rejected on . . .
mainly medical grounds. You see, it's very hard to distinguish
medical, social, and psychological factors at this level. I think
we're very liberal now. We take patients whom we have a very
good idea are going to cause us a lot of problems; cost a lot of
money, and be very difficult to handle. If Ernie came back again
now, and it appeared to us that he couldn't be hemodialyzed,
I think we might accept him now for peritoneal dialysis.
Dr. G: We're in a position today of not having to be confronted
by selection dilemmas very often. . . . We can go a long way
because of our financial condition. But we still have a selection
committee. And I think the thing that scares everybody here is
that we might, if funds were cut, have to go back to the previous
selection process, where you're using such intangible factors to
select a patient because there are no absolute criteria; they just
don't exist.
Dr. F: By the time Ernie was presented to us the second time, in
November 1970, he had received all three types of treatment
that are available, and he had failed in all three. And the
possibility of getting another transplant for him just looked like a

hopeless situation. In fact, the only thing in our minds that would be open to him would be in-center dialysis, which the NKC does not offer.

Dr. G: When Ernie came up the second time, he was on probation. He should have been incarcerated and treatment provided at that point. But we didn't have the facilities, and the authorities didn't want to handle the responsibility of having to take him to a hospital for dialysis under guard. I think that was one aspect of his rejection. Another aspect was the fact that we don't do in-center dialysis anymore. . . . So we take the case of Ernie Crowfeather. He was going to cost what we estimated to be $21,000 a year for in-center treatment, and that would support six people at home, at $3,500 each. We just don't have enough funds to blow them all on one patient when it's very questionable as to whether he can survive the medical and other complications. What is our obligation? How far can we go? One theory is that you spend all the money you have, take everybody in, and when you're broke, you're broke. Another view is that you've got a responsibility to the patients now on the program, that you've got to provide care and treatment for them as on-going patients.

.   .   .   .

Dr. F: I agree that he might be accepted today if his first candidacy came up again. But I think his second application might still be denied, because he'd gotten in so much trouble with the police, for example, and hadn't been good at looking after himself from a medical point of view.

Dr. G: I think this is where Ernie's is a classic case, because it falls into that gray area of decision where you get into so many problems. Whether a person is or can be rehabilitated is a very subjective thing. Can this individual operate at home by himself? You can't tell about a lot of these things until you get into them, and today we can be very liberal because of available financial resources. . . . I can think of two or three people we've taken this year who had a criminal record or were accused of some crime. . . . Since Ernie, we've had another patient who got into legal trouble while he was on dialysis, I think for armed robbery. But I don't see how that alone can jeopardize a person's standing with the Kidney Center. I mean we can't turn him off. This is a commitment that we make to people. Once they get on the program, there's no way that we're going to drop them. We're financially and morally committed to that guy for as long as he lives. . . .

Mr. Z: So far, we've gotten through Russian Roulette without blowing our brains out.

Dr. F: You can outline quite a story from Ernie's side. You know, "This is my last will and testament, and this is what society has done to me." The establishment, the Kidney Center, the

University Hospital, society in general couldn't have responded to his accusations. Everybody was in a defenseless position because he could have presented a very dramatic case. "I have been rejected and denied life-saving treatment because (a) I'm an Indian, (b) I've got a criminal record, (c) I have no money, (d) my wife has left me."

V. The Ernie Crowfeather Campaign Fund: 9 November 1970–1 February 1971

Ernie's second rejection by the Kidney Center seemed to signal the end of his economic and medical struggle to live. With his kidney transplant no longer functioning, and without funds for dialysis, death from uremic poisoning would occur within a few weeks. "Ernie really didn't suffer through his first series of dialyses and the transplant," his primary physician believes. "But when the transplant failed, he became extremely unhappy. He really didn't want to live." His mother and sister, too, feel that Ernie began to lose hope and to abandon the will to live in November 1970. "He'd ask me, 'What are we going to do now, Mom? Am I just going to lie here and die?'"

But once again, the intense way in which those who knew Ernie became involved in his case led to another temporary financial reprieve. This time those who were determined to "save" Ernie went "outside the medical system," launching a massive public fund-raising campaign. Ernie's Indian heritage was the fulcrum of this effort. It motivated the actions of his fund raisers, was the dominant theme of their campaign, and served to rally an extensive local and national response from both Indians and whites.

Three people initiated and guided the Ernie Crowfeather Fund: Dr. N, a young physician of Indian ancestry, who had been a resident at the University Hospital and treated Ernie during his first months there, and who was working at the Indian Health Clinic in Seattle in November 1970; Mrs. J, a social worker with the Washington Indian Center in Seattle, who was herself an Indian; and Mr. D, a Seattle social worker with the American Jewish Committee.

Mr. D and Dr. N had met and become friends through their work with several Indian organizations in Seattle establishing the Indian Health and Dental Clinic. When Dr. N learned of the Kidney Center's decision, Mr. D recalled, "he came to my house that night and told me what was happening to Ernie, and that Ernie would die, and he said, 'What do you think?' And, I suppose because I'm a human being, a social worker, a Jew, and an American, I said, 'Well, we just can't let him die.' I just couldn't understand how they were going to pull the plug on this character and just let him go, no matter who he was. And I suppose the fact that he was an Indian and that he was discriminated against, which I think he was, probably added to it. So Dr. N and Mrs. J and I set out as a committee of three, initially, to convince the hospital to continue his treatment and from there on to raise the money."

Mrs. J had first heard of Ernie in the spring of 1969 after his first rejection by the Kidney Center. "A friend called me and said, 'there is a twenty-seven-year-old guy who is going to die because he has no funds and a bad kidney.' We started thinking about doing something for him, but then he got picked up by a research project, and they did a transplant and the problem was solved. Then, a year later, I went to volunteer at the Indian Health Center, and Dr. N told me there was a young man who would be dead in two to four weeks if he didn't get some funds. When he mentioned Ernie's name, I said, 'Oh, that's the same young man that had the problem last year,' and I told Dr. N I'd like to get involved in an effort to help him. So the three of us got together with a group of the doctors, and then it was determined by the hospital board or somebody that we had to raise $20,000. It was a lot to do, and we did just about everything we could think of to get the money."

The nonprofit Ernie Crowfeather Fund Drive started on 9 November 1970. The University Hospital, after a series of meetings with Dr. N, Mrs. J and Mr. D, had agreed to provide Ernie with dialysis treatments, *if* the fund drive could raise $10,000 by 20 December and another $10,000 by early February. Mr. D and Mrs. J both remember how Ernie's physicians discussed his many personal and medical problems with them, and their fears that, money or not, his prospects were dubious.

Mr. D: When we first began to meet with the doctors at the hospital, they told us what we would be going through and they practically assured us that Ernie was not going to make it, that he was going to become antisocial, that he was manipulative. And we found out that he was. He was a wonder. And we didn't believe it. We really passed it off as being prejudice against

Indians. I think if we had it to do over again, we would have gone about it differently. We wouldn't have gone out and sought public donations. I think we would have focused more on the system, on changing the system. But we didn't have time. We were facing a life and death problem, and that problem was to meet a deadline, to raise $20,000. We didn't have time to really lobby the Kidney Center and the hospital.
Mrs. J: They told us at the outset Ernie was suicidal, and said it wasn't worth the effort of raising the money for him when so many others were in need. But we felt we had to do it, that Ernie was just another typical example of the plight of Indians. . . .
Dr. N said, "Knowing all these things, you must decide. He may be a sociopath, he may be suicidal, he may be wasting our time." I don't know. . . . I think Ernie was great at managing people.

Convinced that Ernie's problems in obtaining treatment were due to his being part Indian, his fund raisers focused their campaign on events that would appeal to the Indian community. On 23 November 1970, the day Ernie's transplant was removed, the *Seattle Post-Intelligence* carried a story headlined "Indian Brotherhood Keeps Ernie Alive." The article described the Crowfeather Fund Drive's activities and featured an interview with Ernie, arranged by his fund raisers in which he talked about his illness, his feelings about being part Indian, and what the fund drive meant to him.

"Two weeks ago," Ernie said, "my doctor noticed that my chemistries had dropped drastically, and informed me that the kidney had failed.

"I've had so many operations that this one doesn't bother me at all. I'm not afraid of the pain. I've got the best doctors I could have. There are so many scars on my abdomen I've suggested they install a zipper."
Ernie approaches most things calmly and with humor. And he acknowledges that his illness has changed the course of his life in fundamental ways.

"I wasn't raised as an Indian," he said. "My father was Sioux, my mother is German Catholic, but I had little contact with Indians as I grew up.

"All my life I was thought of by others as Indian but I found it difficult to identify with Indians. Now I feel something better than proudness—I'm reaching for some other word which would fit. It is Indians who are helping me, and I realize clearly what I have missed. . . . .

"In some ways," he added, "I don't know where I stand. I saw a picture in the papers the other day and had a feeling that I was just an Indian being exhibited. I felt that it wasn't me.

"Don't put me up there on a pedestal, I think to myself, and demand that I fulfill all those obligations. Don't hang those on me like an albatross. If you do that I won't be me. In other words, it boils down to this: am I going to be a good or bad Indian. I can only be me. . . . "

Last week Indian friends gathered at the hospital, and under the leadership of Sioux medicine man, Frank White Buffalo Man, grandson of Sitting Bull, assisted in a Sioux ceremonial healing rite for Ernie, including the ancestral prayer pipe.

After today's surgery, Ernie will require a peritoneal dialysis machine to stay alive.

"That machine is pretty ugly," he said as he pointed to it. "I have—what do you call them?—ambivalent feelings about it. A love-hate relationship. But I know that that machine is my life.

"When I first learned of my disease, my reaction was that it was probably the end. . . .

"Now I believe everything is going to come through and I'm going to live to a ripe old age. I'm learning to live with a new purpose."

Mrs. J and Mr. D remember vividly and proudly the range of fund-raising efforts for Ernie, and the generous response to these appeals.

Mrs. J: We thought it should be an Indian thing, since it was an Indian problem. . . . I think nothing like this has ever taken place before, where we, the Indian community, all became so united. We sort of planned it that way. The Indians had to get behind this one guy. And Ernie's problems, you know, his mental problems, were such typical Indian problems. This society destroys Indians. I don't think Ernie was unusual in his problems. Some of us survive it, and he didn't.

I started by going to a meeting of the American Indian Women's Service Committee, I told them about Ernie, and said "Well, what are you going to do about it?" We . . . set up a press conference. . . . We formed committees, and always had people going around with coffee cans, collecting nickels and dimes. Once we found a $20 bill in a can, and wondered what Indian was rich enough to stick that much in. So while the Indians didn't give a whole lot of money, they all pitched in and really became involved. The Seattle public schools put on an Indian Heritage program, one hour a week, and they'd charge a little admission money and turn it over to us. . . . Whenever there was an Indian meeting in town, I'd go and make an appeal, and they'd resolve to help however they could. . . . The first big effort we made was at a football game during half-time. We collected about $1,400 that day.

We called all the national Indian figures we could think of, and asked them for their help. They all got involved, and they thought of asking the Bureau of Indian Affairs to contribute. I think they gave over $1,000. That December, some of our people went as delegates to a National Congress for Indian Opportunities in Washington, and set up public projects through that meeting. Then, there was a big movement between school kids, who set up various projects and also elderly people who sent in dollars and dimes. We also had things like a two-day jazz and rock concert, and an arts and crafts fair. It really was a wonderful experience, and I think Ernie was delighted with it. The course of his life was changed.

When they first told us we'd have to raise $20,000, I thought we'd never do it, with the depression and all. I thought we might get $10,000, and then help Ernie to get Bureau of Indian Affairs benefits, which he was entitled to. If he went back to the reservation, we thought, he could qualify for medical care, but there just were no facilities there to keep him alive. We tried to get him funded through an Indian Public Health Service Hospital, too. The head of one of those hospitals was asked at a reservation conference, "How come you aren't helping Ernie Crowfeather?" And he said, "Oh, I could help him. But if I take $20,000 and keep Ernie alive, that means your children won't get their vaccinations." And that just took care of it right there. I really took exception to his statement because I figured there goes somebody pitting the reservation Indians against the urban Indians.

But it all turned out okay. We announced around the middle of January that we'd reached our goal, and had a public thank you. We raised just about $23,000.

Mr. D: I think the Ernie Crowfeather campaign probably did more to solidify the urban Indian community than any other single incident I can remember. . . . And I think the public, in general, learned something that most of them didn't know. People were astounded to learn that for a mere $20,000 a life was going to waste. . . . We were able to put Ernie up in front of a TV camera, and get ten pages on him in newspapers, telling people that here's a twenty-eight-year-old Indian who's been rejected by the whole world, and let's not let this character die. Ernie had nothing going for him, and everything going against him, which was great from a publicity standpoint. Crowfeather literally became a household word. People were breaking their backs to send him money.

Ernie's fund raisers omitted two facets of Ernie's case from the publicity campaign. First, Ernie's full history, including his criminal record, suicidal behavior, and difficulties in following his medical regimen, was not mentioned. To a psychiatrist who had worked closely with Ernie, the fund appeal's portrayal of him was "nauseating because it was so sentimental and untrue. . . . It was almost sickening to see the sentimental appeal for saving this poor Indian boy. I'm not saying that any life is not worthwhile. But the whole thing was dramatized and romanticized through wide publicity. The Ernie Crowfeather Fund was a real tearjerker."

Those involved with Ernie's campaign also decided not to dwell on the complex set of social and ethical issues inherent in the operation of the Kidney Center. "In the beginning," Mr. D stated, "the papers started to play this up in terms of Ernie's rejection by the center. But we sat down with a series of newspaper people and told them that they would be doing the center and the public and those who needed the services and the University Hospital a tremendous disservice. We didn't want to hurt the Kidney Center. This wasn't our intention. Our intention was to save Ernie, and to try to change the Kidney Center. We were successful in one and not the other. I think the center has done a good job, and I think the public knows it."

The Kidney Center, as Mr. D realized, was in a potentially vulnerable spot concerning the Crowfeather Fund. Their operation, which is dependent upon generous public support, could have been jeopardized if Ernie was portrayed as a terminally ill patient who had been twice rejected by the "white system," the center, because he belonged to a minority group. When Ernie's campaign started, one of his physicians at the University Hospital stated, "You should have seen the reaction of the people at the center. They were petrified. They didn't know where it would end. All due credit to the Indians and those helping them. They did their job with good restraint, and they didn't point a finger at the center, which they easily could have done—the white man rejecting the Indian. . . . The whole reputation of the center was on the line. It could have been a disaster for them; they were right in the middle of a fund drive."

After Ernie's death, members of the center's staff recalled how they had reacted to the Crowfeather Fund Drive.

Mr. Z: We cooperated. We did that for two reasons. One was selfish—his need for funds occurred at the same time we were launching our fund drive. We had to be careful not to conflict, and we worked with his fund raisers and helped them. The whole thing resolved itself in a very nice fashion. There was no hue and cry that the center did this to us, and now we need some money. The majority of the general public didn't differentiate between the center's drive and the Crowfeather appeal. Ernie's was the first appeal that I know of for someone already rejected by the center. But in the past, center patients had to go out into the community and raise their own funds. So people are very used to this type of appeal, and it had no effect whatsoever on our drive. *Dr. G*: Ernie's people raised the question whether, if they went out and raised money and gave it to the center, we would then accept Ernie. We had to say no. The decision to reject Ernie wasn't specifically a financial one. This is the framework in which we have to operate. . . . I think the publicity about Ernie's case has been very well handled from all standpoints. There were no accusations, no throwing of rocks. But everywhere I go, people ask me about Ernie. Everybody knew about him.

VI. Ernie's Last Chapter: December 1970–29 July 1971

On 6 December 1970, after his transplant was removed, Ernie was discharged once again. He was to return to the hospital for peritoneal dialysis treatments until enough money had been raised, and other preparations completed, for him to begin home dialysis. About Thanksgiving time, he and his wife had worked out a reconciliation and rented an apartment in Seattle so that he could obtain home care.

Ernie's family believe that he was genuinely moved by and deeply thankful for the public's response to his case. "Ernie greatly appreciated the funds raised for him," his mother affirmed. "He saved letters from people, especially schoolchildren, and tears would roll down his cheeks while he read them. He often said to me, 'Mom, if it weren't for the Indians, I wouldn't have this care.' "

Despite his professed gratitude for the funds that enabled his treatment to continue, Ernie did not adhere to the strict routine necessary for a successful dialysis program. Between January and March 1971, while he was on home peritoneal dialysis, he was frequently admitted to the University Hospital. His charts record admissions for "technical problems with dialysis, minor drug overdosage, analgesic and narcotic abuse, and abdominal pain of unknown origin," plus several sign-outs "against medical advice." Ernie's drug dependency had developed over a period of several months as he became increasingly reliant upon pain killers to blot out the discomfort that went with his many infections and various medical tests and treatment. His need for drugs, Ernie's records note, was "a major management problem throughout the remaining months of his life. He was seen on numerous occasions in the Emergency Room requesting pain medication; also on many occasions under false names [he] went to other hospitals requesting and receiving drugs. On 1/31/71 he was admitted for an acute barbiturate overdose."

On 28 February, Ernie entered the hospital with a severe purulent infection around his peritoneal catheter site. A new catheter was inserted for an overnight dialysis, then removed the following morning when Ernie was discharged. Until the infection cleared up, his physicians decided, Ernie again would have to endure "acute catheterization," returning to the hospital every two days to have a peritoneal catheter inserted into his abdomen for an overnight dialysis.

The infection, however, did not respond to medication, and a "large area of Ernie's abdominal wall became involved with a cellulitis" (an inflammation of cellular or connective tissue). With this condition, Ernie could not undergo peritoneal dialysis. His only other treatment option was hemodialysis, a procedure that had not worked well, because of clotting problems, when Ernie first entered the hospital in January 1969.

Ernie was placed on hemodialysis at the University Hospital on 9 March 1971. Subsequently, his physicians arranged a "special contract" with the Veterans Administration Hospital, and Ernie was transferred there for home dialysis training and biweekly treatments. His records chart Ernie's downward spiral after beginning hemodialysis.

He did not attend his dialysis treatments regularly and never showed up for the special training sessions arranged for him. In the interval, he would show up at the University Hospital with multiple physical complaints, some of which were based on medical complications. . . . In addition, he was admitted on many occasions because he had missed one or several of his regularly scheduled dialyses at the V.A. Hospital.

This is one of many UH admissions for this 29 year old Indian male who enters for hemodialysis. Ernie missed his dialysis time at the V.A. Hospital Kidney Center secondary to prior preoccupation with both drugs and alcohol. He spent three days in a stuporous state, claiming that he was not going to undergo further dialysis and wanted to die.

Ernie's friends will not soon forget their ceaseless efforts to get him to utilize the home dialysis machine he was given or to report to the VA hospital for treatment after the machine was removed from his apartment because he failed to use it properly and regularly.

Mr. D: I know that Dr. N was there at Ernie's house at two o'clock in the morning trying to counsel the guy and adjust the machine. I was there in the middle of the night many times, and on the phone, my God, at 2, 4, 7 o'clock in the morning. I know how his doctors at the VA and University hospitals and Mrs. J all tried to help him. If we could have a dollar an hour for what we did, we would literally have been able to stop working.

Dr. A: One of the big failures in Ernie's case, probably the thing that tipped the balance toward his death, came when he just couldn't cut it on home hemodialysis. He was doing fine from the medical-technical point of view. He just goofed it up.

Ernie became increasingly unresponsive to the efforts of his family and friends. He dreaded and avoided his hemodialysis treatments and, as his family saw him, began not to care whether he lived or died.

Ernie's mother: Toward the end, Ernie said if he had it to do over again, he'd never have gone on the hemodialysis machine the first time. He said he'd never relive that suffering no matter how much money he had. . . . He had nightmares about having to go on that machine. I'd hear him crying and moaning in his sleep, and he'd tell he'd dreamt that the tubes were strangling him. It was horrible. . . . Unless you have a child of your own, you can't imagine what it was like to know that his life depended on that machine. I'd have given my life to spare him that suffering.

Ernie's sister: Though Ernie sometimes felt alone, we were with him. Those last few months, when he was so sick, one of us was always with him at the hospital, around the clock. . . . The way he suffered was terrible, day after day. A lot of it may have been self-made—Ernie could have been a lot more comfortable if he hadn't abused the gifts of the heart from so many people. But a lot of his suffering was also due to the operations and tests and dialyses. . . . His lack of responsibility was why he wouldn't learn how to run the home dialysis machine. He was afraid of it, and wanted someone else to be in charge of it. . . . He always hated to go into the dialysis room at the hospital. He'd plead with me, "Don't ever let them do that to me again. . . ." After he lost the transplant, he just started to give up.

In the second week of July a new, excruciating problem was added to the load Ernie was already finding it hard to bear. He learned that his $23,000 fund was almost depleted.

Ernie's sister: Ernie knew that this money was his last resort. People had helped him more than he ever thought possible. He was frightened beyond belief when he was told that the funds were running out. He felt maybe he wasn't worthy of a second appeal. He'd call me, and say, "I'm going to die. The doctors tell me I can only get a few more dialyses unless I raise some money."

Ernie's mother: Ernie was supposed to be on dialysis three times a week. But he said, "I can't afford it twice a week, so what would happen if I went three times a week?" He was always worried about the money part of it. I think that's why he didn't report for dialysis a lot of times; he was trying to stretch out his treatments. . . . When he knew the money was almost gone, he'd lie in bed and say he felt like it was all over for him now, and he couldn't ask all those poor people who'd given him money to do it again. He just gave up, from the way he acted and the things he said. He was an unhappy boy. Those last two weeks, his attitude was. "I don't care. No one can help me anymore."

Ernie's physicians at the University Hospital met with his fund raisers, Mr. D and Mrs. J, to tell them the news and to explore with them the agonizing issue the doctors now faced: given his personal and medical record, should Ernie continue to receive treatment once his funds were exhausted? Mrs. J was bitter and angry because the physicians might now deny Ernie treatment. But slowly she and Mr. D also began to perceive the full facts of Ernie's case and to appreciate the complex problems facing his physicians.

Mrs. J: I knew we had problems with Ernie, but I had no idea how severe they were. I was really distressed that the hospital waited until the money was about gone before they told us. In view of the fact that we went to all the trouble of raising that money, we should have been notified how fast it was being used up. In retrospect, though, I don't think it would have done any good even if we had known. I think Ernie had really become suicidal at that point. The doctors told us there would be another meeting of the hospital board to determine what their responsibility was about giving him treatment if he showed up for dialysis. . . . I said, "Well, are we to be involved in having to decide he's going to die? When I worked so hard to save his life, I don't think it's right; I don't like it."

Mr. D: When Mrs. J and I met with the people at the hospital, we for the first time began to understand some of the painful questions that the doctors have to cope with. And I think we probably made a decision at that point that there was probably nothing more that we could do for Ernie. But it was very tough for us. We're bleeding hearts, both of us.

At their meeting with the University Hospital physicians, Mrs. J also learned that just that day Ernie and his wife had separated again. "I called his wife," Mrs. J related, "and I said, 'Did you know that Ernie hasn't had treatment for a week, and that he's going to be dead if he doesn't go in for dialysis?' And she said, 'Well, I don't know where he is.' She became quite upset, and I told her, 'You'd better find him, and tell him to get treatment if he wants to live, and tell him the hospital is going to decide in the next week or two whether to keep treating him.' Then I called Mr. D and told him, 'I can't buy this, permitting Ernie to die.' I told him to call Ernie's wife, too, and also to call his mother. When he talked to the mother, she told him that at 3 o'clock that morning she had put Ernie and a girl friend on the train to come back to Seattle. So we located the girl friend's apartment, and went there and told Ernie to get a dialysis, which he did."

After this dialysis, Ernie again skipped his scheduled treatment at the VA hospital. Then, on 18 July, "after heavy alcohol intake," he attempted to rob a restaurant at the Hilton Hotel, telling the cashier, "there's a bomb on every floor." He was arrested on the spot, charged with "creating a disturbance," and taken to jail. A few hours later, Ernie began complaining of abdominal pain and nausea. The police took him to a nearby hospital, and he was then sent to the University Hospital for dialysis. "The patient," his chart states, "was given one run of hemodialysis and discharged to the Police Department."

Ernie was in prison for about one week. During that time, he was taken under guard to the VA hospital for dialysis. His sister was with him during his last treatment. "He told me he knew he only had money for two more dialyses. He was just beaten, with no money and divorcing his wife. He said, 'I can't take this any more. I'm not going to be dialyzed again. I'm going to go out and drink myself into oblivion. No one cares any more. The only thing that worries me are all those little kids who sent me money.' "

According to newspaper accounts, Ernie's brief tenure in jail ended when the prison authorities "allowed him to forfeit a $50.00 bond." His release, in part, was prompted by the efforts of Mrs. J. "After the Hilton robbery, I had one of the agency people go down and talk to the probation people, and tell them

Ernie couldn't stay in jail for very long because he had a kidney problem. Then, they just let him out." Upon his release, Ernie disappeared.

While Ernie's friends and family searched for him, his physicians at the University Hospital met "to decide what we were going to do when Ernie came back." They spent long, soul-searching hours over what is perhaps the most complex, difficult issue they can face: the overt termination of a patient's treatment. As it applied to Ernie Crowfeather, however, their discussion was academic. Ernie did not return. He disappeared, taking with him $2,000. This money included a large check for his treatment at the VA hospital, which he had somehow intercepted and cashed.

Ernie's sister: Ernie knew one of us would make him report for a dialysis. That's why he disappeared those last few days, so we couldn't make him do it. Before he left, one of my sisters did take him to the hospital for a treatment. She left him at a motel in Seattle, and he waited awhile and then caught a plane back to Yakima. Then he vanished. I found out that he left some money for his wife, and bought her some clothes, and paid back some of his friends, and just gave some money to other friends. He only had a few dollars left in his wallet.

He called me at my home on 29 July, from a motel in Ellensburg. I'd been going out of my mind for a day and a half, because no one could find him. He told me he'd seen a doctor in Ellensburg the night before, and that day, because he was so sick from not having been dialyzed. Then he said, "I'm so alone. I can't go back to the University Hospital, because they won't help me anymore." I told him he was wrong, that Dr. B would help him. Then I called Dr. B, and told him I'd found Ernie and could I bring him back to Seattle. Dr. B said, "I'll be here." I got to Ernie's motel in Ellensburg as fast as I could, and took him right to the emergency room at the Ellensburg Hospital. He died there, about 11:00 that night.

VII. Reflections

Ernie's University Hospital psychiatrist: When it was all over, I remember I had a certain sense of relief; this death was necessary, was the feeling. There was nothing in it for Ernie. I liked him very much, but I could not feel sad when I heard he had died. I just asked myself, "What was the meaning of his life?"

For a person like Ernie, almost no physician will have the courage to turn off the machine while he is in the hospital. Not because it wouldn't seem like the right decision, but because to explain the decision, if called upon to do so afterward, would be so complicated. . . . If Ernie had made it back here from

Ellensburg, I think he would have been dialyzed again. Fortunately, doctors haven't been confronted with too many Ernie Crowfeathers, yet.

Dr. G of the Kidney Center: If Ernie hadn't died in Ellensburg, if he'd come back, and been presented a third time here, I think we would have rejected him again. I think that just everything Ernie did the last year he lived, after we rejected him the second time, emphasized the fact that the Kidney Center had made the right decision on this individual.

Mrs. J, the fund raiser: It was worth it to me, and I think to all the people who became involved. Ernie was a guy in trouble, and we did something about it.

I think in a way that Ernie had a strong will to live, and a strong will to die. . . . An Indian counselor told me that the strong message she had gotten from Ernie was that he sat by and watched life happen, but he didn't see himself as part of life. That is probably as good a description of Ernie as any.

I felt that everything was done in the system to keep Ernie from living, even the way he was. The recurring theme was that this guy wasn't worth it, why waste time on him when you could save a lot of other people. Who's entitled to say who is to live and who is to die? You know, there's no priority on who should live.

Mr. D, the fund raiser: Ernie really had more than his chance. There were so many of us who bent over backward. He wouldn't accept psychiatric help. He wouldn't even learn how to run the dialysis machine. . . . We couldn't have raised the money again, nor do I think we would have. Ernie didn't want to live, and I can understand that.

Ernie's mother: I think that if Ernie had had some money, and felt more secure, he wouldn't have given up. He had a lot of fight, but he just felt like, here I am, I'm going to die. This worked on him; no one likes to die.

Ernie's sister: Ernie wasn't self-pitying, but he often said, "Why does all this have to happen to me?" I think it might have taken a person like Ernie to go through what he did. . . . Ernie did a lot of living in his life, and I think he died the way he would have wanted to. My mind might be more at ease if I really knew why Ernie abused and hurt himself and others so. I feel there's something unfinished about Ernie's life.

Dr. Belding Scribner: One major thing I think I've learned from Ernie's case is that the selection system has worked, at least in Seattle, because the principals involved are willing to let it work. What is selection, basically? It's the decision by somebody on some grounds that a person will not be permitted dialysis, or a transplant, which says in effect that he must now die. And the system works because the doctor involved, or the family, or the patient himself, recognizes that this is a rational decision, a form of euthanasia, if you will.

But I also know that anybody who wants to beat the system can do it. A lot of people more deserving than Ernie get selected out because they're "dumb bunnies," too "square" to question or try to manipulate the system. Ernie went outside the system to get treated. And this posed a terrible problem for the University Hospital, because we're not supposed to touch anybody who isn't appointed by the Kidney Center. We have no mechanism for funding, and we don't know how to handle somebody who comes in with $20,000 and says, "I want to be treated." If you have money, there's no system. Nobody is going to let you die if you have money.

The selection system probably isn't going to hold up very well much longer. The public, or average guy, is going to become more and more aware of what the selection process really means, and the more awareness there is, the more difficult it's going to be to select. In the long run, it's going to be a lot simpler to put everybody on dialysis, an Ernie included, and hopefully let them kill themselves in due course if that's what they want to do. It's the only rational way to solve this selection problem. Working through this whole issue of selection, at least in this culture, is infinitely more difficult than just putting a few losers on among the 95% that will do reasonably well. Selection then will take the form of advising the patient and his family that we don't think this treatment is right for him, that it would be a fate worse than death to dialyze or transplant him. If the patient doesn't agree, he'll be taken regardless of the expense or the difficulty. The alternative is the route we went for two years with Ernie, which is intolerable for everybody.

When we met to discuss Ernie's case, just before his death, I felt that if anybody was to blame for the jam the University Hospital was in, it was the failure of the penal system to be able to cope with the situation. They abdicated their responsibility completely. If anybody had held up the Hilton and said there was a bomb on every floor, he would have been in a fairly precarious position legally. But they just let Ernie out in a few days, because he was so sick and they didn't want to assume the responsibility for his treatment.[2]

Why can't we figure out a way to terminate a patient when it seems reasonable to do so, when he's indicated that he wants it, too. It really isn't fair to a person to prejudge his ability to cope with dialysis. And yet we do this because we're afraid to get locked into a situation we won't know how to handle. We can't get out once we start. But for some reason, if you don't start a guy, if you don't get really involved with him, the fact you know he is going to die, and then does, doesn't seem to bother you so much. But once you've seen him on the machine, and walking around, then the thought of not dialyzing him and having him die just becomes overpowering.

When we had those last meetings about Ernie, just before he died in Ellensburg, a lot of people spent a lot of time deciding what the hell we were really going to do if he came back. We finally agreed that we would literally have never pulled the plug on Ernie, or anybody else. I said at that meeting, "I really don't think we can kill Ernie. I just can't see the logic of killing Ernie Crowfeather." I know it would have probably been best for everybody, but when I thought about it in the most basic ethical way I am capable of, I said I really don't think we can let Ernie die. It's so foreign to the total effort we make that it just about undoes you to even contemplate how you would go about it. Here's Ernie walking down the street. Sure he robs banks, but he's a nice guy, and people like him. But even liking him isn't important. He's a person who's alive, and you know you can keep him that way. And suddenly you're asked to say, "Okay, this is it. You can't be alive any more."

If Ernie had come back again, we would have treated him. But that would have been begging the question. As long as an Ernie Crowfeather succeeds in beating the system, it indicates that we're not ready to handle the problem of priorities and selection.

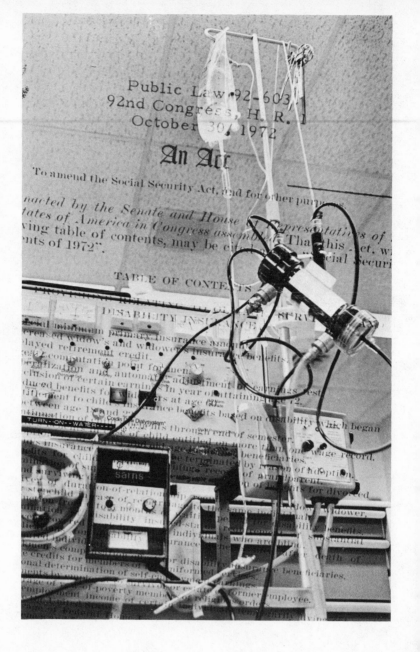

4

*Changing Perspectives on
Transplantation and Dialysis*

10

Transplantation in the 1970s: A Revised Paradigm of Therapeutic Innovation

In certain respects, the evolution of organ transplantation since 1970 has varied from the process of therapeutic innovation we depicted in Part 1, based on the earlier stages of the field's development. The patterns of its movement (and nonmovement) along the experiment-therapy spectrum during the past eight years not only are historically interesting, but also make it more apparent than ever that the experiment-to-therapy process is neither a simple, linear progression, totally conscious, entirely logical and rational, nor altogether biomedically determined.

A primary purpose of this chapter is to update the transplantation picture by focusing consecutively on kidney, heart, liver, and bone-marrow grafting. We not only will consider the most recent phases of organ transplantation but will also compare the evolution that the transplantation of different organs has undergone. Our two major axes of comparison are the medical status of the various forms of transplantation and the medical profession's outlook on them. Medical status includes the nature and outcome of laboratory and clinical activities. By outlook we mean the attitudes, ideology, and goals of the professionals engaged in transplantation: how they view the issues of "patient selection," "clinical management," and "successful and unsuccessful" outcomes; what they define as the state of their field and its major tasks and challenges; and their perspectives on the psychological, social, and cultural dimensions of transplantation. Our analysis demonstrates that a two-way relationship exists between the biomedical aspects of transplantation and its prevailing ethos. This is apparent, for example, in the issues surrounding patient selection. It is also exemplified by the degree to which the medical status of organ transplantation at a given stage in its development determines the nature of the psychological, social, and cultural phenomena confronting professionals and patients and, reciprocally, the extent to which these phenomena influence biomedical attitudes and behavior.

Our analysis has led us to revise and refine the paradigm of therapeutic innovation that we have developed and used in our work on the history and sociology of biomedical research. Our intent has been to work out a more detailed and predictive model of therapeutic innovation that will have theoretical value for the sociology of science and also be useful in making clinical and policy decisions about medical trials.

Virtually all forms of human organ transplantation—kidney, heart, liver, lung, pancreas, and bone-marrow grafts—are still exclusively carried out on patients in the end stage of their diseases, who have failed to respond to more fully established, conventional medical and surgical therapies, or who can no longer be expected to benefit from them. Even renal transplantation is no exception to this rule. For although a few nephrologists have continued to advocate transplants for patients who have not reached end-stage renal failure, the procedure has not so far been carried out on such patients.

Furthermore, exhortations in favor of such trials seem to have waned somewhat, as has the militant way some physician-investigators championed the advantages of renal transplantation, in continuing debate with counterparts who enthusiastically and sometimes passionately favored hemodialysis. A less strident, more balanced and philosophical-sounding tone now predominates in the medical literature:

In recent years, the proper interlocking, as opposed to competing roles of dialysis and transplantation have been recognized and exploited. . . . The new ground rules have permitted either transplantation or dialysis to be considered part of the same continuum of care for renal failure. . . . The mortality should be less and the quality of life should be greater with combined dialysis and transplantation than with either treatment alone. . . . It is self-evident that neither technique is perfect for chronic care. [Starzl, Weil, and Putnam 1977, pp. 6-7]

The optimistic talk among kidney transplanters in the 1960s about how well cadaver organ grafts were functioning after one or two years, and how likely they were to be "good for a decade" has diminished. General recognition of the impermanence of nonrelated cadaver kidneys compared with those transplanted from living related donors has been firmly if somewhat regretfully established. A great deal of energy now goes into efforts to improve transplantation and to place it and the treatments associated with it on a rational rather than an empirical basis. In this connection, tissue and blood typing and several methods of organ preservation are being further explored, as are the effects on transplantation of blood transfusions, presensitization, splenectomy, and chronic dialysis. Various preoperative and postoperative monitoring techniques—largely immunologic in nature or involving radionuclide scanning—are being reported. Above all, attention is focused on the forms of immunosuppressive therapy now in use, and on what Starzl has called their "devastating effectiveness" (Starzl, Weil, and Putnam 1977, p. 7). By and large, techniques of immunosuppression instituted in the mid-1960s are still being employed and examined, for no promising new approaches have been found. There is a considerable amount of collective concern about the many unwanted side effects of chronic immunosuppression and their relationship to patient mortality. The high incidence of neoplasms, especially lymphomas, in transplant recipients is under continuous scrutiny. Attempts to better understand and manage the complications of chronic immunosuppression go on, against the background of what the Thirteenth Report of the Human Renal Transplant Registry calls a general, fieldwide "shift toward earlier reduction of immunosuppression in selected patients so that . . . infectious complications can be controlled" (Thirteenth Report 1977, p. 15). The profound influence on the direction of cancer research that elucidation of the cancerogenic effects of immunosuppression could have, and the "consolation" this could provide are mentioned only occasionally, in a quiet, circumspect way (Billingham 1977, p. xliv). And even less frequently is it claimed that new insights into the mechanisms of glomerular diseases have resulted from the study of the transplanted kidney (Hamburger 1977, p. 1316).

The composite picture of renal transplantation in the 1970s that emerges is of a field still concentrating on persistent clinical problems that began about fifteen years ago—a field that has reached a plateau. This impression is confirmed by the conclusions of the American College of Surgeons/National Institutes of Health

Organ Transplant Registry Report for 1977. The report acknowledges that during the period it covers, 1963 to 1976, some individual centers have made progress in the outcomes of the kidney transplants they have performed, and the mortality in cadaver-graft recipients has decreased. Nevertheless, it goes on to say that "from the international and collective view . . . there has been remarkably little improvement in the results of renal transplantation. This is true when one compares year-by-year statistics and also when results of transplantation from individual institutions are analyzed." Present-day renal transplantations results are described as similar to those that have been periodically reported in the past with regard to the primary criteria of "success and/or failure" used by transplanters: the functional survival of grafts, patient survival, and patient mortality.

There has been, however, a major shift in renal transplantation during the 1970s, in the realm of patient selection. It is one of the most striking and significant ways the present cycle renal transplantation is undergoing differs from the experiment-to-therapy sequence we formulated in chapter 3. As predicted, the selection criteria for renal transplantation have become more inclusive biomedically, socially, and psychologically. But rather than offering kidney transplants to patients who are *less* gravely and irreversibly ill, the selection process has moved in the opposite direction. In the course of the 1970s, the conditions for renal transplantation have been so "liberalized" or "relaxed" (to use the medical profession's own terms), that the procedure is carried out on what Thomas Starzl calls "all risk" as well as "good risk" teminal patients. These include a sizable number of older recipients (in their late fifties and sixties, and even some in their seventies and eighties), and patients with diabetes mellitus, coronary heart disease, and previous malignancies.

The "interlocking" rather than "competing" perspective that now prevails on the roles of renal transplantation and dialysis has contributed to this shift. For the "better appreciation of the interrelationship between transplantation and dialysis" has played a part in motivating physicians to be less "aggressive" in using immunosuppressive treatment to forestall rejection of the transplanted organ. The trend toward "earlier reduction" in immunosuppressive drug therapy grows out of a diminishing tendency for physicians to regard "the prospect of homograft failure with return to dialysis [as] a grim and unacceptable one for many people" (Starzl, Weil, and Putnam 1977, p. 6), along with their greater awareness of the life-threatening complications that can result from chronic immunosuppression:

the sometimes devastating effectiveness of all forms of treatment now in use was attested to by 22 abstracts [submitted to the 1976 Program Committee of the Transplantation Society] detailing the complications of chronic immunosuppression. These included cancer; gastrointestinal ulcerations; viral, bacterial, and fungal infections; hypersplenism; hyperparathyroidism; cataracts; bone diseases; liver malfunction; hyperlipidemia; and vascular disease. The central objective of research in our specialty remains the achievement of graft acceptance with lesser penalties than are now exacted. [Starzl, Weil, and Putnam 1977, p. 7]

I believe that in the past we have overtreated our patients by trying to keep the kidney from being rejected. . . . We have stopped this overly aggressive approach. Now we will save the patient even if the kidney is rejected. . . . Lowering the mortality after transplantation is essential. . . . The first policy should be to obtain the highest patient survival rather than the highest graft survival. [Belzer, in "End-stage diabetic nephropathy 1974," p. S-136]

In some transplant groups, these changes in treatment policy seem to have brought about some decrease in patient mortality as well as graft mortality (Thirteenth Report 1977, p. 15), and this in turn has helped embolden physicians to carry out renal transplants on older and sicker patients with more complex primary and secondary disease states.

As we will argue in chapter 11, however, economic factors rather than biomedical ones have been principally responsible for alterations in patient selection policies. The passage of Public Law 92-603 in 1972, providing Medicare financing for transplantation and dialysis, has fostered not only the suspension of the kinds of psychological criteria that were employed in the 1960s but a relaxation of biomedical contraindications as well.

In our view, the situation has now progressed to the stage where it has become difficult for physicians to "deselect" any patient in irreversible renal failure for a transplant (or dialysis), regardless of how little benefit he or she may be expected to derive from the treatment, how much added suffering it may entail, and what additional problems it may create for allocation of scarce resources.

Within the medical profession, as we will see in chapter 11, patients with advanced diabetes mellitus as well as terminal kidney disease have become an important focus of these "deselection" issues.

Unlike renal transplantation, patient selection for cardiac transplantation has become even more exigent and rigorous. At Stanford University Medical Center, where most of the world's heart transplants are carried out, all patients chosen as potential cardiac recipients are less than fifty years of age ("the younger, the better") and have end-stage cardiac disease with class IV cardiac status, secondary to either angina pectoris or congestive heart failure. Any possibility that they might respond to other intensive medical or surgical therapies has been ruled out. These are gravely handicapped, dying persons, capable only of a "bed-chair" existence, whose life expectancy has been estimated as weeks to months, with a poor prognosis for a six-month survival. However desperately ill candidates may be in these respects, they are considered ineligible for cardiac transplantations if they have other systemic diseases. Active infection of any kind, recent pulmonary infarction, or severe pulmonary hypertension are also regarded as contraindications to the transplant procedure.

Nor is it sufficient that the patient meet these criteria for age, severity of illness, and lack of physical contraindications. To be placed on the list of those awaiting cardiac transplants at the Stanford Center, he or she must meet psychological criteria that the Stanford cardiac transplant group feels provide "reasonable expectation that additional time gained by transplantation would be meaningfully used by the patient, rather than be perceived as simply an extension of the dying process." Has the patient demonstrated emotional stability in response to past and current illness? How did he cope with the coronary care unit, for example? Has he taken medications faithfully and followed medical recommendations? Has he been able to manage risky, independent things well? Does he have any history of psychiatric illness, recurrent situational depression, denial of symptoms, severe family conflict, drug or alcohol addiction? (Addiction is defined as a contraindication for further transplant consideration.) Does the patient have a "strong desire to live," evidenced by family activities and relationships he is eager to resume, work or studies he wants to return to, personal goals he wishes to attain? Does he have a strong, supportive family, willing and able to withstand the apprehension, anxiety, fear, waiting, fatigue, separation, euphoria, disappointment, and grief that the different phases of cardiac transplantation entail? Does the family have enough strength to provide continuing support to the patient as well as to manage the stresses of cardiac transplantation themselves?

The Stanford group systematically collects data on these questions from physicians, nurses, and social workers who have cared for the patient and known his family. But in the extensive and intensive screening to which they subject candidates, they attach particular importance to the information they gather and the impressions they form in the course of face-to-face discussions with the patient and his family. In this psychosocial evaluation, which often lasts several days and is both supportive and probative, the chief social worker plays a key role. The patient and his family are given the opportunity to talk to other transplant recipients and their relatives if they wish, and a special effort is made not only to appraise the quality of their consent to a transplant but to provide them with ample opportunity to decide to abandon the idea.

Finally, only those candidates who can meet the sizable financial costs are considered for the procedure. The Stanford group estimates that the average hospital costs for cardiac transplantation itself are approximately $30,000, while living costs (rent and food) in the Palo Alto area are at least $400 a month for one person. The terms of the grant awarded to Stanford by the federal funding agency stipulate that grant funds can be used only to supplement the patient's insurance coverage for the actual transplant operation and for subsequent follow-up care. These financial criteria are viewed by the Stanford transplant team as more than economic, although they would welcome additional funds for the transportation and living expenses of patients and families. The criteria are also regarded as psychological and social measures of the motivation of the patient and his family to commit themselves to a transplant, with all the risks, sacrifices, and nonmaterial costs it entails, as well as its monetary expenses (Rider et al. 1975, pp. 531-39; Christopherson, Griepp, and Stinson 1976, pp. 2082-84; Christopherson 1976, pp. 58-71; Schroeder 1977; Christopherson, personal interview).

In sum, the only persons considered eligible for heart transplants at present not only are terminally ill with cardiac disease, but have no other major medical problems and are endowed with exceptional psychological, interpersonal, social, and financial strengths and resources. So far as patient selection criteria are concerned, it seems, the only attribute cardiac and renal transplantation now share is that potential patients must be in the end stage of disease. Even here, heart transplant candidates can be said to be closer to death than patients considered for kidney transplants. Why has the selection process for cardiac transplantation become more stringent and exclusive while the selection process for renal transplantation has become more "liberalized" and inclusive?

Though federal funding of renal transplantation has been important in the relaxing and expanding of selection criteria, the major determinants of the guidelines established for choosing cardiac transplant recipients seem to be largely medical. To begin with, there are more clearly defined, undisputed indications in the 1970s than there were in the 1960s that cardiac transplantation is in an earlier stage of development on the experiment-to-therapy continuum than is renal transplantation. Although occasionally a transplant surgeon quietly predicts a reawakening of interest in heart transplantation, or says it will "rise again," one no longer hears the enthusiastic claims for its current therapeutic applicability and value that were so frequently voiced by Christiaan Barnard, Denton Cooley, and like figures in the 1960s. The most positive statements currently made about cardiac transplantation are cautiously optimistic and carefully qualified: "for a very few patients, under very special conditions, heart transplantation can be a rational and socially acceptable therapy, although it is obviously only a transitional and temporary answer to the problem of chronic end-stage heart disease" (Austen 1978, p. 682).

A quasi-moratorium on human heart transplantation still exists throughout the world. For example, only 31 operations were performed in 1976, 21 of them by Shumway's team. And, compared with the 167 transplants from 3 December 1967 through 1970, only 166 were done in the six-year period from 1971 to March 1977. Shumway and his group have carried out 99 of these transplants, and Cabrol in Paris and Barnard in South Africa are the only other surgeons who have consistently done several each year since 1971.

Although Shumway and the Stanford team are scrupulous about "publicly conveying the idea that [they] don't have the exclusive right" to be performing heart transplants (Christopherson, personal interview), the fact that they carry out virtually all such procedures in the United States, and a large proportion of those that occur globally, inevitably means that the medical guidelines they have established for themselves predominate in the field. Shumway's program is based on the kind of clinical research protocol that has been designed not only to investigate and evaluate certain post-transplant problems, but also to identify and control as many factors as possible that might adversely affect graft and patient survival and the psychological and social, as well as the physical, rehabilitation of patients who survive cardiac transplantation for six months or longer. Stanford interweaves sophisticated patient selection and postoperative treatment research with intensive animal studies.

Both because of their selection criteria and because of their commitment to follow their survivors closely and "indefinitely," the Stanford team has performed relatively few heart transplants (126 on 121 patients through February 1977). But their policy of trying to achieve the highest levels of survival and quality of life affects a much larger patient population. In 1976, for example, 276 patients were referred to the Stanford group as potential transplant candidates, and such referrals seem to be increasing. Through contacts with these patients, their families, their physicians, and other medical professionals who have cared for them, as well as through articles and reports, the Stanford group widely disseminates its approach. In addition, they are continually consulted by hospitals and medical centers interested in cardiac transplantation or in possibly starting a program of their own. The Stanford team encourages these inquiries and consultations, partly because they genuinely feel that they have "worked hard, and learned important information" that they "should share with others" in the spirit of a "national resource" (personal communication). It also grows out of their sensitivity to the fact that, because of their specialized and privileged role in cardiac transplantation, they could easily be seen as monopolizing the field in their own interests. They actively try to prevent this. Although they assiduously avoid giving "cookbook formulas" based on their own experience to colleagues who confer with them and above all "avoid answering the question whether another group *ought* to begin such a program," Stanford freely distributes its guidelines and statistical data and invites interested professionals to visit the center for firsthand observation, discussion, and study of patient charts.

Stanford has received a new five-year, multimillion-dollar grant from the National Institutes of Health to continue its clinical research program. Because it is the only cardiovascular surgery group in the world so massively subsidized for human cardiac transplantation, one might argue that federal funding has been a decisive factor in establishing the patient selection criteria now used for heart transplants, as well as for kidney transplants. But evidence indicates that Shumway and his colleagues received their support *after* they had already developed the guidelines and criteria they now use and, to a significant degree, *because* they have established their program on these premises. In this sense, the funding constitutes post hoc approval of the Stanford group's orientation and also provides a special mandate to work with the focused, exclusive, rigorous clinical research model to which they were already committed. Behind this, of course, lies the history of human heart transplants, with its successive "miracle of Cape Town," "international bandwagon," "decline," and "moratorium" phases; its high mortality rate; the failure to develop an artificial heart with the life-sustaining capacities of the artificial kidney machines, as a backup and alternative to cardiac transplantation; and the ever-present fact that although Christiaan Barnard performed the world's first human heart transplant, it was Norman Shumway who developed the surgical method that made it possible.

Like renal transplantation, the field of human heart transplantation, principally under the aegis of Shumway's group, is focused on improving postoperative treatment. Overall improvement is defined primarily as extending the longevity of patients and, second, enhancing the quality of rehabilitation attained by those who have survived more than six months. Though both cardiac and renal transplantation are affected by the fundamental stalemate with respect to the rejection reaction and immunosuppression, cardiac transplantation has not reached a plateau in the same way that kidney grafting has. Under the highly controlled clinical research conditions that Shumway and his team have established, a progressive increase in patient survival has become apparent. According to actuarial statistics calculated for their entire cardiac transplantation series, from January 1968 to February 1977, 121 patients received 127 transplants with one- to six-year survival rates of 53 percent, 44 percent, 35 percent, 24 percent, and 17 percent (personal communication). "Most striking is the change in early survival between patients operated on from 1974 to 1975 and all previously operated patients" (Griepp et al. 1977, p. 197). The one-year survival rate of patients who have received heart transplants since 1974 has become 69 percent, compared with 22 percent in 1968 (personal communication). "Late survival," defined as two years or more, has also increased since the initial 1968 to 1969 period, although "at the present time this difference . . . does not quite achieve statistical significance" (Griepp et al. 1977, p. 198).

The Stanford group has systematically set out to increase the survival of heart transplant recipients, by identifying, manipulating, and managing the major factors responsible for postoperative mortality. They have come far enough along in their clinical research program to be able to single out key elements that they believe account for the "enhanced patient survival" and "decreased patient mortality" they have achieved:

The major factors responsible for decreased mortality appear to be improved management of acute rejection episodes by utilizing endomyocardial biopsy for diagnosis and rabbit antihuman thymocyte globulin for treatment. Improvement in long-term survival has been effected by control of graft arteriosclerosis with a regimen of antithrombotic therapy and control of dietary lipids. Cardiac retransplantation appears to be a reasonable option both in patients with unremitting acute rejection injury and in patients who develop obliterative graft arteriosclerosis in the late postoperative period. [Griepp et al. 1977, pp. 200–201]

With the possible exception of the understanding of the pathogenesis of graft arteriosclerosis the Stanford program has reached, their advances have been very specific, dealing with clinical management, with few direct or even indirect implications for arriving at new insights into the end-stage cardiac diseases for which heart transplants are done, for achieving a more basic, general understanding of rejection, or for attaining what Paul Russell describes as "the long-awaited step of planned specific alteration of recipient responsiveness." The global effect of the clinical progress made in cardiac transplantation is that "the success rates . . . obtained by several experienced teams have now become comparable to those reported for renal transplantation from unrelated donors" (Billingham 1977, p. xliv). In this respect, human heart transplantation has not only significantly "exceeded" the early results in the field of kidney transplantation but has also surpassed those currently reported for liver transplantation.

Comparing the slow, steady improvement in the results of cardiac transplantation with the "holding pattern" trend in renal transplantation, cardiac transplantation appears to be in a stage of development where it has room to "catch up" with renal transplantation, whether or not a "breakthrough" occurs in the realm of rejection and immunosuppression. Furthermore, heart transplantation is currently proceeding under clinical research conditions that are potentially more conducive to improving patient survival than those that surround kidney transplantation. Only a few highly experienced teams regularly do heart transplants; several of these have well-conceived clinical research protocols; the number of transplants performed is highly restricted; and patient selection is not only tightly controlled, but also geared to choosing recipients with the best prognosis for survival. In addition, although the transplanted heart has turned out to be as prone to rejection as the transplanted kidney, it has proved to be a "privileged organ" in certain respects relevant to improving the management of acute rejection. For example, whereas the biopsy technique used by the Stanford group to diagnose acute rejection injury and to monitor antirejection therapy caused a significant incidence of hemorrhagic and infectious complications in the transplanted kidney, it proved "extremely safe" when applied to the heart (Griepp et al. 1977, p. 198).

Finally, as we will discuss more fully, the improvement reported in heart transplantation may also be related to certain social-system attributes characteristic of the few teams remaining in the field, especially the quality of their commitment, solidarity, and morale.

At present, according to transplant surgeon R. Y. Calne, liver transplantation occupies "third . . . place in the 'therapeutic batting order' " (Calne 1977, p. 215), behind renal and cardiac transplantation. With this competitive sports image, Calne refers to the number of liver transplants performed on patients, the duration of their postoperative survival, how long their grafts function, and how well physicians understand and can control the factors that cause the deaths of liver transplant recipients. In all these ways, liver transplantation is closer to the experimental end of the experiment-to-therapy "scale" than either kidney or heart transplantation. But in other regards, such as patient selection, it falls somewhere between the current status of these two other major types of organ grafts. It was on 1 March 1963 that Thomas Starzl performed the first human liver transplant, twelve years after the start of kidney transplants and four years before the start of human cardiac grafts. The relatively modest number of 292 liver transplantations that have been performed over the course of its fourteen-year history is due to a number of factors. Thus far, only 41 surgical teams have undertaken the procedure, compared with the 65 teams that have done 333 heart transplants and the 301 teams that have conducted more than 25,000 kidney transplants. The "heavy, overall mortality" associated with liver transplantation and the "formidable" technical or mechanical problems it has entailed have "retarded the acceptance of this procedure" (Calne 1977, p. 210; Starzl et al. 1976, p. 487).

The procedure's high mortality rate—only 15 percent of patients have survived for a year—has not only discouraged surgeons from attempting liver transplants but also was responsible for the temporary and partial halt from 1964 to 1967, which significantly reduced the total number of liver transplants performed. Thomas Starzl had done five of the first seven grafts, and in the face of the immediate as well as overwhelming mortality of his patients (0 to 23 days), he decided to stop carrying out the procedure on human beings and to "go back to the laboratory" to better understand why it had failed (Starzl, personal communication). From 1964 to 1967 only 22 human liver transplants were done, by teams other than Starzl's. Starzl did not reenter the clinical field of liver transplantation until he was convinced he had made significant laboratory progress in management as well as in identifying the primary causes of recipients' deaths. Once he resumed human liver grafting the number of transplants per year rose markedly (for example, 39 in 1968 and 46 in 1969). Even so, from 1968 through 1975 the average number of liver transplants performed annually in the world has been no more than 19 (with a range of 46 in 1969 to 15 in 1971).

As the foregoing suggests, the field of liver transplantation, like that of cardiac transplantation, is heavily influenced by the approach and outlook of several research physician-surgeons. Their philosophies and policies as well as their techniques prevail. Thomas Starzl is the paramount liver transplant surgeon. He developed the procedure and launched it on human beings, and his group at the University of Colorado Medical Center has done the largest number of orthotopic liver transplants in the world (106 grafts as of February 1976). He took the initiative of calling a moratorium on his own pioneering efforts. And he has consistently defined the ethical as well as the surgical and medical review of his liver transplantation endeavors as his public, professional responsibility. The next most influential surgical group performing liver transplants at this time is probably the Cambridge/King's College team in England, led by R. Y. Calne, R. Waldram, and R. Williams. They have carried out the second largest series of orthotopic liver transplants in the world (50 patients as of May 1976). And, like Starzl and his colleagues, they have been not only "doers" of transplants, but also conscientious observers and concerned evaluators.

The patient selection policies practiced by these two teams are representative of those followed by most liver transplantation groups, which in turn have been significantly influenced by the approaches of Starzl, Calne, and their associates. "In theory," as Calne pointed out, "anyone dying from disease primarily confined to the liver would be a potential candidate for liver transplantation" (Calne 1977, p. 209). And, in fact, liver transplantation has been performed on patients with a wide range of end-stage hepatic diseases. The most common conditions for which liver transplantation has been done are biliary atresia, primary hepatic malignant tumor, chronic aggressive hepatitis, and alcoholic cirrhosis. In addition, it has been tried on a small number of patients with certain inborn errors of metabolism. Although confined to terminal, liver-associated conditions, liver transplantation is applied to a more diverse group of primary diseases than either renal or cardiac transplantation. In this regard, as in all others, the medical criteria of heart transplants are the most restrictive of all: confined to patients dying of inoperable coronary artery disease or congestive heart failure. Even though the patient selection criteria for kidney transplants have become elastic and broadly inclusive, glomerulonephritis still is the primary renal disease with which more than half of the recipients are afflicted. In Starzl's opinion, "None of the diseases for which liver transplantation has been used so far can be categorically excluded as an indication for further trials (Starzl et al. 1976, p. 503). Other surgical groups engaged in liver transplantations are inclined to agree with him on this point.

However, there is one major conviction on which Starzl's choice of recipients has been based that is not shared by all liver transplantation teams. He believes that "children with a wide range of diseases, including biliary atresia" are the "most favorable group of recipients," and that this will be even more true in the future now that microsurgical techniques have "almost completely eliminated . . . the mortality from technical accidents involving vessels that was particularly high in infants with biliary atresia" (Starzl et al. 1976, p. 499). For him, the most important positive conclusion that has emerged from his own experience with liver replacement is that "prolonged survival repeatedly was possible" (as demonstrated by the fact that of the 93 recipients on whom he had performed liver transplants through November 1974, 27 survived from one to six years), and that "many of these patients have been able to return to a full and useful life" (Starzl et al. 1976, p. 487). Twenty of the 27 "survivors" were children. Although Starzl does not feel that the slowly improving "outlook" of liver replacement has yet reached a satisfactory level, he does regard the results with pediatric patients as a far "brighter chapter" in liver transplantation than the "dismal . . . experience with adults with cirrhosis in general and with alcoholic cirrhotics in particular." He also considers the liver transplants he has performed on children to be less "controversial" than the liver replacements he has done on adults with hepatic malignant tumors, for tumor recurrence has been common in patients with primary hepatoma and cholangiocarcinoma (Starzl et al. 1976, pp. 503–4). These are some of the major reasons Starzl has chosen to do more liver transplants on children than on adults. Calne and the Cambridge/King's College group have a different perspective, one that makes them avowedly "reluctant" to do this procedure on children:

Liver grafting is obviously a formidable procedure and the side effects of immunosuppression may be severe. The patients and the relatives require a very full explanation. This may not be possible with children, who cannot appreciate the severity of their disease, the risks of surgery and the unpleasant side effects that will develop, particularly following steroids, and the need for prolonged postoperative hospital surveillance. . . . Following discussions with the parents, it is likely that they will request that every effort be made to save the child. Parents cannot really appreciate the suffering that the child may have to undergo as a result of the graft. For these reasons I am reluctant to advise liver transplantation in young children. [Calne 1977, p. 210]

As a consequence, the Cambridge/King's College series of 50 liver transplants up to May 1976 included only 5 patients aged seventeen and under. One of these was an infant of ten months; the others ranged in age from eleven to seventeen years. Calne affirms that he has "similar views concerning kidney grafting in children."

Apart from these differences concerning child patients, the only "absolute contraindication" for the procedure that seems to be in effect at present is preexisting infection in someone "dying from disease primarily confined to the liver." Experience has shown that "most patients who have received liver grafts, when there has been infection in any part of the body prior to surgery, have died from progressive, uncontrollable infection" (Calne 1977, p. 210). But there are signs in the medical literature that the leading transplant groups may try to institute "more discriminating patient selection" (Starzl et al. 1976, p. 504) in certain respects. Thomas Starzl has expressed the opinion that one of the kinds of progress on which the further development of liver transplantation depends is "reduction of operative and postoperative accident by more discriminating patient selection" (Starzl 1976, p. 504). There are indicators that the criteria used to select adult recipients with cirrhosis or carcinoma of the liver may be tightened up in the future, so that transplant recipients with alcoholic cirrhosis will be chosen from those in a less desperate stage of their terminal disease than previously, and those selected from among patients with hepatic tumors will be free of metastases, though not treatable by the somewhat more conventional means of a partial liver resection. Should liver transplantation evolve in this way, utilizing patient selection criteria that are both stricter and more specific, it will come closer to cardiac transplantation in this regard. At the same time, by choosing certain recipients who are less terminally ill, it would liberalize its selection policy in a way that would advance it further toward the therapy end of the experiment-to-therapy continuum in this one regard than either cardiac or renal transplantation.

Liver transplantation, like renal and cardiac transplantation, is now largely absorbed by the task of "improving results." Under the guiding influence of the several most prominent liver transplant teams, surgeons are striving for "reduction of operative and early postoperative accidents" and for "sharpening the criteria for the differential diagnosis of postoperative hepatic malfunction" (Starzl et al. 1976, p. 504). From the point of view of survival and mortality, liver transplantation is still in a stage of evolution where having a patient live at least one year following the operation is not taken for granted; where the survival of patients for more than a year after transplantation has been reported by only four teams (Starzl et al. 1976, p. 500); and where survival for more than a year is defined as "prolonged" or "chronic" survival. In this connection, Calne has reported that of the 50 patients in the Cambridge/King's College liver transplantation series, 12 survived more than six months; 4 of these lived beyond a year, the longest survivor living five years and three months (Calne 1977, p. 213). The results obtained by Starzl and his group at the University of Colorado are comparable, but somewhat better. Of the 106 patients who received liver grafts in Denver, 26 lived one year or more after transplantation, and (in February 1976) 16 of this group were still alive after more than one to almost six years. The longest survival time of any recipient was six years and three months (Calne 1977, p. 213; Starzl et al. 1976, p. 500).

Although physicians like Starzl do not consider such results satisfactory, they note that there has been a gradual improvement in the outlook for recipients since 1963 (Starzl et al. 1976, pp. 500, 504). For example, in Starzl's own series, the mortality rate has slowly decreased since 1970:

The first 25 recipients who formed the basis of a monograph on liver transplantation included only five one year survivors. The next group of 25 contained six, and the group after that eight. There have already been eight one year survivors among the 18 patients beginning with No. 76. [Starzl et al. 1976, p. 500]

And in a personal interview in the spring of 1977, Starzl reported that only 3 out of the 16 patients on whom he had performed liver transplants during the past year had thus far died. The small, successive increments in the survival of recipients appear to be largely due to improved surgical technique and management.

Here the dynamics of liver transplantation differ markedly from those of renal and cardiac transplantation. The teams engaged in liver grafting have gradually arrived at the conclusion that, in contrast to other types of organ transplantation, neither acute nor chronic rejection has been the main cause of their heavy overall patient mortality. Rejection of the liver accounts for fewer than 10 percent of the deaths in the Denver series, for example, and of the 50 patients in the Cambridge/King's College series, only 4 were considered to have died primarily from rejection. Rather, as indicated earlier, most of the deaths of liver graft patients are now attributed to technical or mechanical problems. Performing liver transplantations has turned out to be more surgically difficult than transplanting either kidneys or hearts, and biliary duct reconstruction has proved the most complex and serious problem associated with the operation. Calne has estimated that "between 30% and 50% of patients have perished as a result of biliary tract disasters," adding that "this figure would probably be higher if patients succumbing in the early postoperative phase had survived long enough to develop biliary complications" (Calne 1977, p. 211). "Even excluding the biliary duct complications," Starzl has gone on to say: "about a fourth of the patients who died left the operating room with situations that were incompatible with survival, such as ischemic liver necrosis, graft vascular thrombosis and uncontrolled hemorrhage. The mortality from technical accidents involving vessels was particularly high in infants with biliary atresia, partly because of the small size of the structure for anastomosis" (Starzl et al. 1976, p. 500).

It is only through an arduous, highly empirical process, costly in patient lives, that surgeons have identified biliary drainage as the "Achilles' heel of liver transplantation" (Calne 1977, p. 211) and developed new bile-duct reconstruction methods that are more adequate and less injurious. The degree to which progress has been made by trial and error is ironically illustrated by the fact that Starzl used what he now considers to be one of the two "preferred methods" for biliary duct reconstruction on several of his first recipients. The technique subsequently "lost favor" with him because of a high incidence of bile fistulas. He "left it" and went on to make another technique his "first choice" for a number of years, but he has now moved away from that method and "come back to" his original one (Starzl et al. 1976, pp. 489, 503; Starzl, personal communication).

What has emerged as the most "interesting" and "surprising" finding made by the transplant groups trying to better understand and systematically reduce the high mortality of liver graft recipients is the seeming rarity of graft loss or patient death from rejection and the resistance the liver seems to have to hyperacute rejection. What is more, the recipients who survive for at least one year after operation have "remarkably stable . . . good or perfect" liver function. Although this seems all the more noteworthy compared with the kidney and the heart, the clinical experience with human liver transplantation is similar to the low incidence of progressive uncontrollable rejection observed in experimental animals, particularly in the pig. Such laboratory studies have suggested that the liver may have a "relatively privileged immunologic status." These laboratory and clinical observations are viewed as "potentially important" as well as "potentially encouraging" features of hepatic transplantation. But transplanters also consider them "perplexing." Why, in this respect, the liver behaves so differently from any other transplanted organ is not something they can yet explain. Furthermore, based on other laboratory observations made in dogs, physicians like Starzl continue to have nagging doubts about whether the rejection of the transplanted liver by human recipients is actually as infrequent as has been supposed: "It may be that some of the structural abnormalities that are presently thought to be nonspecific are actually subtle manifestations of hepatic rejection or recovery from this process" (Starzl et al. 1976, p. 501).

The "critical and, as yet, unanswered questions" regarding whether certain changes in transplanted livers "retrieved for study by death of the recipient or removal at retransplantation . . . could represent ongoing rejection and, if so, how?" present physicians with a clinical dilemma (Starzl et al. 1976, pp. 500–502). On the one hand, they believe "it is possible that many patients have been overtreated with immunosuppressive drugs" (Calne 1977, p. 215), particularly since, "as a final event, almost all liver recipients who die have significant extrahepatic infections" (Starzl et al. 1976, p. 501). If overtreatment is the problem, then the logical "change in management policy" called for would be "lightening . . . immunosuppression" (Starzl et al. 1976, p. 501). But Starzl has not been eager to make this change, both because he has a clinical hunch that hepatic rejection is latently and subtly present in many of their recipients and because "many patients with a graft that is failing early after transplantation respond to increased doses of prednisone" (Starzl et al. 1976, p. 501). Consequently, he continues to use primarily the same triple drug immunosuppression regimen for most of his recipients that he initiated in 1966; azathioprine, prednisone, and horse antilymphocyte globulin (ALG). From his point of view there have been no new developments in immunosuppression since he pioneered his triple drug therapy twelve years ago; nor does he see any forthcoming (personal communication).

In comparison with the Starzl/Denver group, the Cambridge/King's College team has not introduced ALG into their immunosuppression therapy. Their standard treatment has been confined to azathioprine and prednisone, in doses comparable to those used in renal transplant patients. They also have been somewhat more inclined than their Denver colleagues to "attempt to give the minimum dosage of immunosuppressive drugs," thereby cautiously experimenting with the possibility that liver recipients are being "systematically overimmunosuppressed." They report that, with respect to uncontrollable rejection, their most recent results have been "considerably better" than their results with cadaveric renal transplants (Calne 1977, pp. 213, 215).

Along with biliary obstruction, systemic infection, tumor recurrence in patients with primary hematoma, and hepatitis of the homograft, cerebrovascular accidents have emerged as one of the most serious, potentially fatal complications of liver transplantation. The six "crippling" cerebrovascular accidents that have occurred in the Denver series constitute what Starzl views as "the single most common lethal complication intraoperatively and postoperatively, among his adult liver recipients (Starzl et al. 1976, p. 500). The pathenogenesis of this condition is not yet understood, and the autopsies of patients who died from such accidents are being restudied with the hope that preventive measures may be developed for future patients.

But differential diagnosis of postoperative hepatic malfunction, considered by transplant physicians to be "the most critical element" in the care of liver recipients, is still in a relatively crude and tentative state. The need for "more active diagnostic steps," it has been said, not only is essential to making better decisions about postoperative therapy but is also seen to constitute one of the major "kinds of progress" on which the entire "further development of liver transplantation" depends (Starzl et al. 1976. pp. 503–4).

In sum, working under the same general goals of "improvement of clinical management" and "reduction of patient mortality" as are renal and cardiac transplantation, the field of liver transplantation has made clinical progress during the past decade. In this regard, its recent evolution has resembled the gradual progress of heart transplantation rather than the more static state of kidney transplantation. But it has advanced more slowly than human heart grafting, and its overall mortality rate is still considerably higher. As is true for the other fields of human organ transplantation, intensive effort has been directed to "accounting for" the major causes of complications and death and initiating diagnostic and therapeutic steps to cope with them. Thus far, cardiac transplantation has come further in this sphere than liver transplantation. But the physicians who perform liver transplants have been able to establish that the primary problems facing them and their patients are surgical, rather than belonging to the set of rejection/immunosuppression difficulties common to the entire transplantation field. Here its profile differs significantly from that of the field at large. Yet liver transplantation is not exempt from difficulties related to immunosuppression. The connected questions of whether more liver recipients are subject to subtle forms of rejection than has been apparent, and whether many patients have been overtreated with immunosuppressive drugs remain unanswered in the face of the equivocal data that exist. And in the "nonradical" framework within which liver as well as heart and kidney transplanters are now proceeding, they have not been eager to risk altering the established immunosuppression drug therapy programs. Physicians' clinical and ethical scruples, and the lack of impending new developments in immunosuppression, reinforce the status quo in this domain.

In the 1970s, bone-marrow transplantation (BMT) has joined renal, cardiac, and liver grafting as a major clinical development in the transplant field. It is only since 1968 (some ten years after the first human trials of the procedure were carried out), that a number of programs have been organized to perform BMT regularly on patients with severe combined immune deficiency, bone-marrow aplasia (aplastic anemia), or acute leukemia and to systematically study its effects. By 1977, a total of 350 patient-recipients had been reported to the International Bone Marrow Transplant Registry. It was estimated that another 250 patients not listed in the registry, but in many cases recorded and described in the medical literature, had also received transplants. Some forty teams were known to be conducting BMTs at a collective overall rate of 12 per month. Thus,

the sum total of bone-marrow grafts performed has already surpassed the number of cardiac or liver transplants that have been
done, and their "accession rate" is far greater.

Yet BMT is in an earlier stage of clinical trial than the transplanting of kidneys, hearts, or livers; and it is still confronted with a
number of problems characteristic of the "black years" in the
development of a therapeutic innovation. "What needs to be
scrutinized severely . . . is not the problem of BMT," writes
Georges Mathé, a pioneer in the area, "but rather its indications
and protocols" (Mathé et al. 1977, p. 157). Some of these "indications" problems are comparable to those that were particularly
acute and prominent in earlier phases of renal transplantation;
others are like those with which liver transplantation is currently
grappling. In addition, BMT is dealing with donor/recipient selection phenomena that have no exact counterpart in previous transplantation experience.

BMT has passed through several phases in the history of its early
clinical trials. Experimentation with bone-marrow grafts began in
the late 1940s, when researchers were studying possible means of
treating victims of radiation warfare. In 1958, while the "International Bone Marrow Transplantation Club" formed by the
investigators in this area was still working with rodents, Mathé and
his team in Paris and Thomas and his colleagues in Boston
"embarked on man" (Mathé et al. 1977, p. 155). In both sets of
trials, following the protocol used in the laboratory, the transplants
were performed after total-body irradiation. Mathé and Thomas
demonstrated the feasibility of such grafting, but their "optimism"
was soon replaced by distress because the recipients developed
"terrible secondary disease, similar to the worst observed in
mice" (Mathé et al. 1977, p. 155). This was a syndrome that had
unexpectedly erupted in some of the animals who had received
genetically nonidentical bone-marrow cells and was characterized by
severe weight loss, dermatitis, hepatitis, and gastroenteritis. It
subsequently came to be known as graft-versus-host disease
(GVHD) when it was discovered that this lethal syndrome, a type of
rejection in reverse, was related to an immunological attack of donor
lymphocytes against the recipient. Mathé and his colleagues soon
came to consider this secondary disease as a "stumbling block" to
BMT, "within the framework of medical ethics" as well as biomedically. However, the investigative progress made during the 1960s

in identifying and characterizing the human leukocyte antigen (HLA) locus gave them "renewed hope," for the HLA system was shown to be a genetically inherited, critical determinant in the fate of human tissue grafts. From this discovery, the possibility of performing bone-marrow transplants between HLA-matched family members (particularly between siblings, who have a 25 percent chance of being HLA-identical) became a reality. In 1968–69 the first such HLA-matched bone-marrow transplants were tried in a few centers. The recipients were several children with fatal, congenital immune deficiency diseases who received what were reported to be "successful transplants" from a brother or sister who was an HLA-identical donor. The possibility of bone-marrow graft in man" was considered to have been "confirmed" by these trials, and since then numerous transplant teams have entered the field, performing a steadily increasing number of human bone-marrow grafts.

According to Mathé, the protocols for BMT with severe aplastic anemia and acute leukemia have "not changed substantially" since the clinical trials of the late 1960s (Mathé et al. 1977, p. 157). At the same time, as van Bekkum points out, so "many different treatment procedures" are being used in connection with bone-marrow grafting in patients suffering from severe combined immune deficiency, that "few reliable conclusions" can be drawn from the results of the 68 BMTs for this condition done between 1968 and 1977 (van Bekkum 1977, p. 149). Furthermore, as has been indicated, a considerable number of the same forty teams working in the bone-marrow transplant field do not report their recipients to the registry. In these several regards, BMT has not attained the overall level of standardization and collaboration that characterizes other areas of transplantation (albeit with some variability between them). However, there are signs that, in a self-consciously organized way, bone marrow transplanters are trying to achieve greater uniformity and cooperation. "It is . . . encouraging," writes van Bekkum, "that the majority of transplanters involved in the treatment of SCID [severe combined immunodeficiency disease] have formed a club [the SCID section] under the auspices of the International Cooperative Group on Bone Marrow Transplantation in Man and of the International Society for Experimental Hematology, and that members of this club are making serious attempts to devise and adopt common clinical protocols" (van Bekkum 1977, p. 149).

These difficulties of integrating and unifying the clinical trials of BMT teams are associated with a basic problem of patient selection. This problem stems from the fact that the three main diseases for which bone-marrow transplantation is performed—immuno-deficiency, aplastic anemia, and acute leukemia—"have little in common, but they share many of the difficulties encountered in the use of bone marrow grafts" (van Bekkum 1977, p. 147). These shared complications include the lack of suitable compatible donors for many patients; the development of graft-versus-host disease in a majority of patients in whom a bone-marrow transplant is estab-lished; and a prolonged period of posttransplant immunodeficiency. Fifty percent or more of the candidates for bone-marrow transplan-tation are considered ineligible, because in the field's present state of development, the grafting of incompatible bone marrow results in fatal graft-versus-host disease. Even among patients grafted with compatible sibling marrow, there is a high incidence of GVHD, which is responsible for the death of 25 to 50 percent of the patients in whom a take of bone marrow is obtained. This death rate is increased by the effects of the "conditioning" with immuno-suppressive drugs and, often, total body irradiation before bone-marrow grafts for aplastic anemia or acute leukemia. Even in the germ-free isolation environment in which patients are placed after irradiation, these conditioning procedures make prospective re-cipients highly susceptible to potentially fatal infection, owing to the drastic extent to which their immune systems have been suppressed. A number of the infections to which they are vulnerable are of unclear etiology or involve unidentified viruses; and, if they survive the grafting, patients continue to be prone to serious infection for six to twelve months after transplantation. Thus a "vicious cycle" is created by the steps taken to enable the recipient's body to accept and retain the donated marrow: a cycle that, especially in patients who undergo total body irradiation, closely resembles that experi-enced in the earliest, blackest years of kidney grafting.

In the light of these and other "serious hazards," and the consequent high morbidity and mortality associated with BMT, physicians in the field are generally agreed that it should be a "procedure of last resort" (Fawzy, Wellisch, and Yager 1977, p. 5), restricted to "patients who are truly doomed if they are aplastic, and to leukemic patients who are truly chemoresistant" (Mathé et al. 1977, p. 157).

There is also consensus that marrow transplantation is still a sufficiently "experimental procedure" (Fawzy, Wellisch, and Yager 1977, p. 5) and enough of a "complex clinical undertaking" that, ideally, it should be performed "only by physicians who have experience with problems of transplantation and with intensive supportive therapy" (Storb et al. 1977, p. 184).

But the field is still in that "black years" stage when even physicians with the highest qualifications for doing human BMTs implicitly ask whether they are justified in carrying out this procedure, no matter how hopelessly ill the recipients may be or how unresponsive to other therapies. A pioneer leader like Mathé, for example, not only has verbally raised the question, "Has the prognosis of panaplasia and of leukemia been significantly improved by bone marrow transplantation?" but has set up a clinical experiment to address himself to it. From 1971 to 1975, at the Institut de Cancérologie et d'Immunogénétique in Villejuif, he selected 17 patients with advanced aplastic anemia who met the clinical criteria for BMT used by registry members and by the University of Washington School of Medicine in Seattle (which, as of July 1976, had performed the largest number of marrow grafts in patients with aplastic anemia—73 in all). Rather than doing BMTs on these 17 patients, Mathé gave them "unlimited intensive hematologic care," including indefinite isolation in aseptic units and unlimited platelet and white-blood-cell transfusions. His published results showed that there was "no difference between the cumulative survival of our severe panaplasia patients managed by unlimited intensive care, and that of patients with identically severe aplasia, who have been treated with a BMT from a matched sibling donor." "Some of my friends may not understand why I present this data," Mathé went on to say, "after having spent 10 years of my life convincing other clinicians to work on BMT. Yet, I must question the indications at this time" (Mathé et al. 1977, pp. 156–57). Rather than recommending a moratorium on the procedure, Mathé advocated that the criteria for the selection of recipients be made even more restrictive. He also made an appeal for changes in the clinical protocols used for bone-marrow transplantation that would allow transplanters to "attempt the immunorestoration of immunodepressed patients"; and, because experiments in animals suggest that protection against GVHD mortality may be obtained by using third-party antigens, he "encouraged" his colleagues to make a "renewed effort" in the laboratory to carry out HLA-*mis*matched bone-marrow transplants under certain special conditions (Mathé et al. 1977, pp. 158, 167).

Mathé's clinical experiment notwithstanding, there seems to be overall consensus among transplanters that BMT has increased survival in the treatment of severe aplastic anemia (a disease that would normally be rapidly fatal, with a prognosis of less than three months). In "the Seattle experience," for example, of the 73 patients with aplastic anemia, 31 survived "with normal marrow function between 6 and 62 months," and 28 were reported to have "returned to normal activities." The mortality among the 42 patients who died was especially during the first three months after transplant and was largely due to complications associated with graft rejection, GVHD, and infection. While the Seattle group states that "it is clear that therapeutic advances have to be made in regard to the three major problems responsible for most mortality," they conclude that the "survival in hematologic remission of approximately 43 per cent of the patients with severe aplastic anemia treated by bone marrow transplantation" is "superior to the results following conventional therapy" (Storb et al. 1977, pp. 183–84).

Although (with considerable caution and ambivalence) physicians have reached this judgment about the results of transplantation in selected patients with aplastic anemia, their outlook on "the clinical applicability role of bone marrow transplantation in acute leukemia is unresolved" (Gale 1977, p. 7). During the past twenty years, intermittent attempts have been made to treat resistant acute leukemia using "supralethal therapy" followed by "rescue" with bone-marrow transplantation; but not as many marrow grafts have been performed on leukemic as on aplastic patients, and the results have been judged "equivocal" at best and "discouraging" at worst. It has never resulted in the prolonged, disease-free survival of more than several patients refractory to conventional treatment. For example, of the 30 patients with acute leukemia on whom the UCLA Bone Marrow Transplantation Group performed grafts from 1973 to early 1977, only six (20 percent) were reported to be alive without leukemia more than one year after transplant, and the median survival of transplanted recipients was no more than 169 days. Deaths have tended to occur early in the posttransplant period from infection, or later (six to twenty-seven weeks) from "opportunistic infection," interstitial pneumonitis, or both (Gale 1977, p. 4; UCLA

Bone Marrow Transplant Group 1977, pp. 159–60). To our knowledge no formal moratorium on bone marrow transplantation for acute resistant leukemia has yet been called or publicly suggested. But in the results obtained so far, and in the language that transplanters use to describe them ("significant obstacles remain and require intense clinical investigation," etc.), one senses that the question whether to continue marrow grafting for leukemia hangs in the balance.

The selection problems with which bone-marrow transplant teams are currently grappling are not confined to the choice of appropriate recipients and disease states. They also include a number of biologically and morally difficult issues concerning the selection of bone-marrow donors, revolving around both related minor donors and the possibility of using unrelated donors. Because the grafting of incompatible bone marrow at present invariably results in fatal GVHD, transplant teams have not experimented with bone-marrow transplants between siblings who are not genetically matched. Yet their inability to do so continues to distress and challenge transplant teams, not only because for lack of suitable donors they must turn away an estimated 50 percent or more of the candidates for bone-marrow transplantation. The possibility of conducting and studying a number of BMTs between selected compatible donors and recipients who are not siblings or even related has been seriously considered, and four such procedures have been reported in the literature (O'Reilly, Dupont, et al. 1978). However, for reasons that have not been extensively spelled out in the literature but that appear to be ethical as well as technical, the transplant community seems hesitant to ask for live bone-marrow donations from genetically matched donors who are not family members. In addition to the problems of rejection, infection, and GVHD, there is the restraining fact that donor bone marrow must be obtained in an operating room under general anesthesia. To be sure, it is a relatively simple procedure; it entails no more than several days of hospitalization for the donor; fewer than 10 percent of his or her total marrow cells are taken; and the donor's body replenishes the marrow by regeneration in two or three weeks. But, as is the case with live unrelated kidney donations, this gift seems to exceed what the medical profession feels justified to ask of those who are not kin. Thus, the team who carried out one such BMT with an unrelated donor took the unusual step of stating in their case report that "we are indebted to the donor, whose steadfast personal commitment to this patient allowed for the ultimate successful outcome" (O'Reilly, Dupont, et al. 1978, p. 1317).

In its outlooks and goals, human bone-marrow transplantation has not yet arrived at the "improvement of clinical management" stage of development shared by kidney, heart, and liver transplantation. It has only recently moved far enough from the laboratory into the clinic to "confirm the possibility of bone-marrow grafting in man" between suitably matched siblings (Mathé et al. 1977, p. 155).

Although the number of teams working in the field of bone-marrow transplantation has been steadily increasing since 1968, collectively performing a sizable number of marrow grafts, they have not been inclined to make extravagant claims about what they have thus far accomplished clinically. Many factors have contributed to their sobriety: the long road, fraught with trial and error, that they have had to travel to reach the still relatively "black" period in which they now find themselves; the gravity and heterogeneity of the conditions they treat with marrow grafting; the high degree of biomedical uncertainty about aplastic anemia, acute resistant anemia, and severe combined immune deficiency that still exists; the life-threatening side effects of the preoperative "conditioning" to which they subject recipients; and the relative youth of many of their patients. But it is their discovery of the "terrible" graft-versus-host disease and their stressful clinical experience with it that have been the greatest deterrents to overoptimism or easy affirmations on the part of bone-marrow transplantation teams. A strong current of organized skepticism and probative questioning underlies whatever positive results physicians working in the area have thus far reported. The possibility that a formal moratorium will be called has still not been precluded, particularly a moratorium on bone-marrow transplantation for acute leukemia. And transplanters have reemphasized that at this juncture human bone-marrow grafting is justified only in patients who are otherwise "doomed."

At present there is a little talk of imminent "breakthroughs" or dramatic "spinoffs" among teams engaged in bone-marrow transplantation. Rather, the more modest allegation is made that "some degree of satisfaction may be derived from the fact that knowledge of normal and abnormal immunology and physiology is being increased during endeavors to provide new therapeutic approaches for the patient with otherwise fatal disease.'' And this knowledge is seen as consoling in the face of the "many discouraging complexities associated with marrow transplantation" (Thomas et al. 1975, pp. 901–2).

In spite of a number of dissimilarities in the evolutionary history of renal, cardiac, and liver transplantation, and although the grafting of each of these organs is in a different stage of development, these three fields of human organ transplantation have a common outlook on the prospects and problems before them. The current orientation of human bone-marrow grafting, in contrast, must be considered apart.

One of the most striking features of the perspective shared by kidney, heart, and liver transplanters is the somber recognition that no fundamental progress been made during the past ten years in the scientific understanding and the clinical management of the central problem of uncertainty in transplantation: rejection and related immune responses.

I sense that many clinicians these days are beset by confusion and uncertainty about transplantation. The spectacular successes achieved for certain patients by transplantation of several organs are there for all to see. . . . Our confusion is fed by our growing perception of the immune response to foreign cells as one of immense complexity and our uncertainty about the fact that the overall survival figures of organ transplants . . . seem to have improved very little. Perhaps for a truly substantial improvement in transplant survival the long-awaited step of planned specific alteration of recipient responsiveness will have to be realized. I still consider this the most important single topic in transplantation and one that is by no means devoid of hope for the future. [Russell 1977, p. 1327]

A far more serious question that I have heard voiced is this: Are we in fact making progress toward the solution of the clinical problems? Admitting that the key problem is still that of immuno-logical rejection, are immunologists perhaps too preoccu-pied with beautiful but highly artificial models that have as much relevance to clinical transplantation as landing on Mars has to climbing the north face of the Eiger? Why is it, these skeptics ask, that clinical transplantation continues to depend on the use of the same immunosuppressive agents as it did a decade ago? [Brent 1977, p. 1344]

"Confusion and uncertainty," "growing perception of immense complexity," "disappointment," "climbing the north face of the Eiger" rather than "landing on Mars": the language used by transplanters in the 1970s to describe the state of the field and their attitudes toward it contrasts sharply with their rhetoric in the 1960s. In that more "heady" decade, they spoke and wrote often about impending "leaps forward" in understanding the biological mechanisms underlying graft acceptance and rejection; imminent "breakthroughs" in piercing the immunologic "barrier" and in "overcoming" the rejection reaction; the "spinoff" implications of both the negative and positive effects of immunosuppressive therapy for a wide-ranging "assortment of diseases"; and the "exciting leads," "new approaches," and "solutions" that studying the immunological problems of transplantation promised to provide for the understanding, prevention, and cure of autoimmune diseases, neoplasms, and the very conditions for which renal and cardiac transplantations were done.

A sense that "the days of impressive breakthroughs are over and clinical results tend to accumulate slowly" now predominates in human organ transplantation. This "adjustment of earlier attitudes" (Starzl, Weil, and Putnam 1977, p. 6) is expressed by transplant teams in informal, daily-round discussion as well as in their publications and in the papers and addresses they deliver at medical meetings:

We are being conservative and less euphoric about the likelihood of seeing a big . . . major breakthrough. . . . We do not feel that we are on the threshold. [Personal communication, Stanford Cardiac Transplantation Team, April 1977]

Liver transplantation is a terribly difficult undertaking, much like climbing Mount Everest. [Starzl, personal communication]

The "climbing Mount Everest" imagery depicts transplant endeavors in the 1970s as a slow, difficult, step-by-step effort to overcome enormous obstacles. This orientation constitutes a new phase of the courage to fail ethos, one that is less expectant and aggressive but no less audacious than the outlook of the 1960s. Transplanters know that certain of their attitudes and goals have altered, but they are not completely aware of the fact that the vocabulary, imagery, and ideology of the field have undergone such systematic and collective changes. Nor do they necessarily recognize that this general modification in their outlook may be contributing to the "dead-center position of immunosuppression," and to the failure to develop "radically new methods . . . in the last 8–10 years" (Starzl, Weil, and Putnam 1977, pp. 6–7). For, as Brent and Russell have both pointed out, transplant physicians have become more cautious about rapidly translating laboratory findings on animals to clinical trials on patients, more "reluctant" to experiment with established immunosuppression protocols that produce "tolerable . . . although far from perfect results," and less inclined to "accept the risks that must inevitably accompany the introduction of new methods" (Brent 1977, p. 1345; Russell, personal communication).

As the foregoing implies, the prevailing ideology of renal, cardiac, and liver transplant physicians in the 1970s reflects the routinization that has come to characterize their clinical behavior. Starzl has described this "trend" as the "relegat[ion]" of "progress to the shuffling of details and to the adjustment of earlier attitudes and policies" (Starzl, Weil, and Putnam 1977, p. 6). Within this more conservative framework, transplant teams are now primarily focused on the goal of improving clinical "management" of transplant patients. Their attention and energies are directed toward the better handling of acute and chronic rejection; the achievement of graft acceptance "with lesser penalties than are now exacted"; the resolution of technical and mechanical problems associated with transplant surgery; the "standardization" of procedures like biliary-duct reconstruction; and the "control" of postoperative recurrences of patients' underlying diseases. In their view, the central objective of these efforts is to progressively "increase [and] enhance patient survival."

From its outset, human organ transplantation has been confronted with psychological and social phenomena that are inherent in the various stages of a therapeutic innovation. In addition, transplant teams, patients, and their families have been faced with a number of unique psychological and social experiences and problems. These grow out of the fact that the transplanted organ must be donated by a fellow human being—known or unknown, related or unrelated, alive or dead—and that such gifts of life are scarce resources that must be allocated to those who need them according to some system of priority and eligibility. In turn, these gifts of life and allocation features of transplantation have opened onto still larger questions, societally, culturally, and existentially phrased, such as: How much of a society's inherently scarce resources ought to be invested in medical and surgical undertakings like organ transplantation, and in the health-illness-medicine sector more generally? How vigorously ought we or ought we not to intervene in the human condition in the ways human organ grafting involves? To what extent and in what manner do we have the moral obligation to give of ourselves to our "brothers," our "sisters," and our "strangers"? And, What are the proper definitions and ultimate meanings of human individuality, personhood, life, and death? The whole range of psychological, social, and cultural questions that organ transplantation has encountered coincides with a number of the issues related to biomedicine that are central to "bioethics," the new interdisciplinary field of inquiry and action that began to emerge in the mid-1960s. In fact, transplantation (separately and along with hemodialysis) is one of the chief advances in biology and medicine on which bioethics has concentrated its attention. It has been a key case, evoking and epitomizing some of major questions of value and belief with which bioethics has been essentially concerned (Fox 1976, 1977).

Organ transplantation has undergone a general progression from primary absorption in the biomedical aspects of the procedure to increasing involvement in its "human" facets; from preoccupation with microdynamic, psychological, and social concerns to interest in macrodynamic, societal, ethical, and existential issues; from questions focused on the experiences and problems of organ transplant recipients, donors, and their families to those faced by medical personnel who belong to transplant teams; and from phenomena situated in the microcosm of the transplant unit, within the hospital, to those in the world outside the transplant community and the medical center, which are not exclusively relevant to the grafting of human organs.

Characteristically, transplant teams' awareness of what they are prone to call "psychosocial factors" and their active involvement in them has begun with concerned interest in the process of decision-making and the quality of consent that organ transplantation entails for recipients, donors, and their families. These decisions have been seen as inherent to stage one of the transplantation procedure, and attempts to evaluate them have usually led to further consideration of the stresses associated with later stages and to how patients react to and deal with these stresses. Such explorations have typically been conducted in a psychoanalytically oriented, psychiatric framework, whether psychiatrists, social workers, transplant nurses, or physicians have been chiefly responsible for them. At present, the most classic examples of this approach are to be found in the field of bone-marrow transplantation. That marrow grafting is in an earlier stage of development than kidney, heart, and liver transplantation seems to have contributed to its greater psychiatric concern with the stresses experienced by recipients. In addition, the preparatory immunosuppression that bone-marrow transplantation patients undergo with total body irradiation or very high doses of chemotherapy or both, their "entry into isolation" ("the point of no return," in the words of two psychiatrists), and the "cruel threat" to their lives that graft-versus-host disease poses ("the turning of the transplant against [them]"), which is unique to bone-marrow grafting, have all been conducive to analyses of the psychic stresses to which this form of organ transplantation subjects recipients (Brown and Kelly 1976, pp. 442, 444).

Ordinarily, it has been in a somewhat later stage of the evolution of a transplant procedure that teams have become more explicitly and systematically appreciative of the role certain social factors play in the attitudes and behavior of transplant recipients. The Stanford heart transplant group, for example, is notable for the attention they have paid to these dimensions of the transplant experience, for the importance it attaches to them, and for the ways it has based patient policy on such insights. According to Lois Christopherson, chief social worker for the Stanford Department of Surgery and the Cardiac Transplant Team, they have repeatedly observed that some of the recipients and their families form a "very close group . . . a supercluster" (personal communication). When this occurs, the patients characteristically ask, "Why can't we have a transplant club?" The Stanford team does not actively encourage such proposals. Unlike certain renal transplantation and dialysis teams, who are impressed with the supportive value of patient groups, the Stanford unit feels that, on balance, this clublike identification with fellow recipients and their relatives has more disadvantages than advantages. In their view, it reinforces and helps to perpetuate what the Stanford group terms the "transplant aura": a tendency for recipients to put their "primary emphasis . . . on transplantation status" rather than on "self-selected, meaningful life activities." In this respect, the "supercluster" or club runs counter to the inclination of many patients to resume their preoperative activities: "Most recipients whose previous activities had been satisfying to them soon found categorization as a heart recipient to be superficial and to interfere with the cultivation of other, more meaningful roles" (Christopherson, Griepp, and Stinson 1976, p. 2084). Emergence from the "transplant aura," the Stanford group believes, "importantly ease[s] the stresses placed on the family unit during the recipient's critical illness and postoperative convalescence. . . . The patient's return to activities that were enjoyed prior to serious illness and his resumption of family responsibilities diminish[es] disruption of family roles and allow[s] other family members to return to their normal patterns of interaction" (Christopherson, Griepp, and Stinson 1976, p. 2084).

The Stanford group also has come to regard "dissociation from fellow recipients" as "helpful" to patients in dealing with deaths of other cardiac recipients and with indications, usually in the form of infections, of [their] own susceptible state":

The return of recipients to homes located in geographically distant and separate parts of the country allowed resumption of previous social relationships and diminished the likelihood of interaction with one another. Only a few close friendships grew from shared transplant experiences; the majority of recipients avoided such associations because the illness or death of a recipient with whom they closely identified would be doubly painful. [Christopherson, Griepp, and Stinson 1976, p. 2084]

It was not until cardiac transplantation had reached the point where there were a substantial number of recipients for the Stanford team to observe, who had survived the procedure for one year or more and achieved a significant degree of "physical and psychosocial rehabilitation," that they identified and began to make policy decisions about such social phenomena as the "transplant aura" and the "transplant club." Thus far, they have emphasized what they consider to be the harmful consequences of a continuing transplant patient subculture more than they have stressed its possible benefits.

It is generally only after a transplant field has progressed considerably beyond its early clinical experimental phases, and after particular teams have worked in the area for a certain period of time, that they crystallize what they have learned about the relationship between the dynamics of their group and their own as well as their patients' ability to cope with the transplant situation and function reasonably well within it. For instance, based on their fifteen years of team experience, Starzl and his colleagues have concluded that "major input by a well-trained chief is obligatory for the success of a kidney transplant program. Attempts to maintain transplant side-shows without such a major commitment have usually failed" (Starzl, Weil, and Putnam 1977, p. 1). The Stanford heart transplant group has reached a similar conclusion. On the basis of their experience, they believe that the ideal chief has a clear conception of his role; does not go beyond it; has the capacity to delegate authority as well as responsibility to selected members of the team; has a sense of perspective and of humor; and though critical of his colleagues and of himself fosters team unity, purposiveness, and high morale. In addition, the Stanford group feels that the fact that a number of its members have worked together since the first human heart transplant was performed at their medical center, and that they have collectively created an atmosphere in which they can learn from their own mistakes, makes not only their team functioning but also their patient care "all the better" (personal communication).

Somewhat earlier in the development of human bone-marrow transplantation than has usually been the case with other forms of organ grafting, systematic concern has arisen over the problems the medical staff faces in the special hospital subculture of a transplant unit, and how their reactions affect both their own behavior and that of patients and their kin. At UCLA, for example, "in response to a clearly perceived need . . . a three-tiered program of psychosocial care has been instituted through the . . . Psychiatric Consultation–Liaison Service [that] . . . focusses on helping the medical team, along with bone marrow transplant patients and their families" (Fawzy, Wellisch, and Yager 1977, p. 5). It appears that the exceptional degree of strain bone-marrow transplantation entails for the staff has precipitated a somewhat earlier and more intensive preoccupation with the attitudes, feelings, and social system of the medical team than was true for renal, cardiac, and liver transplantation when they were in comparable stages of development. The accelerated awareness of bone-marrow transplant groups about the social as well as the psychological dynamics of their own functioning, and their organized attempts to deal with and utilize these insights, may also have been influenced by the fact that when marrow grafting began to be done more extensively, many renal, cardiac, and liver transplant teams had already reached this kind of consciousness about psychosocial factors and were discussing them more openly.

The overall evolution of kidney, heart, liver, and bone-marrow transplantation toward an increasing involvement in more societal, ethical, and existential issues seems to grow in part out of the progression through which a therapeutic innovation and those associated with it tend to pass as they gradually expand their concerns beyond the immediate problems. In the case of human organ transplantation, several more general social and cultural phenomena influenced this progression, particularly the implications and consequences of the emergence of a bioethics movement and, as we shall see in chapter 11, the passage of the Public Law that now finances the care of patients with chronic renal failure. In turn, some of the psychological and sociocultural concomitants of transplantation have affected its biomedical parameters; for example, its patient selection and deselection policies and the reluctance of kidney transplanters to radically alter their established protocols.

This detailed comparative overview of the evolution undergone by human kidney, heart, liver, and bone-marrow transplantation, and of the medical status they reached in the late 1970s, illustrates the complex, multivariant nature of therapeutic innovation. It is apparent that the medical profession attaches special significance to patient mortality and survival rates as primary indicators of where the various forms of transplantation fall on the experiment-therapy continuum. The profession also regards the kinds of medical uncertainties and unknowns with which these transplant subfields are faced, and the criteria they use for patient selection, as important measures of how experimental or therapeutic they are. But our analytic survey of the transplant situation has shown that a wider range of factors is associated with the developmental stage of the grafting of different organs than those that are emphasized by the medical community.

All these factors are not of equal consequence, however, nor is their relationship to each other, and to the overall question of experiment-therapy status, entirely logical. For example, the number of kidney, heart, liver, and bone-marrow transplants performed is a crude "box score" datum that is only roughly correlated with other more sensitive and telling indicators of their respective positions on the experiment-therapy spectrum. The kidney transplants that have been done outnumber by the thousands all other forms of organ grafting. Quite appropriately, renal transplantation has not only been performed regularly by a sizable number of teams for the longest period of time, but also has moved further away from the experimental pole and closer to the "conventional therapy" end of the spectrum than have cardiac, liver, and bone-marrow transplantation. And, although bone-marrow transplantation is still in an earlier, more experimental, "black years" stage of evolution than the grafting of other organs, to date more bone-marrow transplants have been carried out in patients than either heart or liver transplants.

Other indicators we have identified seem to be more powerfully and consistently related to the experiment-therapy status of organ transplantation subtypes. For example, it has been shown that the biomedical, psychosocial, and bioethical approaches that characterize the fields of cardiac and liver transplantation are significantly influenced by several transplant physicians and their teams, and that their influence has been institutionalized in a number of ways. This appears to be a reliable and valid correlate of the fact that the grafting of these human organs has moved beyond the "black years" stage but is still accompanied by a high mortality rate and major unresolved "clinical management" problems.

As the foregoing suggests, the indicators that have emerged from our study of transplantation should not be weighted equally or considered one by one, as discrete variables. They constitute the sort of matrix that is appropriate for cluster analysis. And, ideally, their applicability to the processes and stages of therapeutic innovation more generally ought to be further tested on cases other than organ transplantation.

Our analysis has disclosed several alternative phase-movements between the "early clinical trials" and the "established therapy" points on the experiment-therapy spectrum. The transplantation sequence has suggested that after a medical innovation has moved past early clinical experimentation into what might be termed the "pretherapeutic" stage of its development, patient selection may take one of several forms. Trials with a procedure or drug may advance directly to the stage where it is used in the treatment of progressively less critically ill patients. This is the postexperimental/pretherapeutic pattern of patient selection that we originally postulated. But we have found that at least two other possibilities exist. The therapeutic innovation may be extended to terminally ill patients with a wider, more inclusive range of serious diseases and medical problems than was characteristic of those who were the subjects of earlier clinical trials. This is currently the case with renal transplantation and the "all risk" patients who have become its recipients. There is a third alternative patient selection trend that has become apparent. This is exemplified by the field of heart transplantation, which continues to choose recipients from among patients who are dying of end-stage cardiac disease as it did at its inception but has now gone on to select the "best risk" patients—psychologically as well as biomedically—within this otherwise "doomed" category.

Along with these "intermediary" phases of patient selection, the changes in ethos that the transplantation endeavor has undergone make it seem more likely that an ideology and goal-set of "climbing Mount Everest," "improving clinical management," and "reducing patient mortality" constitute one of the orientations that can be expected among the medical profession after an innovation has advanced considerably beyond its "black years" and before it attains the status of standard therapy. This perspective—relatively conservative, low-key, patiently hard-working, routinized, and clinically focused—stands in marked contrast to the phases in ideology and goals that often precede it: the exuberant, aggressive, frequently hubris-ridden outlook that characteristically prevails in the very first period of early clinical trials, and the expectations of "imminent [basic science] breakthroughs" and "favorable spin-offs" that are likely to follow once physicians have faced problems of uncertainty, limitation, and unwanted side effects that their clinical experimentation has engendered as well as disclosed. It remains to be seen to what extent the "Mount Everest" stage is particular to the transplant situation, largely as a consequence of a distinctive, if not unique, impasse that the field has reached in understanding and dealing with its most fundamental problem—rejection and other immune responses. But, given the inherently cautious yet deeply committed nature of this stage, and the degree to which it involves turning away from the laboratory to concentrate on clinical improvement, it presents a number of questions that our study has not resolved. What further shifts in ideology and goals, brought about by what kinds of events, might help precipitate the "breakthroughs" in knowledge that were expected in an earlier stage and that could propel toward established therapy status a therapeutic innovation that has reached this evolutionary point? If such a spurt forward does *not* take place within what the medical profession defines as a reasonable period of time, will the therapeutic innovation be abandoned even by those sober pioneers who have remained committed to it? And if the advances in knowledge and technique that are forthcoming lead away from an innovation while it is in the pretherapeutic phase of development, how receptive or resistant to this change in direction will those medical groups be who have been the most involved with the innovation?

Finally, our reconsideration of the experiment-therapy paradigm in the light of the evolution of human organ transplantation during the past decade has confirmed our view that not only biological and medical, but also psychological and social factors are systematically involved in the unfolding of such an innovation. The sequence we have identified is one in which the medical team's preoccupations become less exclusively biomedical and less oriented toward individual patients as an innovation advances beyond early clinical trials, and their focus shifts from microdynamic psychological considerations to progressively more macroscopic social and cultural concerns.

A full-scale analysis of the policy implications of our findings lies beyond the scope of this chapter and this book. But we would like to suggest in broad outline what some of these questions might be. It seems to us that the most basic policy issues are related to the degree to which the process of therapeutic innovation is a latent one, developing in patterned ways that are not necessarily planned or recognized by the medical profession, patients, and the various persons and groups who are more indirectly responsible for, or affected by, particular new medical procedures and drugs.

The case of organ transplantation has provided at least two striking examples of the phenomena that can result from the partly unconscious and undirected nature of this collective process. The first is the general, only half-conscious way the ideology and goals of transplanters have changed. This shift has involved a reallocation of transplant physicians' energies: the deflection of some of the attention they previously invested in the laboratory to clinical problems of technique, treatment management, and patient survival. Is this change in orientation an inherent or even inevitable concomitant of a certain juncture in the pretherapeutic development of any medical innovation? Or has it occurred largely in response to the "dead center" status of the particular problems of rejection and immunosuppression that transplantation faces? How commonly does this kind of impasse in basic knowledge occur in the evolution of a therapeutic innovation? Is such an impasse a consequence as well as a cause of the tendency of research physicians to turn away from the laboratory toward the clinic in the pretherapeutic stage?

The second example, to which we turn in the next chapter, concerns the powerful effect Public Law 92-603 has had on the patient selection policy of many renal transplant teams. Objective evidence indicates that physicians have not only relaxed and liberalized their criteria for choosing kidney transplant recipients but in many instances have virtually ceased to use them. Does this mean that if and when the federal government extends its financial coverage to the medical care costs associated with other diseases, it will significantly reduce "gatekeeping" and triage on the part of physicians? How desirable or undesirable—biomedically, socially, and ethically—would such a development be, for patients and the public as well as for physicians and the medical team?

Further empirical research, both historical and sociological, is needed to answer such policy-related questions. And in the final analysis perhaps the most basic, general question that needs to be investigated is how relevant or irrelevant, helpful or harmful it would be to make all those who participate in clinical research more aware of the therapeutic innovation process with all its intended and unintended consequences. Would this knowledge, for instance, permit them to guide and alter the process in ways that would mitigate the suffering of the "black years"; reduce the possibility that episodes like the heart transplant "bandwagon" will occur; make physicians less medically and morally reluctant to call moratoriums on their own clinical trials; lead to different balances between laboratory and clinical efforts at different stages of the therapeutic process; make it less probable that physicians' biomedical reasoning about patient selection will be so directly and significantly affected by changes in the political economy of health care delivery; and make it more likely that the psychological, social, and cultural aspects of the process will be handled with greater insight and deliberation? We think so, and we believe that these developments would render the process of therapeutic innovation more rational, flexible, governable, biomedically fruitful, ethical, and humane.

11

The Democratization of Dialysis:
Public Law 92-603

"As long as an Ernie Crowfeather succeeds in beating the system," Belding Scribner reflected in 1971, "it indicates that we're not ready to handle the problem of priorities and selection." A year later, Congress sought to resolve this problem by the passage of Public Law 92-603, the Social Security amendments of 1972. Through the provisions of PL 92-603, end-stage renal failure patients acquired what is perhaps their most unusual characteristic: they became the first, and thus far the only, victims of catastrophic illness singled out for special coverage of their treatment costs by the federal government.

Since we wrote the first edition of this book, the major developments associated with dialysis and renal transplantation have been social, political, and economic rather than biomedical ones, centered on the passage and sequelae of PL 92-603. By largely removing financial barriers to treatment, the federal government in effect has become the new gatekeeper of renal transplantation and dialysis. The government's assumption of this complex role has had pronounced effects on dialysis and transplantation and has raised a number of critical issues that have implications far beyond the confines of these therapies alone. In the five years since the passage of PL 92-603, these effects and issues have been seen at three intersecting levels. The most macro-level is that of the federal government. Why renal disease should have been singled out for special coverage, and the implications for federal financing of other catastrophic illnesses, constitutes one cluster of questions generated by the events leading to the passage of the 1972 law. More fundamentally, how valid is the premise that lowering the financial barriers to expensive therapies like dialysis and transplantation ipso facto resolves the issues encapsulated by the term "the allocation of scarce resources"? And, even if one looks at economic factors alone, what does it mean, societally, to endorse and act upon the value that medical care is a "right" for all persons in all circumstances?

Moving to the second level, how has the passage of PL 92-603 affected the delivery of dialysis and, to a lesser extent in numbers of patients, transplantation? The mushrooming numbers of end-stage renal failure patients receiving treatment since the advent of federal funding, and the regulations governing that funding, have intensified clinical, psychosocial, and economic debates about types of dialysis care, particularly home versus center treatment. And with the availability of federal monies, the rapid growth of proprietary dialysis centers has generated important economic and ethical questions about the "property" of profit-making in the treatment of diseases such as chronic renal failure.

Third, at the most micro-level, how has PL 92-603 affected patients and the physicians and other medical professionals who care for them? As we think of the issues dealt with in earlier chapters, such as patient selection, the stresses experienced by the providers of transplantation and dialysis, and the quality of life issues posed for and by recipients of these treatments, it seems to us that those involved in dialysis and transplantation today are confronted by many of the same problems as their predecessors, albeit in sometimes more refined and subtle forms. And to these have been added new questions and difficulties, resulting from the new, post-1972 socioeconomic and political context in which transplantation and dialysis are carried out.

Lives and Dollars: The Passage of PL 92-603

With the passage of PL 92-603 on 30 October 1972, Medicare insurance coverage for transplantation and dialysis was extended from those over sixty-five years of age covered by the original 1965 Medicare law to more than 90 percent of the United States population. The extension was provided in two ways. First, persons under sixty-five eligible for Social Security cash benefits because of an incapacitating disability such as end-stage renal failure became eligible for Medicare *after* a twenty-four-month waiting period. Second, and more important in terms of the numbers of patients it affected, section 2991 of the law extended Medicare coverage to those under sixty-five otherwise ineligible for cash disability benefits.

Section 2991, as Rettig observed in his analysis of the policy debate surrounding its enactment, is significant not only because it extends Medicare coverage for end-stage renal disease treatment to almost the entire United States population. "It is significant also because it is a concrete instance of the willingness of the national legislature to pay a very substantial price to preserve the lives of a very small number of individuals" (Rettig 1976*a*, p. 2). In analyzing the passage of PL 92-603, focusing particularly on section 2991, Rettig has traced a series of events and debates that began in the early 1960s, when the costs of dialysis treatment and the related scarcity of facilities became starkly apparent. Though the issue of paying the costs of dialysis was recognized as critical, the federal government's policy through the 1960s was restricted to providing research, demonstration, and training funds. "Traditionally, payment for treatment of illness has been the responsibility of the patient or the local community," noted a 1964 Senate Appropriations Committee report dealing with artificial kidney programs. "If the Federal Government were to share the full cost of lifetime treatment for all who suffer from these chronic diseases and conditions, the financial burden would be excessive," a federal official observed (quoted in Rettig 1976*a*, p. 10).

By 1972, however, a number of factors had altered the government's position toward direct patient-care financing for end-stage kidney disease. These included a growing experience with transplantation and dialysis that, in turn, led to an increasing number of physician and patient advocates for expanded government financing; the 1967 Gottschalk Committee report (see chap. 7); Veterans Administration funding of dialysis for veterans; funding for community dialysis centers through the 1970 Regional Medical Programs Service; and the advocacy of catastrophic illness insurance by such politically powerful figures as Russell B. Long, chairman of the Senate Finance Committee (Rettig 1976*a, b*). Two other factors have played critical roles in many types of health legislation. The first was active and persuasive lobbying for patient-care financing by "vested interest" groups such as the National Association of Patients on Hemodialysis and Transplantation, and the National Kidney Foundation; officials of the latter organization, indeed, helped to draft the language of the amendment that became section 2991 of PL 92-603. The second, and the most emotionally powerful and persuasive factor, was "the importance of identified lives."

The policy debate preceding the enactment of Sec. 2991 does not reveal an automatic reflexive response by the government to the victims of end-stage renal disease. Rather, it suggests a "tipping process" at work. Specifically, it appears that publicity of lives lost for the lack of scarce medical resources had to occur, including specific dramatization of identified lives. Beyond this, it was necessary for the cumulative effect of an increasing number of government programs to be felt. Finally, the number of patients being kept alive had to increase to the point where they simply could not be ignored.

Publicity included dramatization of particular identified lives. In 1965, Dr. Theodore Tsaltas, the Philadelphia physician who was dialyzing himself, testified before the House Committee on Appropriations to great effect, testimony later seen on the NBC TV documentary. In 1966, on a visit to Seattle, Representative John E. Fogarty, chairman of the House committee, observed Mr. Ernie Morelli dialyzing himself in his home. In November 1971, Mr. Shep Glazer, of New York City [vice-president of the National Association of Patients on Hemodialysis and Transplantation], testified and was dialyzed before the House Ways and Means Committee and apparently contributed to the willingness of Representative Wilbur Mills (D-Ark.) to support a kidney disease amendment to Medicare. [Rettig 1976a, pp. 34-35]

After a decade of inconclusive debate, the government's role in financing the treatment costs of dialysis and transplantation was legislatively resolved suddenly and rapidly in the fall of 1972. Although part of the bill known as HR 1, the end-stage renal disease provisions were not related to that legislation's long and stormy history. Neither the House nor the Senate heard testimony on renal disease during the nearly year-long hearings on HR 1's proposed amendments to the Social Security Act, although the House Ways and Means Committee did consider renal disease in separate 1971 hearings on national health insurance.

The end-stage renal disease amendment was not considered until the provisions of the entire H.R. 1 bill were being debated seriatim on the Senate floor. On a Saturday morning, hardly a normal legislative workday, September 30, barely one month before the November [presidential] election, Senator Vance Hartke (D-Ind.) was recognized at 11:30 a.m. to propose an amendment on chronic renal disease. Thirty minutes of time was allocated to the immediate consideration of the kidney amendment. . . . With nearly half of the Senate absent, the measure was adopted by a vote of 52 "Yeas" and 3 "Nays."

The remaining steps of the legislative process were traversed with comparable speed. The conference committee of the House Ways and Means Committee and the Senate Finance Committee met for only a single day to consider differences on the entire bill. The kidney disease amendment received no more than ten minutes' discussion and the Senate proposal was accepted in its essentials with a slight modification in one provision. Both House and Senate accepted the conference committee report on October 17, and President Nixon signed H.R. 1 into law as Public Law 92-603 on October 30, 1972. [Rettig 1976a, pp. 38-39]

As Rettig's study shows, the 1972 end-stage renal failure legislation was prompted by many factors, growing out of a decade of policy debates within the medical-scientific community and the legislative and executive branches of government. In part because of the legislative drive to enact HR 1 before the November 1972 presidential elections, the Congress's rapid action on the amendment was far from a model of thorough and deliberate examination of an expensive and possibly precedent-setting piece of legislation. In terms of economics alone, it is clear that Congress acted on the basis of hasty and drastically low cost estimates, as *New York Times* reporter Richard D. Lyons stressed on 11 January 1973 in a story headlined "Program to Aid Kidney Victims Faces Millions in Excess Costs."

Original cost estimates ranged from $35 million to $75 million in the first fiscal year of operation. The debate record in both houses shows that the highest estimate was $250 million in the fourth year. Yet calculations made by Federal experts after passage set first year costs at $135 million, rising to $1 billion annually a decade from now. [Lyons 1973]

Not surprisingly to those familiar with federal financial forecasting, the second round of cost estimates cited by Lyons also proved to be low. During the first year (1973-74), treatment costs under PL 92-603 were $240 million. Accurate data on the number of transplantation and dialysis patients and their treatment costs and outcomes have been unavailable since the termination of the National Dialysis Registry in 1975 and the Renal Transplant Registry in 1976, with responsibility for data gathering and reporting transferred to the Social Security Administration. Based on imprecise data, the dialysis and transplant population was estimated to be 37,000 persons at the end of 1977, at an annual cost (Medicare and VA) of about $1 billion, and the NIH had projected a $3 billion cost for Medicare-reimbursed treatment by 1984 (Rennie 1978; Friedman, Delano, and Bhutt 1978).

The influential *New York Times,* in response to Lyons's story, worried editorially in January 1973 that section 2991 was another "chapter in the growing history of Congressional fumbling with health matters . . . the point is not that victims of renal disease are unworthy of help, but that Government resources have to be allocated to meet many needs . . . society has a right to expect that the legislators will understand what they are doing and know the magnitude of commitment they are making when they pass special interest legislation, whether for kidney disease sufferers or anybody else ("Medicarelessness" 1973).

The type of decision on allocation of resources represented by the renal disease provisions of PL 92-603 also concerned the National Academy of Sciences' Institute of Medicine, which in March 1973 appointed a six-member panel to review the "implications of a categorical catastrophic disease approach to national health insurance." While recognizing the "strong medical, economic, and political reasons" for the "special consideration" granted to kidney patients under PL 92-603, the panel also paid heed to counter-arguments that the treatment costs under the law "are uncontrollable" and that the law "creates an inequitable distribution of medical resources" (*Disease by Disease* 1973, pp. 2–5). The panel was concerned, however, not with PL 92-603 per se, but with the law as a precedent for moving toward national health insurance on a disease-by-disease basis. The panelists reacted unanimously and negatively to this prospect.

We are in unanimous agreement that coverage of discrete categories similar in kind to end-stage renal disease would be an inappropriate course to follow in the foreseeable future for providing expensive care to those who are unable to afford it. Among the many reasons for not following this disease-by-disease approach, we feel that two are particularly compelling:
The first of these relates to the effect that coverage of particular designated diseases would have on the total allocation of medical resources and the influence of that allocation upon equity. . . .
The second argument against the disease-by-disease approach to

national health insurance is the indeterminate volume of diseases of this kind and the unpredictability of costs associated with these . . . the committee believes that an immense skewing of medical resources may result, along with the creation of incentives for the development of even more technologies that would be highly expensive. [*Disease by Disease* 1973, pp. 6–7]

While the renal disease amendments to PL 92-603 may have been enacted hastily and on the basis of imprecise cost estimates, and while the legislation may have set a dubious precedent for a catastrophic-disease approach to federal financing of patient care, it seems unlikely that Congress would have voted otherwise in 1972 or that its members were unaware of the implications of their actions. In the case of end-stage renal disease, Rettig argues convincingly,

the enactment of Sec. 2991 was the near-inevitable outcome of a whole series of federal government actions which occurred prior to 1972. While it was not inevitable that the end-stage renal disease provision be passed in 1972, the prior commitment of the federal government to R&D, demonstration, and capacity-building within DHEW, and to patient care financing of eligible veterans meant that sooner or later the decision would be taken. [Rettig 1976*a*, p. 45]

That the decision was taken in 1972, the record indicates, owed much to the fact that Congress knew there were identified and identifiable lives at stake. The legislation's proponents had delivered a clear message: "lives had previously been sacrificed for dollars but that situation should now be changed" (Rettig 1976*a*, p. 44).

Delivering Treatment: Some Unresolved Issues

As one looks at the delivery of treatment for end-stage renal failure in the 1970s, there are two major sets of issues, prominent in the 1960s, that have been intensified rather than diminished or resolved by the passage of PL 92-603. The first set of issues, which bears on the relationship between transplantation and dialysis, has to do with the supply of and demand for donor kidneys. The second set of issues, which has evoked a continuing clinical, psychosocial, and economic dialogue since the early 1960s, concerns the comparative merits of center and home dialysis.

Scarcity and Due Process

One of the major problems of scarcity associated with end-stage renal failure—the availability of donor organs—has not been and cannot be alleviated by an infusion of treatment funds. In the greater New York City area during 1972, for example, 1,500 patients were undergoing dialysis compared with only 167 who obtained transplants, primarily (63 percent) from cadaver donors (Friedman and Kountz 1973). With the upsurge in treatment candidates since Medicare funds became available in 1973, the shortage of donor organs has become all the more acute, and the uremic patient's most likely treatment will be dialysis unless or until a suitable donor kidney is found (Comptroller General 1975, pp. 27–29).

Although largely ignored in the literature since PL 92-603, an increasing pool of transplantation candidates for whom there is a serious scarcity of donor organs presents allocation issues not unlike those of the 1960s in their ethical and legal dimensions. For although funding is no longer a major factor in patient visibility and eligibility, selection for receipt of scarce donor kidneys still must be made. And dialysis, as we shall see, presents even more complex allocation issues, centering on whether every person with end-stage renal failure should be maintained on an artificial kidney simply because funds are available.

That selection for renal transplantation continues to operate in essentially the same fashion as we described in earlier chapters, and that certain types of selection still operate for dialysis, raises a fundamental issue in constitutional law that has received little attention in medicine generally, and particularly in the area of scarce, lifesaving resources. That issue, left unresolved by the 1972 Medicare amendments, is whether the procedural safeguards offered by the Constitution's guarantee of due process should operate in the decision to deny a scarce medical resource.

Judge A. Leon Higginbotham, Jr., one of the few legal scholars to have addressed this question, holds that due process should operate at the institutional level in such decisions.

(1) . . . since the substantial proportion of hospitals are government owned and operated, and most remaining hospitals have important connections with government, there is sufficient state action to make the due process clause applicable; (2) . . . denial of treatment

is a deprivation of life within the meaning of the due process clause; and (3) . . . established procedures, which leave room for arbitrary and discriminatory decisions, are constitutionally invalid. [Higginbotham 1975, p. 1736]

Following from this argument, Judge Higginbotham then proposes a basic framework for allocating lifesaving medical resources, viewing dialysis and transplantation as paradigmatic. The procedural safeguards he suggests include hearing and notice, the use of impartial decision-makers and of patients' representatives, and a record of the proceedings and an opinion detailing the facts and opinions used in making the decision (Higginbotham 1975, pp. 1744-49).

In the future, Judge Higginbotham notes, the problem of scarcity that has been experienced in the treatment of end-stage renal failure "is apt to rise with particular force in the area of artificial hearts" (Higginbotham 1975, p. 1735, n.6). How artificial hearts might be allocated in the future, and the due process and other issues raised by such a system, has been explored by Annas through the medium of a hypothetical Supreme Court decision in the year 2002, *Minerva* v. *National Health Agency* (Annas 1977). Thinking of the implications of PL 92-603, Annas's provocative scenario involves the passage of a National Health Insurance Act in 1982, which creates a National Health Agency with the sole authority to allocate scarce and expensive medical resources. In 1990, the Supreme Court upholds an agency decision to prohibit the use of dialysis machines and close all dialysis clinics, based on a cost-benefit analysis. Then, in 1998, following a burgeoning demand for artificial hearts, the agency promulgates regulations for the allocation of no more than twenty thousand hearts per year.

The regulations prohibited the manufacture, sale, or implantation of an artificial heart without a permit from the Agency; prohibited individual purchasers from being recipients of artificial hearts without a permit from the Agency; and provided that permits to recipients be issued only by the Agency's computer, which would pick qualified applicants at random from a master list. This regulation is challenged by Dr. P. Minerva, a thoracic surgeon, and two of her patients, Z. Themis and Z. Dike. Themis did not meet the Agency's qualifications standards as he is less than fifteen years old; Dike, while meeting the standards, has not yet been chosen by the computer. The plaintiffs challenge the regulations as being a violation of their right to privacy, and challenge both the qualification criteria and the random selection procedure as being violations of their rights to equal protection and due process under the fifth amendment to the U.S. Constitution. [Annas 1977, p. 60]

How does the court rule in *Minerva?* Annas's paper needs to be read in its entirety to appreciate the majority and minority opinions he constructs. Suffice it here to say that in a five-to-four decision, with the five justices in the majority all possessing artificial hearts implanted before the lottery was begun, the Supreme Court upholds the validity of the National Health Agency's allocation system. That computerized lottery system in the year 2002 strikes some familiar echoes of dialysis selection in the 1960s:

(1) To be placed on the National Waiting List for Artificial Hearts, the candidate must meet the following criteria: He or she must
   (*a*) be more than 15 years old but less than 70 years old;
   (*b*) be capable of living at least 10 additional years if the implant procedure is successful; and
   (*c*) not be a chronic alcoholic or a drug addict.
(2) Individuals certified as meeting the criteria in part (1) by a physician certified by the National Health Agency as a qualified thoracic surgeon shall have their names immediately placed on the National Waiting List for Artificial Hearts. Individuals will be selected from this list at random at the rate of 400 a week. Individuals will be notified of their selection by telegram which will indicate the date and place of the implant procedure. All transportation costs will be paid by the National Health Service. Individuals shall remain on the list until they die, or until such time as they fail to meet any of the criteria set forth in part (1). [Annas 1977, p. 62]

Where to Dialyze? The Home versus Center Debate

The increased number of dialysis patients, their more heterogeneous medical and socioeconomic status, and the aggregate costs of treatment in the wake of Pl 92–603 have intensified the need for informed decision-making about how dialysis care can best be organized and delivered to provide the best medical and social-rehabilitative care for the greatest possible number of patients at the lowest feasible costs. Because Medicare will not pay for chronic in-hospital dialysis, debate since 1972 has focused upon the relative merits and costs of center and home dialysis. Home dialysis is considerably less expensive than center dialysis, costing an average of $5,000–10,000 per year for the former in 1974 compared with

$22,000 for the latter (Scribner, personal communication). But though costs are a crucial factor, particularly on a national scale, one must also consider patient outcomes, and here the data are less unequivocal.

Seattle's move from an in-hospital to a center to a home dialysis program, as we saw in chapter 7, was motivated by an urgently felt need to expand treatment capability and to lower costs. But the program has continued, in part, because of the Seattle physicians' conviction that most patients, medically and psychosocially, do better on home treatment than in-center treatment. The Seattle experience with home dialysis has been supported, on a larger scale, by a five-year study (1967–71) of patients from twelve home dialysis training centers conducted by the Health Services and Mental Health Administration. In following 628 patients, Gross, Keane, and McDonald's cumulative rehabilitation data showed 81 percent of survivors engaged in "some activity" and 62 percent "carrying on full-time activity." These figures, they concluded, "support home dialysis as an effective remedy" (Gross, Keane, and McDonald 1973).

Based upon their experience in Seattle, Scribner and his colleagues have argued forcefully, in publications and in congressional testimony, that public financing of dialysis demands nationwide implementation of home dialysis programs. "For the great majority of patients who are supported by public funds," Blagg and his colleagues at the Northwest Kidney Center wrote in 1972, ". . . the only available alternative to self-dialysis should be transplantation . . . patients supported by public funds should not have [the] choice [of institutional dialysis], since [it] represents an inefficient use of limited resources" (Blagg et al. 1972).

Despite their arguments for the medical, social, and economic advantages of home dialysis, its proponents have witnessed a precipitous decline in the percentage of patients on home care between 1972 and 1976, while the dialysis population has grown fivefold. In 1972, 40 percent of all dialysis patients in the United States were being treated at home, whereas in 1975 only 4 percent of new dialysis patients received home training, and by 1976 the total percentage of home care patients had shrunk to an estimated 12.9 percent. This decline in the United States contrasts strikingly with the trend toward an increasing percentage of home dialysis patients in most European countries; in Great Britain, for example, home patients have increased from 50 to 80 percent between 1972 and 1976 (Delano 1977; Oberly and Oberly 1977; Scribner 1976).

Why, as some physicians engaged in home dialysis fear, may home treatment be a "dying entity" in the United States? The reasons are several and, proponents of home programs argue, flow primarily from the impact of PL 92–603 on dialysis. Although home dialysis in 1973 was a manifestly less expensive form of treatment than center dialysis, the implementing regulations for section 2991 discriminate economically against patients who opt for home care. Thus, for example, the regulations provide that Medicare pay 80 percent of dialysis costs, whether at home or in a center. For in-center patients private insurance usually covers the other 20 percent of expenses or, if the patient has no such coverage, his or her bills are commonly not collected. Home dialysis patients have found that, irrespective of third-party coverage, they are regularly billed for the 20 percent not covered by Medicare; in addition, Medicare does not cover home supplies needed by the patient, which cost upward of $1,500 per year, nor does it reimburse them for the period of in-center training for home care. The regulations also contain financial disincentives for transplantation, the most striking of which is coverage for only twelve months after the transplant, despite an unremitting need for medication, checkups, and so on.

What end-stage renal failure patients have found, in effect, is that home dialysis and transplantation still entail personal expenses that, while greatly lessened by PL 92–603, can present a severe financial drain.

The most detailed accounting we have seen of the costs of home dialysis and transplantation was provided for us by Mr. and Mrs. James D. Campbell, who at present are graduate students at the University of Missouri. Analyzing the expenses incurred by Mr. Campbell's fifteen months on home dialysis and his subsequent transplant, they found, was a lengthy and arduous task, but one that was revealing to them and that they believe should be shared with others, since there is a lack of such comprehensive information.

As shown in the financial case history reproduced here, Mr. Campbell's treatment costs over a forty-three-month period totaled $46,000. Most of these costs eventually were reimbursed by Medicare and other sources, but the Campbells still had to pay some $4,600 from their own funds. While this outlay was significant for them, it was a cost they were able to bear and one they bore

Table 6. One Patient's Home Dialysis and Transplantation Financial History: June 1, 1973–Dec. 31, 1976

Total Amount Billed

1. Hospital bill	$24,163.45
2. Physician charges	4,038.66
3. Personal expenses	7,031.06
4. Leasing fees for dialysis machine (12 months)	3,000.00
5. Home dialysis supplies (12 months)	7,800.00
Total	$46,033.17

Total Credits

1. *Hospital bill*	
a. Medicare	$14,880.28
b. Blue Cross	4,857.65
c. State papers (county social service)	2,821.32
d. Waived hospital fees	513.00
e. Personal payments from patient	445.06
f. Major Medical	320.34
g. State Renal Disease Commission	180.80
Total hospital credit	$24,018.45
2. *Physician charges*	
a. Waived physician charges	$ 1,199.40
b. Medicare	935.60
c. Blue Shield	869.00
d. Personal payments from patient	152.76
Total physician credit	$ 3,156.76

3. *Personal expenses* (other than hospital & physician)

   a. Personal payments from patient $ 4,019.92

   b. State Renal Disease Commission $ 3,011.14[a]

         Total personal expense credit $ 7,031.06

4. *Leasing fees for dialysis machine*

   a. Medicare $ 2,400.00

   b. Blue Cross   600.00

         Total leasing credit $ 3,000.00[b]

5. *Home dialysis supplies*

   a. Medicare $ 6,240.00

   b. Blue Cross   1,560.00

         Total supplies credit $ 7,800.00[b]

         Total credits $45,006.27[c]

Total Credits by Source

Source	Amount	Percentage Paid
Medicare	$24,455.88	54%
Blue Cross/Blue Shield	7,886.65	18%
Patient	4,617.74	10%
State Renal Disease Commission	3,191.94	7%
State papers	2,821.32	6%
Waived fees	1,712.40	4%
Major Medical	320.34	1%
	$45,006.27	100%

Breakdown of Hospital Charges

Miscellaneous charges	$14,008.09
(includes approximately 50 dialysis treatments)	
Board and room	3,872.50
Laboratory fees	3,670.25
Prescription drugs	1,537.86
X-rays	906.75
IVs	168.00
Total	$24,163.45

Breakdown of Hospital Credits

Medicare	$14,880.28
Blue Cross	4,857.65
State papers	2,821.32
Waived fees	513.00
Patient	445.06
Major Medical	320.34
State Renal Disease Commission	180.80
Total	$24,018.45

[a]The State Renal Disease Commission helped by reimbursing certain personal expenses during 26 of the 43 months. Blue Cross/Blue Shield insurance premiums plus prescriptions obtained through a drug bank program were covered completely the entire 26 months; mileage, meals, and lodging connected with trips to the hospital and clinic were covered for 15 months.

[b]Amounts were obtained from a VA Hospital which did the billing for the leasing and supplies. Medicare and Blue Cross portions were figured at 80% and 20%.

[c]As of 12/31/76 the difference between the total billed and the total credited was $1,026.90. Of that, $145.00 was in hospital fees and $881.90 was in physician charges.

Physician Charges

Total	$ 4,038.66

Breakdown of Physician Credits

Waived fees	$ 1,199.40[d]
Medicare	935.60
Blue Shield	869.00
Patient	152.76
Total	$ 3,156.76

Personal Expenses

	Dialysis		Transplant			Totals
	1973	1974	1974	1975	1976	
Blue Cross insurance premiums	195.35	309.60	154.80	532.20	722.40	1,914.35
Prescriptions (nonhospital pharmacies)	535.06	107.57	26.76	688.87	408.22	1,766.48
Transportation to hospital, parking, meals, motels	220.00	220.00	350.00	423.31	263.28	1,476.59
Setting up home for dialysis[e]	649.54	155.37				804.91
Lab fees (other than those on hospital bill)		58.25	27.60	92.60	194.96	373.41
Moving expense[f]	261.72					261.72
Utilities for home dialysis	55.00	123.60				178.60
Medicare premiums		54.00	27.00	54.00		135.00
Phone calls to hospitals		50.00	70.00			120.00
Totals	1,916.67	1,078.39	656.16	1,790.98	1,588.86	7,031.06

Of Interest

Dialysis total = $2,995.06; $2,995.06/15 months = $199.67 per month
Transplant total = $4,036.00; $4,036.00/28 = $144.14 per month
Total personal expenses of $7,031.06/43 months = $163.51 per month average personal outlay
Taking $4,019.92 (amount from above table not reimbursed by State Renal Disease Commission) plus $445.06 (amount paid on hospital bill) plus $152.76 (amount paid to physicians), the total nonreimbursed patient cost was $4,617.74/43 months = $107.39 per month.

[d] A portion of these waived fees occurred during the one-year period that state papers were in effect since a requirement for eligibility is waiver of physician fees. Occurred one year post-transplant, after Medicare coverage ended.

[e] Includes such equipment as reclining chair, special plumbing, storage shelves, cabinet.

[f] Move from one-bedroom apartment to two-bedroom rented house to accommodate home dialysis.

willingly, given their commitment to his treatment and to the active, fulfilling life he has achieved. But as "consumers," they faced numerous problems and dilemmas in financing Mr. Campbell's treatment, beginning with the discovery that many gaps were left both by Medicare and by private insurance; Medicare, for example, covered only 54 percent rather than the supposed 80 percent of treatment costs.

One of the first problems the Campbells encountered was finding out what types of aid they were eligible for and where and how to obtain that aid, then familiarizing themselves with the rules and regulations of different agencies and companies.

The next obstacle is meeting eligibility requirements. Often this requires a patient and family to give up what they may consider to be very private information. Financial statements, tax returns and means tests all imply an invasion of financial privacy which many people are unaccustomed to and may thus refuse aid that they are entitled to. In addition, the eligibility requirement may have limited time and benefit requirements (such as Medicare and Major Medical benefits).

If one passes the eligibility requirements in terms of income level and need, the problem of aid is by no means permanently solved since many agencies and companies require continual proof of eligibility. . . . In the case of a disabled kidney patient, the problem of eligibility can be compounded by the fact that many agencies and/or companies require the individual to be "totally" disabled to be eligible for aid. The term "total disability" is at present problematic in that there is no clear agreement as to what constitutes a total disability. . . . One of the major problems, then, facing the disabled kidney patient and his physicians who must certify his disability is the fact that agencies and companies do not as yet have a mechanism for dealing with patients who are functioning at a 70% to 80% level.

Another problem concerns private insurance coverage to supplement Medicare. Some patients may not be able to qualify for any insurance coverage and/or may obtain coverage, but at an extremely high premium rate. For example, our Blue Cross/Blue Shield premium rose approximately 50% in one quarter as a result of being placed in a "high-risk" group. The net result of such action can often force patients who need aid the most to be unable to meet these constantly rising premiums and thus be forced to lose insurance coverage.

Although we attempted to utilize the sources of aid that we were entitled to during this period, we observed many other patients and families who refused aid they were entitled to for a number of reasons, many of which stem from the above problems we have outlined. Also, there is the fact that financial problems are just one more item on a list of many problems which a renal patient must cope with. In the midst of multiple life changes and the physical effects of chronic illness, many may find it difficult, if not impossible, to contend with all the necessary requirements now needed to obtain financial aid. [Campbell and Campbell 1977]

To physician and patient proponents of home care, the decline in home dialysis patients, the financial disincentives to home treatment written into the Medicare regulations, and the soaring national costs for dialysis are inextricably linked with the growth of proprietary dialysis centers. The range of ethical and economic issues associated with the establishment of profit-making dialysis centers were first thrust before the public eye through a series of articles in the Boston *Globe* by investigative reporter Richard A. Knox, published between July and October 1971. Knox's articles dealt with the operation of the Babcock Artificial Kidney Center in Brookline, Massachusetts, incorporated as a proprietary corporation in February 1970 by a group of physicians from Boston's Peter Bent Brigham Hospital, an institution that had pioneered renal transplantation and dialysis in the 1950s and 1960s. That corporation, National Medical Care, Inc., has grown into the largest proprietor of dialysis in the United States and is an extraordinarily lucrative enterprise for its management and shareholders. In 1971, when National Medical Care became a public stock company, it had earnings of $0.27 per share. In January 1977 another corporation sought to acquire National Medical Care by a $143 million stock exchange, worth $31.83 for each share of National Medical stock.

In an October 1976 "Special Situation Survey," Forbes Investors Advisory Institute attributed the "phenomenal growth" of National Medical Care to the enactment of PL 92–603, which caused the number of dialysis patients to "zoom" from some 6,000 in 1972 to 25,000 in 1976. With this increase in patients, National expanded from fifteen centers administering 77,000 dialysis treatments in 1972 to forty-eight centers giving 388,000 treatments in 1975, handling about one in six of all hospital and center patients in the United States. The company's revenues have grown apace, from $18.7 million in 1972 to $77.9 million in 1975. Reducing all that dialysis entails to a money-making opportunity, Forbes pointed out that "What is exciting here is not only National's growth, but also the fact that this growth is *not* dependent on the course of the economy. . . . According to the Social Security Administration, the number of people taking dialysis treatment should *double* by 1980. Because of its commanding lead in this field, National should benefit mightily from this" (National Medical Care, Inc. 1976).

The physician-founders of National Medical Care have argued, with validity, that the establishment of propriety centers in the early 1970s met acute needs for chronic dialysis center facilities in areas such as Massachusetts. At the same time, however, reaping profits from the victims of a disease such as end-stage kidney failure is ethically repugnant to many. For while there has been an unmet need for dialysis capabilities, that need can and has been met by the establishment of nonprofit facilities that provide treatment at a far lower cost per patient per year, a savings not only to patients and families but to public and private insurance carriers as well. As of 1977, the proprietary facilities had refused to divulge to the government their data on treatment costs which, as Rettig observed, "directly tests the resolve of the Social Security Administration to move to audited costs as a basis for establishing reimbursement rates for dialysis treatments" (Rettig 1976*b*, p. 23). However, the widely quoted average cost of $24,000 per patient per year for in-center dialysis, of which a significant percentage is paid to proprietary operations, contrasts sharply with the nonprofit Northwest Kidney Center's 1976 average cost per patient of $8,825.

The imposition of stricter cost-accounting and reimbursement procedures by the federal government may reduce the profit factor and costs to patients in proprietary centers, such centers may meet increasing competition from nonprofit centers, and proposed legislation such as HR 8423 may redress the economic disincentives to home dialysis and transplantation at a savings of tens of millions of dollars annually to patients and to public and private insurers (Stange and Sumner 1978). But since the inception of home dialysis, the question of home versus center treatment has involved far more than cost differentials, and removing cost inequities will not alone end the controversy about the relative merits of different treatment sites.

In the early 1970s, discussion centered on the question whether certain categories of patients, principally disadvantaged inner-city residents, could be trained for and fare well on home dialysis, matching the experience of the Northwest Kidney Center. Countering charges that the decline in numbers of home-treatment patients was linked with the growth of proprietary centers, Dr. Eli Friedman of New York's Downtown Medical Center observed in 1973 that Brooklyn is not Seattle:

> In Brooklyn not only are there virtually no community nephrologists (for a population of over two million) but the neighborhood practitioner is progressively becoming extinct. Much of Brooklyn, the Bronx, Philadelphia, Detroit, Newark and Chicago look like Germany after World War II, with few of the on-line social rehabilitation programs that make the state of Washington a good place to live in.
>
> Thus, an alternative explanation for the falling percentage of patients on home dialysis may be that the extension of maintenance hemodialysis from its pioneering in Seattle to inner-city America has met with unexpected problems worthy of exploration. These difficulties are real and not reflections of physicians' greedy desire to milk fees. [Friedman 1973]

More recent outcome studies and clinical experience, however, have altered the perspective of nephrologists like Friedman, bringing them into far closer accord with the views of Scribner and his Seattle colleagues on the use of home dialysis. Now, they agree, overall survival statistics argue in favor of home dialysis, for "the average home dialysis patient survival at five and six years is 74 percent (range 52–88 percent) while the average of center patients alive at the same point is 52 percent (range 52–53 percent). Home dialysis patients' survival is equal to live donor transplantation and superior to cadaveric transplantation" (Delano 1977, p. 5).

Data on various subgroups of home dialysis patients further indicate that outcome is related to age and diagnosis, including general health status, rather than to demographic characteristics per se or to the range of delivery services available in a given area. One widely cited study, conducted by the Regional Medical Programs Service, looked at cumulative five-year mortality figures among 1,063 patients trained for home dialysis at twelve centers between 1967 and 1973 (Roberts 1976). Significantly lower survival rates were found among several categories of patients. First, only 34 percent of patients aged fifty years or older lived five years, compared with 53 percent of those aged thirty to forty-nine and 63 percent of those under thirty. Second, patients with renal failure secondary to complicating systemic diseases such as diabetes and hypertension had significantly lower survival rates than patients with glomerulonephritis, pyelonephritis, and polycystic disease.

Third, when the patients' general health and activity status at the start of home dialysis was rated from a good risk of 1 to a poor risk of 5, "there was a consistent trend toward lower cumulative survival with each 'poorer' health status." Finally, "the differences in survival of the two centers with the highest and lowest 5-year cumulative survival were markedly different." The center with the highest survival rate (85 percent) was in a suburban area with a large middle-class population that included a high percentage of patients who were older but had generally good health. In contrast, the center with the lowest survival rate (30 percent) drew primarily upon an indigent inner-city population that included many patients with a poorer health status.

Findings such as the above have led Friedman to sharply recast his view of why the proportion of home dialysis patients has been steadily decreasing. "It has become clear," he wrote in a 1978 paper, "Pragmatic Realities in Uremia Therapy,"

that the fraction of uremic patients on dialysis at home reflects physician bias rather than regional differences in patient populations . . . in the United States . . . more than 75 percent of patients on dialysis in the state of Washington and 60 percent of patients in Indiana receive this treatment at home at the same time that fewer than 15 percent of patients in the Northeast perform self-dialysis. The explanation for this discrepancy must be physician bias since objective studies show home patients to have lower morbidity and better rehabilitation than center patients. Delano and I have dealt with the question of whether indigent, undereducated patients are suitable for home hemodialysis. In our experience, many of them are. [Friedman, Delano, and Bhutt 1978, p. 370]

The probable role of physician bias in the choice of treatment setting and the roles of age and other complicating illnesses in determining a patient's course on either home or center dialysis underscore the fact that financial access and even equity for treatments such as chronic dialysis cannot provide for equity in treatment outcomes—American values of equality, universalism, and social justice notwithstanding.

Whether all individuals *ought* to receive a treatment such as dialysis, irrespective of any other factors besides meeting the medical criteria of having a given disease and the guarantee of federal funds to meet treatment costs, remains the central medical-ethical and public policy issue raised by the passage of PL 92–603. And it is also a central concern for those most immediately engaged in the use of such therapies as providers and patients, as they are being forced to consider anew the old issues of patient selection and quality of life.

Gatekeeping under PL 92–603: "Deselection" and the "Invisible List"

From the echelons of Washington policy-makers to the decisions that must be made by physicians and patients, one of the most pivotal and complex of the medical and moral issues generated by PL 92–603 is its bearing on the question of who should receive dialysis or transplantation. The messages physicians have received from Washington have been ambivalent in this respect, for there are unresolved differences of opinion between government agencies. In June 1975 the government's financial "watchdog" agency, the General Accounting Office (GAO), issued a report to Congress on dialysis and transplantation under PL 92–603. As indicated in a portion of the report's title, "The Need for More Vigorous Effort," the GAO concluded in part that not all patients "were getting the treatment needed, in part because doctors were not referring patients for treatment or dialysis facilities were rejecting patients because of stringent acceptance criteria" (Comptroller General 1975, pp. i, ii). At least implicitly, the GAO viewed treatment criteria as no longer tenable in the face of Medicare funding and accordingly recommended to Congress: "That the Secretary [of HEW] act now to encourage the liberalization of existing criteria for treatment at facilities not accepting patients because of age suitability for home dialysis, diabetes and other diseases by establishing guidelines for treatment under the Medicare Program" (Comptroller General 1975, p. 66).

In its commentary on the GAO report, however, the Office of the Secretary of Health, Education, and Welfare, under whose aegis the Medicare program operates, disagreed with the assumption that public funding should in itself require that all end-stage renal failure patients be treated by transplantation or dialysis. In commenting on the above GAO recommendation, the secretary's office stated:

We concur in principle. However, we believe that this recommendation gives the impression that the criteria of the type listed should not be used to exclude patients from dialysis. While we agree that whole categories of patients should not be excluded because they have been labelled as diabetic or are over a certain chronologic age, etc., we do not agree that every patient with end-stage kidney disease should be dialyzed. The purpose of Public Law 92–603 is to assure that patients will not be excluded from dialysis because of economic factors; it is not to require that every patient with kidney disease receive either dialysis or transplantation. [Comptroller General 1975, p. 66]

There is a range of opinion, too, among individual physicians and dialysis groups about how and to what extent treatment criteria ought to be "liberalized" now that economic barriers to selection have largely been removed. The medical profession, by and large, was acutely uncomfortable with the necessity of selection in the face of scarce dialysis resources in the 1960s, and all users and observers of selection criteria in those years could point to their various shortcomings—the uncertainties of biomedical criteria, the arbitrariness of "first come, first served" and random lottery methods, and the ways that economic and psychosocial criteria were apt to favor those already financially and socially privileged.

But the unease that physicians felt about "playing God" in their role as the primary gatekeepers of dialysis has not, we have found, been done away with by financial accessibility to dialysis; or, perhaps more accurately, it has been replaced by new sources of disquiet about their roles and the treatment they are offering.

Although a major precipitant, the passage of PL 92–603 is not the only factor that has contributed to what we believe is a shift of atmosphere and emphasis among those engaged in dialysis. (Several of these factors have been traced in the previous chapter with respect to renal transplantation.)

One reason some professionals and patients have lost zeal and expectancy about dialysis is the plateau that renal research has reached in the 1970s. The optimistic sense of an "imminent" research breakthrough in understanding normal and abnormal kidney function has diminished, and the routinization of many of the once-challenging technical problems of maintenance dialysis has dampened the pioneering spirit that infused many participants during the 1950s and 1960s.

There have been, to be sure, important technical advances in the 1970s. These include progress in developing a compact, portable "suitcase" kidney, the growing use of the generally more durable and long-lasting A-V fistula in place of the cannula shunt, and bovine and dacron heterografts that may permit dialysis for those whose blood vessels cannot tolerate a fistula or a shunt. Important advances also have been made in managing the problems of anemia, nutrition, bone disease, and peripheral nerve disorders that affect dialysis patients, and physicians "do better" at dialyzing patients with complicated multiple disease states. But these advances notwithstanding, there is the recognition that, after almost two decades of intensive clinical and basic research, "existing data are as yet inadequate to establish rational guidelines" for "adequate" dialysis therapy (Burton 1975).

Another phenomenon has contributed to the "dialysis atmosphere" of the 1970s, and in particular to what we sense as a greater difficulty among professionals in reaching consensus on the old and new questions that confront them. A "third generation" of physician-dialyzers is now at work. Though some of them were trained by the physicians who pioneered the artificial kidney and the dialysis process, many have only a distant sense of what that work was like a decade ago. That some of this new generation have never personally dialyzed a patient, and indeed are amazed to learn that this was a regular task for their progenitors, seems to us a significant barometer of a new era in dialysis and of the physician-patient relationships it may entail. There also is the new, younger generation of dialysis nurses, who remain, by and large, deeply involved with and committed to patients. But we have noted a tendency among nurses relatively new to the field to be somewhat less vulnerable to the strains associated with their work and less apt to engage either in doubting questions about their enterprise or in expressions of hope than are nurses who have been involved in dialysis for many years. At the same time, some of the nurses who have worked for a longer period with dialysis make invidious comparisons between the present and what they view as the "good old (pioneering) days" of dialysis.

But, far more than the state of knowledge and art and a succession of generations, the passage of PL 92–603 has shifted the emphasis and atmosphere of dialysis in the 1970s. The complex, often agonizing dilemma that, we believe, has most affected dialysis in this decade was stated simply and eloquently by two Tufts–New England Medical Center nephrologists in announcing the center's plan to open a nonprofit, self-care dialysis facility (a delivery mode that many feel will be increasingly used because it combines the most advantageous features of both home and in-center dialysis). In 1977, they explained, Massachusetts had only 94 dialysis beds for some 700 patients, nearly half of which were operated four shifts a day by Boston's proprietary Kidney Center. Both now and to meet the projected increase to 1,400 patients within five years, there must be an expansion of dialysis facilities. For, stated the physicians, *"with payment guaranteed under Social Security, there is no way—morally—to turn anyone down anymore"* (McLaughlin 1977; italics added).

There seems to be widespread consensus among physicians that the minimizing if not the elimination of psychosocial selection criteria has been a highly positive trend, one that began before PL 92–603 but that has been greatly accelerated by Medicare funding. Many physicians still believe, however, that certain more biologically and clinically based criteria *should* be used, if not to refuse dialysis to a candidate then at least to discourage him or her from beginning a course of palliative treatment that, it is medically presumed, will not be truly beneficial. As in past years, the chief medical contraindications are being too old or too young, and having other severe or life-threatening conditions such as diabetes, cardiovascular disease, metastatic carcinoma, liver disease, and organic brain syndrome.

But what is in fact progressively occurring, impelled by financial access, is that virtually *all* criteria of negative selection are being slackened if not abandoned. For, as expressed above by the Boston nephrologists, physicians now feel morally unjustified in denying treatment to virtually any patient with end-stage renal failure, whatever reservations they may have about the patient's prognosis. When we revisited Seattle in the spring of 1977 we found, pre-eminently reflective of this trend, that the Northwest Kidney Center's "Admissions and Policy Committee" no longer exists. Belding Scribner and his colleagues, however, remain deeply concerned about the problem of "how not to dialyze" certain patients. Reflective of this concern, the Northwest Kidney Center now has what Scribner called a "deselection committee" in reserve, to back up if necessary a physician's decision not to put a patient on dialysis (Scribner, personal communication).

For medical professionals, medical-moral questions about whether all candidates ought now to receive dialysis are inevitably accompanied by concerns about the medical, psychological, and social course of many of their new patients. And these concerns, in turn, have raised anew, and on a larger scale, the same intense questions about the quality of life and the meaning of treatment termination that prŌviders and patients have grappled with since the advent of chronic dialysis.

As has been documented in Roberts's analysis of home dialysis patients, and by other studies of both home and in-center patients, socioeconomically disadvantaged patients, the elderly, and those with other grave systemic illnesses or generally poor health status are not nearly as likely to have favorable prognoses in terms of either rehabilitation or survival as are more affluent, younger, and healthier patients. The socioeconomic democratization of dialysis under PL 92–603 has, on the one hand, accorded with the general value consensus that income, social class, and associated racial, ethnic, and religious factors ideally should not deter patients from receiving dialysis. At the same time, we have found that staff members of the several dialysis units we have visited since 1973 have been both surprised and deeply troubled by the dramatically poorer course of a significant percentage of socioeconomically disadvantaged patients. In some instances, the staff felt guilty because these patients were not doing well, creating staff morale problems that further negatively affected the patient's course on dialysis. At one university hospital dialysis center we visted, for example, the nurses had gone through an emotionally wrenching time of blaming themselves for having unconscious prejudices against poor minority patients from the inner city, and for their inability to communicate effectively with such patients. The nurses had attributed the relatively poor course of these patients to the staff's personal limitations and failings, rather than to more "objective" medical, psychological, and social factors.

Dialysis staff also are troubled because many of their patients with complicating illnesses do nct do well on chronic dialysis, which raises in their own minds questions about the medical wisdom, the humanity, and the ethical and economic justifiably of having accepted such patients for treatment to begin with. The largest category of dialysis patients with often severe, systemic illnesses are diabetics, who "probably represent 30% to 40% of the total annual number of new candidates for regular maintenance dialysis" (Shapiro, Leonard, and Comty 1974, pp. 5–8). The range of problems experienced by these patients, and their growing number, has thrown into sharp focus the medical and ethical question whether it is appropriate to place all end-stage renal failure patients on chronic dialysis.

The experiences of many diabetics who receive dialysis, and of the staff members who care for them, were chronicled at a 1974 symposium by physicians from the Minnesota Regional Kidney Disease Program, which has the largest and reportedly the most successful series of diabetic transplant and dialysis patients ("End-stage Diabetic Nephropathy" 1974, pp. S-137; S-13-14; S-150, S-99).

Dr. C. M. Kjellstrand: We have seen the handwriting on the wall of two bad ways of treating a diabetic, cadaver transplantation and dialysis. If you separate the two curves, you will see that they end at zero at three years. If you take a patient from cadaver transplantation who will be dead in three years and put him on a treatment of dialysis, he will also be dead in three years. Zero plus zero always equals zero.

Drs. F. L. Shapiro, A. Leonard, and C. M. Comty: Diabetic dialysis patients do require a larger commitment of staff time, both during and between dialysis treatments. This requirement not only increases the cost of regular dialysis but it could adversely affect the quality of care being provided to other patients in programs with limited personnel and facilities.

The psychosocial problems involved with providing dialysis treatment to diabetic patients . . . associated with the high percentage of visual disorders and medical complications, can adversely affect the morale of the dialysis nursing staff who treat the patients on a chronic basis as they witness the all-too-often slow decay of the patient.

Drs. Comty, Leonard, and Shapiro: A high incidence of psycho-social problems has been observed in a group of 497 diabetic patients with end-stage renal failure treated by repetitive hemodialysis. The causes of the problems appear to be directly related to blindness, with loss of employment and role reversal in the male patient. Further, the average patient spends at least 2.6 days of each month inhospital with complications, in addition to a regular dialysis schedule involving treatments three times a week, either at home or incenter. In addition to these demands on him, the diabetic patient has other demands such as regulation of his diet, fluid intake and insulin therapy. He is further incapacitated by loss of sexual function which may cause a major breakdown in marital relationships. The dialyzed diabetic patient also places a large burden on society since only 25% of the patients are self-supporting, and others are supported entirely by some form of medical assistance.

The question addressed by these statements, which have been reiterated by other physicians as they dialyze other categories of "less than ideal patients," was posed at the 1974 symposium at the end of a panel discussion on neurologic complications of diabetics on dialysis.

Dr. Cahill: There are several more questions, but there is just one I am going to ask and I'm not going to ask any of the panelists to answer. The question is, and I will just paraphrase it, "For a person who has had 20 yr. of relatively disturbing disease and who is on his last leg, so to speak, is it morally and ethically justified to spend the last 4 yr. in a transplant or dialysis program, realizing the grim morbidity of even the best treatment?" I think that is a good remark on which to conclude and that is why we are all here.

For many patients, and for those who initiate and manage their chronic dialysis, the financial democratization created by PL 92–603 has exacerbated the quality-of-life issues that this mode of therapy has evoked since its inception. Liberal selection policies are not unique to the years since 1972, but their increase and the consequent influx of often complexly ill patients has magnified the problem of selection and "deselection." In 1971, Belding Scribner saw that selection would evolve much as it has since the passage of PL 92–603: "Selection . . . will take the form of advising the patient and his family that we don't think this treatment is right for him, that it could be a fate worse than death to dialyze or transplant him. If the patient doesn't agree, he'll be taken regardless of the expense or the difficulty" (Scribner, personal communication). And then, for some patients, there will be the usually agonizing decision of whether or not to terminate treatment. With increasingly liberal, inclusive selection policies, the issue of "deselection" will be faced more frequently, and physicians and patients will have to reach accord on the procedures by which dialysis will be withdrawn. One such accord is that which has been evolved for Minnesota's Regional Kidney Disease Program (RKDP), out of what its physicians militantly call a "trial by combat" approach of accepting for dialysis all patients who are dying of uremia and have "a desire to live."

We consider regular dialysis a relatively successful form of palliative therapy and will offer it to informed patients who desire therapy. *Because of our "trial by combat" approach*, we initiated a written agreement between the patient and the RKDP which is completed when dialysis is begun. This agreement explains that dialysis will be provided for as long as the patient desires the treatment or until, in the opinion of the medical staff, dialysis is no longer indicated because of supervening severe medical complications, such as cerebral insults or atrophy, disabling cardiac problems or inability to adjust emotionally to the stress of medical complications and dialysis. We have discontinued dialysis in nine hopeless patients, allowing them to die of uremia in the past five years. [Shapiro, Leonard, and Comty 1974, p. S–8]

Changing the economic factor in the allocation of scarce, life-saving medical resources, as we have seen in the five years that have elapsed since the passage of PL 92–603, can have profound effects, both intended and unintended, on the use of a therapy such as dialysis. At the same time, we have seen that the infusion of economic resources has not resolved, and cannot resolve, some of the most complex medical, ethical, and social issues attending the use of such a modality and in many instances exacerbates those issues. If one views PL 92–603 as the progenitor of future legislation, whether in some form of national health insurance or specific to given catastrophic diseases, there surely are lessons to be learned from the issues that have been framed by the passage of PL 92–603 and the effects it has and has not had at both macro and micro levels.

At a macro-societal level, however much we might wish to avoid it, we must eventually face and deal with the ethical and economic questions of how much of our resources we *ought* to and *can* commit to the extensive number of chronic and catastrophic illnesses that afflict our citizens. During the turbulent decade of the 1960s, dialysis and transplantation were sometimes invoked in connection with the national debate about the war in Southeast Asia. If we really believe in health and life, some argued, then why have we been willing to invest so much in a war in Vietnam and unwilling to commit funds to those with end-stage renal failure? Now, in the 1970s, others ask, "Why are we spending so many resources on forms of treatment like dialysis, rather than investing more in the delivery of basic medical services for the entire population?" The irony that dialysis has now acquired a status like that of Vietnam does not escape those who argued for renal disease treatment funds in the 1960s.

And if the government elects to support treatment costs, as it has done for end-stage renal failure, those involved in the policy decision and its implementation need to think through the implications of becoming the economic gatekeepers. Do they want to, or should they, in effect become the primary medical and ethical decision-makers as well? What seems to us to have been one of the most significant consequences of PL 92–603 is the extent to which government funding of dialysis has contributed to the slackening, if not the elimination, of *biomedical* as well as psychological and social criteria of judgment and selection. It highlights the degree to which this kind of medical decision-making can be influenced by economic and political factors.

Finally, if our ethics are to be guided by economics, so that it is seen as morally indefensible to deny a treatment like dialysis to any patient who is financially eligible, we must be prepared to deal with the increasingly numerous quality of life issues that will be posed. We end this chapter with excerpts from two letters written by a young woman on dialysis shortly before her death. To us they are a haunting reminder of all that can be involved in the decision to embark on a treatment like dialysis.

[10 September 1974] I even find myself looking at the obituary notices more often, just to see if someone I know may have passed away . . . and it makes me more sick to be "correct" in finding a familiar name. And you can tell how the other patients, although just casually conversing after such an occurrence, are really so very hurt and afraid—as if an invisible list exists whose names are crossed out and such an exclusive list includes your name.

[9 October 1974] I really hate dialyzing now, more than ever. . . . I'm so tired of putting up a front for everybody—the brave, independent soul. I'm tired of putting in my own fistula needles and they actually do hurt; I'm tired of cleaning the machine by myself; I'm tired of trying to arrange my dialysis schedule to fit my family's convenience as well as my own; I'm tired of becoming friends with patients and some die and they all get sick; I'm tired of hearing all the problems patients and staff seem to always have; I'm tired of hearing about the transplant failures or even the jealousy of a transplant success; I'm tired of hearing about all the hopes for all sorts of miraculous medical advances—they'll never come.

12

The Societal Meaning of
The Courage to Fail

The importance of hemodialysis and human organ transplantation lies as much in their social and cultural significance as in their medical and surgical value. These therapeutic innovations are associated with key structural attributes of modern medical research and practice and with the values and beliefs on which these attributes are based. Furthermore, dialysis and transplantation have been extensively practiced and brought to public notice at a historical juncture when there are indications that the kind of modern society in which they have been developed is moving into a new evolutionary phase. Some of the metamedical phenomena and issues connected with dialysis and transplantation are integrally related to modern societal patterns and to alterations they are at present undergoing.

There is a sense in which medicine, even in its less heroic, more everyday activities, is always committed to intervening in ultimate problems of the human condition. Its latent existential functions concern birth, life, physical and psychic suffering, disability, and death.[1] In the practice of modern medicine, the physician ushers life in and ushers it out. Through contraception and abortion, he helps determine whether or not human lives will come into existence. He pronounces death. He diagnoses human malaise. He administers to those deemed physically or psychologically ill. And he tries to forestall as well as to cure the forms of anguish—labeled sickness—with which he has been trained to deal. From this perspective, organ transplantation and chronic hemodialysis are merely two of the more recent techniques that medicine has devised to sustain life and fend off death. As such, they seem to fit without controversy into modern medicine's institutionalized commitment to doing all it can to prevent death. In turn, trying so energetically to prevent adventitious death expresses a broader cultural pattern: the dynamic meliorism or activism that characterizes modern Western, and particularly American, society.

Nevertheless, dialysis and transplantation have not simply been heralded as lifesaving developments. They have also become focuses of fundamental reflection and discussion on the assumptions about death and attitudes toward it on which modern medicine and research are based. The advent of hemodialysis and organ transplantation has highlighted the active, undaunted striving of modern medicine to control death and its growing ability to do so. At the same time, it has increased awareness of the bivalent nature of death, and of the poignant conflicts entailed by this progress in staving off death and prolonging life.

In various ways, dialysis and transplantation have heightened consciousness of how imperfect and approximate medical understanding of life and death and the distinction between them still is. The development of transplantation has contributed significantly to medical discussions over whether we need a better definition of death than cessation of respiratory and cardiac function. In turn, these deliberations have revealed the indeterminate and relatively arbitrary nature of the conceptions of death institutionalized in modern medicine. It has also become plainer that the essential nature of death—the fundamental explanation of how and why it occurs, and whether it is an immutable part of life and the human condition—still eludes medical science. The introduction of the concept of "brain death" and its implications have only begun to be explored. But this at once symbolic and organic transposition of the primary site of death from the heart and lungs to the brain has already created new ambiguities about what constitutes life and humanness as opposed to mere existence. For example, if we accept cessation of the information processing capacity of the brain as the basic functional criterion of death, then how alive and how human are any persons with severe cerebral impairment?

This is closely related to the difficult "quality of life" considerations that both dialysis and transplantation have raised. However great the internal and external pressures to save life, should physicians invariably do everything they can to treat dying patients by chronic dialysis or transplantation? Is the interlude of survival thus given to patients and their families always sufficiently meaningful, and free of physical and psychic suffering, to be called full human life? How should one appraise the time and experience granted the person who has received a heart or liver transplant but who never recovers sufficiently to leave the hospital? Or the bone-marrow recipient whose "new life" lasts no more than six months? Or the kidney recipient who rejects one donated organ after another? Or the patient on dialysis who does not feel physically well and suffers psychically and spiritually from his bondage to the "miraculous monster"? Does the "quality" of the prolonged lives of such patients justify the original medical decision to offer them dialysis or transplantation or the decision to continue? And what if the patient wishes to terminate the treatment and die a so-called natural death? What are the physician's medical and moral responsibilities and prerogatives? Should he try to strike some kind of balance between his commitment to maintain life and protect its sanctity and his concern for the quality of life of his patients and their kin? If so, what should the balancing logic be, and where will it lead?

The problem of arriving at a rational, ethical, and humane equation is complicated by a number of other elements. Certain factors push the medical profession toward trying to provide dialysis and transplantation to all whose lives might possibly be extended. Because medical decisions about dialysis and transplantation occur in the emotive context of personal, face-to-face encounters with patients and their families rather than in a more impersonal, distant, and statistical way, it is difficult for physicians to foreclose these therapeutic options.

Furthermore, physicians testify that once they have begun to treat a patient with an "extraordinary" life-sustaining procedure like dialysis or transplantation, it is extremely hard for them to stop, even if they recognize that they are compounding the patient's suffering rather than relieving it. It would have been easier to withhold the therapy in the first place than to allow a patient not to continue on the artificial kidney machine, to withdraw immuno-suppressive therapy after he has received a transplant, or to decide not to carry out successive renal implants on a patient who has rejected previous ones. From a strictly rational point of view, physicians acknowledge, there may not be that much moral difference between stopping heroic efforts to save life and not starting them. But initiating such treatment seems to emotionally bind the physician to his terminally ill patient in such a way that to then desist and passively relinquish the patient to death becomes over-whelming, beyond the legal aspects it entails. It exposes physicians to feelings of betrayal, guilt, defeat, and grief that they find almost too much to bear.

The great medical uncertainty still involved in dialysis and transplantation also inclines physicians to offer them to the termi-nally ill patients who seek their care rather than to deny them such a possibility or to advise them against it. On both biological and socio-psychological grounds, it is difficult to predict which patients will do well and which will not; thus, many physicians are prone to give patients the benefit of the doubt by not disqualifying them. At least in American society, they are reinforced in this tendency by the belief, shared by medical professionals and patients and their families, that if the afflicted person can be kept from dying there is always the possibility that a "breakthrough" may provide a more effective treatment or even a cure. This orientation is further strengthened by the general cultural disposition to actively prevent or delay death whenever possible, and by the correlative extent to which the physician's obligation to maintain life usually comes to prevail over his responsibility to ease death. And in some instances, the drive to achieve or maintain either a personal or an institutional reputation for trailblazing and record-breaking with dialysis and transplantation also powerfully influences physicians to intervene.

In the realm of dialysis and renal transplantation, the passage of PL 92–603 in 1972 represents a new set of economic and political pressures that have made physicians feel medically and morally compelled to offer these treatments to all patients with end-stage renal failure. In the 1960s the allocation question these therapies raised was, Why is our supposedly affluent and just society unable or unwilling to provide the resources necessary to keep those afflicted with terminal kidney disease alive? The resolution of this question, through the passage of PL 92–603, has created other questions of allocation and equity. Is it medically and morally proper to dialyze or transplant *all* these patients because monies are available, whether or not they will benefit from treatment? On a societal level, should we be investing this much on such catastrophic illness and in such costly, life-maintaining but not curative, "pre-therapeutic" treatments?

Beyond this, how much of our material and nonmaterial resources should we be utilizing in the health-illness-medicine sector of our society? And, in the face of the unchoosing and deselecting problems that the "democratization" of dialysis and renal transplantation has paradigmatically raised, what modes of decision-making will lead to the most medically and ethically appropriate consequences for patients and for society?

The development of life-prolonging treatments like dialysis and transplantation has made the existential dimension of the physician's role more manifest. It has also increased the strains and dilemmas associated with these role facets and pointed up their relationship to much broader value considerations in the society at large. This process of amplification is itself an important phenomenon. It involves a greater professional and public awareness of the problems of meaning that occur in the medical domain, and an increased tendency to openly discuss and seek counsel on them. The emergence of bioethics is perhaps the most organized and important expression of these concerns, which do not seem to be purely a consequence of scientific and technical advances that dialysis and transplantation represent. Nor does it appear to be confined to medicine. Rather, it is one manifestation of a broader and deeper cultural shift toward a more overt, collective preoccupation with ethical and existential issues. Medicine has become a particularly strategic focus of these societal concerns.

We believe that chronic hemodialysis and organ transplantation have received so much public and professional attention because together they constitute a paradigm of these essentially moral and religious problems with which modern Western society is grappling.

This aspect of the social and cultural meaning of dialysis and transplantation is also integral to the questions these procedures have raised about the bases and significance of human solidarity. The nature and importance of our relationship to one another is a core issue in every society, system of ethics, and religion. Dialysis and transplantation have reemphasized how central it is to medicine as well. This has occurred in a period of generalized crisis over whether and how an advanced modern society like our own can achieve a more trusting, intimate, inclusive, and transcendent form of solidarity.

Both the increase in human experimentation over the past twenty years and this solidarity crisis have contributed to the marked attention being given to the relationship between the physician-investigator and his patient-subject. The numerous commentaries on this relationship are strikingly bifurcated. On the one hand, a great deal of apprehension is expressed about the ways research physicians can mislead, exploit, or injure their subjects in the name of patient welfare, scientific progress, or public good. On the other hand, in its ideal form this same relationship is heralded as the prototype of the new solidarity toward which modern man is groping. A vision is invoked of a society conducive to the establishment of relationships in which individuals of diverse backgrounds and conditions—brought together by their suffering, competence, hope, courage, sense of adventure, quest for knowledge and meaning, and desire to serve—collaborate, in equality and trust, to realize "distinctively human . . . noble," melioristic goals (Mead 1970, p. 165). The qualities and values celebrated here are traditional precepts of the Protestant ethic and American creed on which modern American society was founded. They are not merely being reaffirmed. It is implied that, animated by these values, the more extensive institutionalization of collectively oriented, participant-collaborator relations could transform the society, moving it into a new, more advanced evolutionary stage that is "beyond modern." Yet the socially structured ambivalence about this is palpable, for this same alliance between physician-investigator and patient-subject is also recurrently portrayed as the relationship par excellence through which the rights and integrity of the individual can be unduly sacrificed to the needs and demands of other persons and of society in general.

Nowhere is this ambivalence more conspicuous than in the discoveries that physicians and patients, donors, and their families have made about the dilemmas and paradoxes of the gift as they occur in the context of organ transplantation. Organ donation is an ultimate expression of a sublime value in our society: the Judeo-Christian injunction to give of one's self to others, sacrificially if need be, that they may live and flourish. Because it is an act of the highest moral value, ideally organ donation should be what the philosopher Hans Jonas terms a "supererogatory gift . . . beyond duty and claim . . . reckoning and rule," characterized by "true authenticity and spontaneity" (Jonas 1970, p. 16). It should also be transcendentally fulfilling and liberating. For many donors and recipients and their kin this does seem to be the case. But at the same time, the sheer existence of organ transplantation as a lifesaving option, the current medical supposition that a live, well-matched donation optimizes the outcome, and the institutionalized arrangements that have been developed to facilitate organ exchange all place certain people under constant pressure to make such a gift. In this respect organ donation, a gift that in principle surpasses coercion and constraint, is also conscripting and obligating.

The bonds of kinship have exerted a powerful influence over organ donation, soliciting and in some instances, such as between twins, compelling the gift. This has not been as surprising and unsettling to the medical profession as the factors that seem to induce living, unrelated donors to offer an organ to a named person or an "unnamed stranger" (Titmuss 1971, p. 242). Is this the most wholesome, disinterested, universalistic form of giving possible? Or is it a driven, pathologically self-mutilating act? The psychodiagnostic and ethical difficulties of ascertaining what the "true" motives for wishing to give an organ are and ought to be have brought physicians face to face with the question of how much "faith" they collectively have in the "altruistic principle," and how much they believe in the need and capacity of human beings to relate to each other, both as their "brothers' keepers" and as their "strangers' keepers" (Bevan 1971). It has also confronted them with the related issue of whether controls ought to be exercised over proffering gifts of the magnitude, and with the attributes, of organ donation. Should such gifts be encouraged and fostered? Should they be monitored and selectively restrained? Can we say, as Richard M. Titmuss suggests, that "the notion of social rights—a product of the twentieth century—should . . . embrace the 'Right to Give' in non-material as well as material ways"? (Titmuss 1971, p. 242). If so, then is any attempt to restrict or deter the gift of an organ a violation of that right? Or is surveillance of this act necessary, in the name of upholding other critical modern Western values like the "integrity of personal bodily individuality" and the "sanctity of life" (Callahan 1969) while preventing the forms of "voluntary self-degradation and dehumanization" (Kass 1971, p. 783) that are their antitheses?

Perhaps the most troubling aspect of the gift relationship for the medical team and donors, recipients, and their relatives is a particular sociopsychological consequence of the "three obligations"—"giving, receiving, repaying"—that Mauss has designated as its constituent "elements" (Mauss 1954, p. 37). Giving, receiving, and return giving tend to draw those who participate in this exchange-cycle into a closer, more involved relationship. In organ transplantation, the meaning of what is interchanged is so extraordinary that donor, recipient, and kin can become bound to one another, emotionally and morally, in ways that are as likely to be mutually fettering as to be self-transcending. We have come to think of this facet of organ donation and receipt as the potential "tyranny of the gift." The custom of keeping the identity of the cadaver donor and the live recipient unknown to each other and to their kin, which the medical profession now observes, is a normative response to their gradual recognition of this phenomenon. Another such pattern, subsumed under the medical team's gatekeeping functions, is the attempt to screen out live related donors whose gift of an organ might lock the giver and the receiver into a creditor-debtor relationship harmful to their own equilibrium or to that of their family. Clinical experience with organ transplantation, then, has led the profession to govern the gift as much on psychological and social as on biological grounds. This regulatory behavior has evolved independently of physicians' predisposing philosophical perspective on "the question of obligation and spontaneity in the gift," its meaning and likely consequences (Mauss 1954, p. 63). Although physicians involved in transplantation tend to be skeptical about how often "avowed altruism" is the primary "motivation for irreversible acts of self sacrifice of denial" like organ donation (see Bieber 1969), they were initially inclined to encourage such gifts as necessary to the ongoing of modern medicine and as morally elevating to it. Before their exposure to the "double bind" consequences of organ donation, they would have thought that it had the same positive, pragmatic, and symbolic significance as voluntary gifts of blood. But, in contradistinction to Titmuss's thesis about the virtues of such gifts over all other modes of donation, the transplanters have learned that the gift can be "treacherous," producing the kind of social and psychological "disability" that reduces the "quality of life" for both the donor and the recipient (Lederberg 1971).[2]

"The theme of the gift, of freedom and obligation in the gift, of generosity and self-interest in giving reappear in our society like the resurrection of a dominant motif long forgotten," Marcel Mauss wrote (Mauss 1954, p. 66). Organ transplantation is one recent development that has again brought such issues of gift exchange and social solidarity prominently into view. Transplantation and hemodialysis also center on problems of uncertainty, meaning, life and death, allocation and scarcity, and intervention in the human condition. This is where the ultimate significance of these therapeutic innovations and their "courage to fail" ethos is to be found. And these questions, with which the "new biology" and medicine more generally are preoccupied, are a part of a changing modern society that is increasingly concerned with such ethical and existential matters in many different domains.

Notes

Preface

1. Our recognition of the applicability of Mauss's conception of the gift to transplantation and dialysis and as a central theme in our society antedated the publication of Richard Titmuss's study *The Gift Relationship*, in which he applies Mauss's formulation to a comparative study of blood donation systems in England and the United States (Titmuss 1970).

Chapter 1

1. Normative constraints, both biomedical and ethical, also preclude the live-donor transplantation of a vital single organ, such as the heart or liver, whose removal would bring death to the donor. As far as we know, this premise has not been challenged. Apparently there is latent consensus among the medical profession and the lay public that the donation of an unpaired organ by a live individual would not only exceed the limits of acceptable gift giving, but would constitute a deliberate act of suicide by the donor and of premeditated killing by the physician. Heart transplant teams have discovered that this question of accepting a vital unpaired organ from a living donor is not merely academic. For example, especially during the first year of Stanford's heart transplant program (1967–68) when the implants were so heavily publicized:

    a number of individuals contacted the medical center by mail, telephone, or in person expressing a wish to donate their hearts. In most instances they appeared to be profoundly depressed and suicidal and viewed heart donation as a process which would make their suicide a meaningful event and perhaps relieve some of their guilt [Christopherson and Lunde 1971a, p. 29].

2. Kidney Transplant Registry data show 165 living unrelated donor transplants performed from 1953 through 1969. No figures, however, exist concerning the number of candidates who, for whatever reasons, were not accepted as unrelated living kidney donors. The Ninth Report

of the Human Kidney Transplant Registry noted that, according to
their data through April 1970, "living unrelated donors are no
longer used."

3. In Catholic religious orders, for example, the restriction on giving and
receiving gifts enforced by superiors is partly a consequence of the vow
of individual poverty each of its members has taken. But it also grows
out of the recognition that the exchange of gifts by persons symbolizes
and reinforces particularistic relations between them. Traditionally, in
such religious orders, close personal relations were discouraged in the
name of a more universalistic, total commitment to God, the church,
and mankind in general.

4. Pseudonyms are used for the patients and doctors in these cases.

5. These donation patterns that we would predict given the structure and
dynamics of a modern kinship system are borne out by data from the
Eighth Report of the Human Kidney Transplant Registry. In 1967
through 1969, living related donors served for 43 percent of all kidney
transplants. Among this 43 percent, the donor-to-recipient kinship
relation was as follows: mother (donor), 13 percent; father, 8 percent;
brother, 11 percent; sister, 9 percent; other blood relative, 2 percent.

6. According to statistics compiled by the Kidney Transplant Registry, less
than 1 percent of all kidney donations in the United States have been
from children to their parents. As Simmons, Fulton, and Fulton (1970)
suggest, other elements limiting the number of available children who
could donate have been the necessity, in most states, of obtaining a
court order for a minor to donate a kidney, and the fact that "younger
kidney recipients were favored in the earlier, more experimental stages
of kidney transplantation; only now in some centers are persons in
their fifties being transplanted."

7. Some observers feel that the stresses accompanying what we have
identified as the gift-exchange aspects of organ transplantation are so
great that the procedure is dubious on sociopsychological grounds.
Dr. Robert S. Morison, for example, has stated his apprehension over
what he regards as the excessive degree of mutual dependence,
protection, and identification that may grow up between donor and
recipient, with what he feels are deleterious consequences for the family
social system as well as for the individuals involved. He has gone so far
as to suggest the establishment of a "taboo" against live organ transplantation between close relatives, analogous in some ways to the incest
taboo (personal communication).

8. Similar feelings about the artificial heart were expressed by Mrs.
Haskell Karp, whose husband received the first total implant of an
artificial heart on 4 April 1969 and then was given a human heart
transplant on 7 April: "I see [Mr. Karp] lying there, breathing, and
knowing that within his chest is a man-made implement where there
should be a God-given heart." After the human transplant, Mrs. Karp
was reported as saying, "As long as he has a normal heart, I now feel
that he has returned from the dead."

9. According to the Eighth Report of the Human Kidney Transplant Registry, there have been no reported "living donor deaths related to nephrectomy. . . . One documented death in a maternal donor has been presented. This was due presumably to pulmonary embolism within eight days following the donor nephrectomy." The registry also notes, however, that the live donor runs a slight but definite risk of various postnephrectomy complications, "including operative site infection, infection of the urinary tract, acute tubular necrosis of the kidney, and phlebitis. Each of these complications has an incidence of 1% or less." As in any operation, too, the live donor faces the risk of anesthesia-related death. And he must weigh the long-term possibilities that his health and life may be jeopardized by his losing function in his remaining kidney through an illness or accident.

Chapter 2

1. For the first systematic sociological discussion of "the uncertainty factor" in medicine and its significance for the physician and patient see Parsons 1952, chap. 10; see also Fox 1957, pp. 207–41; and Fox 1959, pp. 28–43.

2. "Rejection" is caused by the immune reaction, in which the body recognizes that a transplant of living tissue from any source but an identical twin is foreign. The body's defensive tissues then seek to destroy the graft by producing antibodies which react with the antigens or foreign proteins of the transplant.

3. Although matching programs rapidly became available, a prominent medical geneticist estimated in 1968 that less than one-third of the country's transplant centers were doing adequate histocompatibility tests.

4. Terasaki describes the three major possible results of matching tests, in order of desirability, as follows: "When the lymphocytes of both members of a [donor and recipient] pair react the same to a group of antisera . . . , *conformity* of the antigen is said to be present. The absence of an antigen in a donor which is present in a recipient is defined as *compatibility*. When an antigen is found on the donor lymphocytes but not on those of the recipient, a *mismatch* exists" (Terasaki, in Starzl 1969, p. 23). On the Terasaki Scale, matches are graded A, B, C, D, and F; A matches occur only between identical twins, and B matches are quite rare.

5. The HL-A system (Human Leukocyte Antigen System) is a complex genetic system that is a major determinant of histocompatibility. The other major determinant of histocompatibility in man is the ABO blood group antigens.

6. An antimetabolite is a drug that interferes with normal metabolism by entering directly into a metabolic reaction. For a good review of the work of Schwartz and Damashek and other early studies on the use of immunosuppressive drugs, see Moore 1965, chaps. 7–8.

Chapter 3

1. This concept was first developed by Robert K. Merton and Elinor Barber (1963).
2. In the case of identical twins, where no rejection problem threatens, Goodwin and Martin wrote as early as 1963 that "successful transplantation of kidneys . . . [approximately 30 identical twin transplants had been performed since 1954], which only a short time ago was a perilous surgical experiment, is now an established surgical procedure and should be done whenever one twin is fatally stricken with renal disease" (*Urological Survey* 13:229).
3. Personal communication, John J. Bergan, M.D., Director, Organ Transplant Registry. The Human Kidney Registry is now being maintained as part of this overall ACS/NIH Registry.
4. The following statements are drawn from: Cardiac transplantation in man (1968); Cardiac and other organ transplantation (1968); *Cardiac replacement* (1969).

Chapter 5

1. The word moratorium is derived from the Latin *moratorius*—"serving to delay"—and is defined in the *Oxford English Dictionary* as "a legal authorization to a debtor to postpone payment for a certain time." In press accounts of cardiac transplantation, often quoting physicians, the following words and phrases appeared synonymously with moratorium: *halt, diminish, stop, stop entirely, slow the tide, set aside for the time being, cease, boycott, suspend, defer, slow down, languish, decline, abandon, pause, quit.*
2. Dr. David disapproves this statement, feeling that it is unfair to the institute.
3. That the donor shortage has been a problem at many institutes was noted in a *New York Times* editorial a year after Cooley's remarks: "the present and presumably temporary near-cessation of heart transplant operations reflects, in part, the lack of donors of this vital organ" (Heart transplants tomorrow 1970).
4. We first analyzed the clinical moratorium phenomenon through a detailed case study of the development of mitral valve heart surgery from 1902 to 1949, which involved a cessation of the procedure from 1928 to 1945 (Swazey and Fox 1970).

   The phenomenon has occurred in areas of human organ transplantation besides heart implants. Human liver transplantation, for example, was begun in March 1963 by Dr. Thomas Starzl and his colleagues in Denver. The survival time of the first seven liver recipients, five in Denver and one each in Boston and France, ranged from zero to twenty-three days. A three-year moratorium on human liver transplantation ensued, until Starzl's group resumed the procedure in 1967. Starzl tersely accounted for the 1963–67 halt when he told us: "We went back to the lab because we could not make it work. If the patient doesn't live, it doesn't work."

5. A clinical moratorium is revealed to the medical profession in various ways. Dr. Elliot C. Cutler, who began human mitral valve surgery in 1923, signaled a moratorium on the procedure through the subtitle of a 1929 paper on surgery for chronic valvular heart disease: "Final Report of All Surgical Cases." The Montreal Heart Institute made its decision known to the profession and to the lay public through a press release. In other instances, as at certain hospitals performing heart transplants, an "unofficial, gentleman's agreement" to halt the procedure was reached, and was made known only through informal, face-to-face communication. Finally, some research groups publish a retrospective statement that a moratorium had been in effect, after or as they have relaunched clinical trials. This is the style in which Starzl's team handled the liver transplant moratorium.

6. For the best recent statement by a sociologist of the concept of social circles and appropriate methods for studying their influence see Kadushin 1968.

7. We realize that this increase in coverage is partly a consequence of the general growth of the mass media in the past two decades and of the increase in reporting developments in the life sciences.

8. A similar burden of proof falls on the nonphysician (for example, clergyman, lawyer, journalist) who advocates calling a clinical moratorium.

Chapter 6

1. Typical of the first press release accounts was that on page 1 of the *Houston Post*, 5 April 1969, headlined "Man Given Mechanical Heart in Saint Luke's Operation." The story reported that the artificial heart "was developed by Drs. Cooley and Liotta during the past four months. It is a modification of a working model first developed by Dr. Liotta in 1959, while he was still in his native land, Argentina."

2. In light of our earlier discussion of research physicians' criteria for success and failure, it is interesting to note the measure of a "successful attempt" and of "animal survival" in this instance. "We consider survival in this particular experimental situation when the dog regains spontaneous respiratory movements and the survival duration ends when it is impossible to maintain adequate spontaneous respiratory movements."

3. Letter from Denton Cooley to Mr. Jonas Rosenthal, *McCall's* Public Relations Department, 6 November 1969; this letter was released to the press by *McCall's*.

4. Discussion of the Cooper–McCollum correspondence is drawn from personal communications from M. E. DeBakey.

5. Baylor's new and more stringent requirements that all research protocols involving human experimentation be submitted for peer review also reflected the college of medicine's concern over a widely publicized operation that took place at Methodist Hospital on 22 April 1969. According to the initial publicity releases, "the world's first complete human eye transplant" was performed by Dr. Conrad D.

Moore, assistant director of the Institute of Ophthalmology, Texas Medical Center, and an assistant professor of ophthalmology at Baylor. Mr. John Madden age fifty-four, was reported to have received a new right eye from a donor who had died on 21 April of a brain tumor. Dr. Moore stated that his decision to attempt the transplant was made after Madden's own eye was destroyed following an unsuccessful corneal transplant attempt. He also told reporters that he had not sought permission to perform the operation from the Baylor research committee because "I don't think it has anything to do with human experimentation. We're not endangering the life of the man or the organ. In a sense we're replacing tissue we've transplanted before, but in a more complete sense."

As soon as the operation was reported by the mass media, eye specialists around the world voiced their doubts about the possibility that Mr. Madden might acquire vision in the transplanted eye. On 26 April, the Houston Ophthalmological Society's Executive Council issued a formal statement in which they expressed their professional judgment that the transplant could not succeed because: (1) the optic nerve does not regenerate once it has been cut, (2) it is "technically impossible" to sew together the blood vessels that supply the transplanted eye, and (3) within a few minutes after the donor's death, his eye's retina is no longer viable—it too dies. The council went on to declare that "it is extremely unfortunate that thousands of blind people may have been given a false sense of hope," and that "total eye transplantation and the publicity given to it are both very unfortunate."

In response to the criticisms of the transplant, Moore revised the original report at a 26 April press conference. He declared that he had left the recipient's optic nerve and a portion of the retinal lining intact, transplanting only the front portion of the donor's eye. He went on to say that the procedure used had been developed in experiments with cats in 1958 while he was a resident in ophthalmology at New York University Medical Center. The chairman of the Ophthalmology Department at NYU, Dr. Goodwin Breiner, however, promptly rebutted his assertion, stating that although Moore had taken a postgraduate basic science course at NYU he had never been a resident there. Nor to Breiner's knowledge had any animal experiments such as Moore described ever been done in the twenty years he had been at NYU.

In the wake of Moore's conflicting reports about the eye transplant and the uncertainties concerning prior animal experiments, a joint committee from Baylor College of Medicine and Methodist Hospital was formed in April to "review the events of the operation." A second committee, composed of trustees and faculty of Baylor Medical School, was appointed on 1 July by L. F. McCollum to review again the reports and findings concerning both the artificial heart implant by Cooley and Moore's eye transplant.

On 13 May, the press reported that, as predicted, Mr. Madden had not had sight restored via the transplant, although his new eye did have some feeling and movement. The following month, on 10 June, Moore was expelled from the Houston Ophthalmological Society, because he had engaged in "ophthalmic practice not in keeping with the standards of this community." (Quotations drawn from: Eye man: three weeks in the dark 1969; Specialists say eye transplant is doomed 1969; Surgeon denies total eye transplant 1969; Kass 1969; Doctor in eye transplant ousted by medical group 1969.)

6. The best-known of these codes are the Nuremberg Code and the World Medical Association's 1964 Declaration of Helsinki, which also sets forth a Code of Ethics for Human Experimentation. In the United States, a Public Health Service document issued 1 May 1969 and entitled "Protection of the Individual as Research Subject," states the regulations that must be followed in investigations with human subjects if a project is to be funded by the various national institutes of the Public Health Service. This agency funds approximately 35 percent of all biomedical research in the United States.

7. In *Experimentation with Human Subjects*, the volume published out of the "continuing seminar" on this subject held by the American Academy of Arts and Sciences over the course of 1966–67, this precept emerged as a central theme. It was especially stressed and developed by Margaret Mead and Talcott Parsons, as well as by Paul Freund (Freund 1970).

8. This phrase is used by DeBakey and his associates at the end of their co-authored article "Orthotopic Cardiac Prosthesis: Preliminary Experiments in Animals with Biventricular Artificial Heart" to acknowledge and describe the part Liotta played in the experiments on which their published report was based. It is interesting that although Liotta had been coauthor with DeBakey in a number of previous articles, he was cited only in the acknowledgement section of such a key publication. This seems all the more significant because many other members of the Baylor–Rice Artificial Heart Program are included in the roster of authors: Hall, Hellums, O'Bannon, Bourland, Feldman, Wirting, Calvin, Smith, and Anderson (DeBakey, Hall et al. 1969, p. 142).

9. See, for example, the subtitles of Thomas Thompson's article "The Texas Tornado vs. Dr. Wonderful" (*Life*, 10 April 1970).

10. This phrase appears in a letter, dated 2 September 1969, written to DeBakey by Cooley.

11. Excerpted from a letter written by Cooley to BeBakey, 2 September 1970.

12. This is the first of four papers prepared by the Research Group on Human Experimentation, Barnard College, Columbia University, for the American Sociological Association Sessions on the Sociology of Science, at the American Association for the Advancement of Science Annual Meetings in Chicago, December 1970. With grants from the Russell Sage Foundation, under its program on the Social Aspects of Biology, Barber and his co-investigators in the research group (John J.

Lally, Julia Makarushka, Daniel Sullivan, and others) have been conducting an extensive study of "the social control mechanisms that operate to produce the existing standards of ethical concern and practice among American biomedical researchers who use human subjects." The final results of this study have now been published: See Bernard Barber, John J. Lally, Julia Makarushka, and Daniel Sullivan, *Research on Human Subjects: Problems of Social Control in Medical Experimentation* (New York: Russell Sage Foundation, 1973).

13. This is not to imply that, in contrast, the medical school training that physicians receive in research ethics is exemplary, or necessarily adequate. In her paper "Learning to be Ethical," Julia Makarushka reports that of the 308 physician-investigators that she and her colleagues in the Barnard College, Columbia University Research Group on Human Experimentation interviewed, fewer than half said they had received any formal training in the ethical problems of human research in medical school (Makarushka 1970).

14. The case was filed in the United States District Court for the Southern District of Texas, Houston Division, by "Shirley Karp, Individually, as Executor of the Estate of Haskell Karp, and as next friend of Joel Karp and Martin Karp, Minors, and Harry Michael Karp." Its civil action number is 71–H–369.

15. *Karp* v. *Cooley*, 348 F. Supp. 827 (1972), p. 832 (S.D. Texas).

16. Ibid., p. 827.

17. Ibid.

18. California, New Mexico, and the District of Columbia, for example, are singular in requiring only lay testimony on the issue of informed consent rather than adhering to the prevailing view that expert medical testimony is necessary.

19. We are deeply indebted to the Honorable A. Leon Higginbotham, Jr., U.S. district judge for the Eastern District of Pennsylvania, for the help he gave us in formulating the analysis and critique of the court's ruling that follows.

20. Plaintiff's brief on appeal to the U.S. Court of Appeals for the Fifth Circuit, pp. 4–5.

21. *Karp* v. *Cooley*, 349 F. Supp. 827 (1972), p. 836 (S.D. Texas).

22. See Order of Judge Singleton, filed on 6 July 1973.

23. Ibid.

24. *Karp* v. *Cooley*, 349 F. Supp. 827 (1972), p. 836 (S.D. Texas).

25. Ibid.

26. Plaintiff's brief, pp. 33–34.

27. Ibid.

28. Plaintiff's brief, p. 41.

29. *Karp* v. *Cooley*, 349 F. Supp. 827 (1972), p. 836 (S.D. Texas).

30. The series of stories written by John Quinn for the *New York Daily News* and Judith Randal for the *Washington Star*, upon which we have extensively drawn, are exceptions to this rule.

Chapter 7

1. The first artificial kidney had been constructed in 1914 by Drs. Abel, Rowntree, and Turner at Johns Hopkins University. Their device, constructed from discarded glass tubing and rubber stoppers, was built and used solely for basic research into the process of dialysis and its biochemical and physiological correlates. For an account of Kolff's early work, see Thorwald, 1971.

2. In October 1972, after our manuscript was completed, Congress enacted H.R. 1, the Social Security Amendments Act. Under the provisions of H.R. 1, the majority of dialysis or transplantation treatment costs for patients with terminal kidney diseases will be paid for through Medicare. Some implications of this legislation are discussed in our final chapter.

3. Established in 1929 by the founder of the Atlantic and Pacific Tea Company and incorporated in 1942, the John A. Hartford Foundation's assets in the mid–1960s were approximately $342 million. The foundation's stated purpose has been to further medical research, "especially the clinical aspect, in voluntary, non-profit hospitals." The foundation's particular concern is "to reduce the lag between findings in the laboratory and their application in the care and treatment of patients." Funding the initial phases of an innovative artificial kidney center thus was entirely compatible with the foundation's general orientation and goals (Lewis 1967, p. 588).

4. It is pertinent to a study of the dynamics of a community-supported kidney center to note that Seattle has one of the best-organized and most effective nonprofit community blood banks and cross-matching agencies in the country. R. M. Titmuss points out that in this respect Seattle is recognized in the United States as "exceptional. . . . Among the large urban and metropolitan areas only a minority of places—like Seattle—appear to have no chronic shortages of blood" (Titmuss 1971, p. 65).

5. Home dialysis was first attempted in 1963 by Dr. John Merrill and his renal team at Boston's Peter Bent Brigham Hospital. In contrast to Seattle's chronic dialysis programs, Merrill's group has continued to view both hospital and home dialysis as temporary procedures "until homotransplantation is available." This commitment to transplantation was stated to us by a member of the renal unit in 1970: "The Brigham is not running a chronic dialysis program, although some patients are on dialysis for two or three years until a kidney is available. Our philosophy is to get the patient transplanted."

   The Brigham group's decision to "explore in a preliminary fashion the feasibility of [home dialysis]" was prompted by a joint medical-lay conference sponsored by the AMA and the National Kidney Disease Foundation in June 1963. One of the participants concluded that a "number of research-oriented centers" should begin to develop comprehensive prophylactic and treatment programs for renal disease, including the use of hemodialysis, peritoneal dialysis, and transplantation. Given the problem of obtaining federal or private funding for the construction of university hospital treatment centers, Merrill and his co-workers believed that "it seemed possible that facilities might be constructed in the community to deal with this problem" (Merrill et al. 1964, pp. 468–70).

At the time of their first published report, Merrill's dialysis research team had performed thirty home dialyses on three patients over periods of nine, four, and three months. The patients were first dialyzed twice a week at the Brigham, "until it was felt that their clinical situation was stable." They then went on a weekly schedule of one in-hospital dialysis and one treatment in the home, monitored by a nurse and a physician from the hospital's dialysis research team. That Merrill and his fellow clinical investigators felt it necessary to flank their first home dialysis patients with expert medical personnel indicates both their cautious approach to this innovative treatment and their apprehensions about possible technical problems and medical emergencies that might confront the patient and his family. At the same time, there is no evidence in their first publications that they anticipated the range of psychological and social problems that subsequent experience showed to so frequently accompany chronic home dialysis.

The "chemical and clinical results of home dialysis," Merrill and his colleagues reported, "were in every way comparable to those carried out in the hospital." "Although the patients were not completely rehabilitated, they were able to work six hours a day between dialyses." These results, and the "Seattle experience" of performing over 2,800 dialyses without the supervision of a physician, encouraged the Brigham team to "assume" that home dialysis could be conducted with "community facilities and local personnel," such as a nurse or a "responsible member of the family" trained in the techniques of dialysis (Merrill et al. 1964).

6. Several months after beginning chronic dialysis, this patient developed systemic lupus erythematosus, from which she died after thirty-four months on home dialysis.

7. In the national survey of dialysis patients conducted by Katz and Proctor, 75 percent of their study population were found to be male, 79 percent married, and 59 percent between the ages of thirty-five and fifty-four. Their sample of 689 patients represented 81 percent of the estimated dialysis patients in the United States in the latter half of 1967 (Katz and Proctor 1969, p. 2, 27).

8. Peritoneal dialysis is used for both acute and chronic renal failure, as an alternative to hemodialysis. In this method, a catheter is inserted through the patient's abdomen into the peritoneum, the serous lining which covers the abdominal cavity and viscera. The peritoneum, like

the artificial kidney, acts as an inert, semipermeable membrane, allowing removal of undesired fluids and solutes from the body and the introduction of desired solutes. Until recently, the major problems encountered in long-term peritoneal dialysis were devising a semi-permanent access to the peritoneum, and the almost invariable occurrence of an often fatal abdominal infection. The Seattle dialysis research unit began trials with home peritoneal dialysis in March 1964, and as of May 1970 had utilized this home-treatment method with twenty-four patients (Tenckhoff and Boen 1965; Miller and Tassistro 1969; H. Tenckhoff, personal interview).

9. The following discussion and quotations concerning the fund-raising and public relations work of the Northwest Kidney Center are drawn from fund-raising information sheets and other literature distributed by the center.

Chapter 9

1. According to the most recent system of nomenclature adopted by the American Psychiatric Association, the "antisocial type" of "sociopathic personality" that was attributed to Ernie is now termed an "antisocial personality." The second edition of the American Psychiatric Association's *Diagnostic and Statistical Manual of Mental Disorders* uses this term for "individuals who are basically unsocialized and whose behavior pattern brings them repeatedly into conflict with society" (p. 43).

The classic work on this type of personality disorder, formerly designated as "constitutional psychopathic state" or "psychopathic personality," is Dr. Hervey Cleckley's *The Mask of Sanity* (St. Louis, Mo.: C. V. Mosby Co., 2d ed., 1950, pp. 355–56). According to Cleckley, the sociopath's clinical profile has sixteen dominant characteristics: "1. Superficial charm and good 'intelligence'; 2. absence of delusions and other signs of irrational 'thinking'; 3. absence of 'nervousness' or psychoneurotic manifestations; 4. unreliability; 5. untruthfulness and insincerity; 6. lack of remorse or shame; 7. inadequately motivated antisocial behavior; 8. poor judgment and failure to learn by experience; 9. pathologic egocentricity and incapacity for love; 10. general poverty in major affective reactions; 11. specific loss of insight; 12. unresponsiveness in general interpersonal relations; 13. fantastic and uninviting behavior, with drink and sometimes without; 14. suicide rarely carried out; 15. sex life impersonal, trivial, and poorly integrated; 16. failure to follow any life plan."

2. This indictment of the penal system by Dr. Scribner and some of his associates is sociologically interesting and significant. In the sociological view, both sickness and crime are forms of deviance, because they entail nonconformity to "normal" social expectations and responsibilities. One of the major distinctions between them is that whereas illness is defined as "not the fault" of the individual, and thus as semilegitimate,

behavior that is considered criminal is not exempted from condemnation and incurs punishment rather than treatment. Typically, in modern Western society, serious illness is cared for in a hospital, whereas crime is dealt with in a prison. As our society moves progressively toward defining many actions that were once deemed criminal either as illness or as the consequence of social evils, and as our concept of dealing with those who have engaged in crime becomes more oriented toward personal rehabilitation and social reform, the distinctions between crime, sickness, and injustice become more blurred. The case of Ernie Crowfeather is complicated not only by these changing definitions and the ambiguities they create, but also by the fact that at the same time he was guilty of criminal acts, gravely ill, and receiving a type of extraordinary treatment not routinely available in a prison hospital. In a sense, Ernie ended up "commuting" between prison and the University and VA hospitals as much because of indeterminacy regarding which institution had primary responsibility for his care, as because of the complexity of his medical condition. The irony of his predicament is that had chronic dialysis and renal transplantation not yet been devised, Ernie would not have been alive either to receive treatment or to be sentenced to jail.

Chapter 12

1. This insight and its conceptualization are partly a consequence of discussion and interchanges about the sociology of medicine and of the professions that have continually occurred between one of the authors (Fox) and Talcott Parsons over more than twenty years.

2. Since we prepared this edition of *The Courage to Fail,* an extensive study has been published of adult and minor kidney transplant recipients and donors and their families at the University of Minnesota Hospitals from 1970 to 1973. *Gift of Life,* by sociologists Roberta Simmons and Susan Klein and transplant surgeon Richard Simmons, presents questionnaire and interview data on transplant candidates, potential donors, and families, and one year follow-up data on those involved in medically successful grafts. (R. G. Simmons, S. D. Klein, and R. L. Simmons, *Gift of Life: The Social and Psychological Impact of Organ Transplantation* [New York: John Wiley, 1977].)

Bibliography

Abram, H. S. 1968. The psychiatrist, the treatment of chronic renal failure, and the prolongation of life. *Amer. J. Psychiat.* 124: 1351–58.

———. 1971. Psychotic reactions after cardiac surgery: A critical review. *Sem. Psychiat.* 3:70–78.

———. 1972. Psychological dilemmas of medical progress. *Psychiat. Med.* 3:51–58.

Abram, H. S.; Moore, G. L.; and Westervelt, F. B. 1971. Suicidal behavior in chronic dialysis patients. *Amer. J. Psychiat.* 127: 1119–1204.

Advisory Committee of the Human Kidney Transplant Registry. 1969. An analysis of the incidence of early transplant failure data from the Human Kidney Transplant Registry. *Transpl. Proc.* 1, pt. 1 (March): 197–205.

Alexander, S. 1962. They decide who lives, who dies: Medical miracle puts a moral burden on a small committee. *Life* 53 (9 November): 102ff.

Altman, L. K. 1970*a*. Infections in hospitals stir concern. *N. Y. Times,* 9 August.

———. 1970*b*. Three years of heart transplants: Twenty-three live. *N. Y. Times,* 3 December, p. 28.

Altruism rediscovered (editorial). *New Eng. J. Med.* 284 (18 March): 612.

American Medical Association's House of Delegates' statement on heart transplantation. 1968. *JAMA* 206 (16 December): 2631; for the full statement, see *JAMA* 207 (3 March 1969): 1704–6.

Amos, D. B. 1967. Transplantation: Opportunities and problems. In *Research in the service of man,* Conference sponsored by the

Subcommittee on Government Research, 27 October 1966, pp. 177–81. Washington, D.C.: U.S. Government Printing Office.

Anderson, F. R. 1969. The physician, the terminal patient and the law. *Lex et Scientia* 6, (April–June): 55–76.

Annas, G. J. 1977. Allocation of artificial hearts in the year 2002: Minerva v. National Health Agency. *Amer. J. Law and Med.* 3: 59–76.

Appel, J. Z. 1968. Ethical and legal questions posed by recent advances in medicine. *JAMA* 205 (12 August): 101–4.

Army sets up dialysis and transplantation centers. 1970. *JAMA* 214 (5 October): 36.

Arnold, J. D.; Zimmerman, T. F.; and Martin, D. C. 1968. Public attitudes and the diagnosis of death. *JAMA* 206 (25 November): 1949–54.

Artificial heart. 1973. *N. Y. Times,* 8 September.

Artificial heart is implanted in man. 1969. *N. Y. Times,* 5 April 1969, p. 1.

Artificial heart is performing well. 1969. *Philadelphia Inquirer,* 6 April, p. 1.

Artificial heart patient's condition good. 1969. *Boston Sunday Globe,* 6 April, p. 12.

Artificial Heart Program Conference: Proceedings. 1969. Washington, D.C., 9–13 June 1969, ed. Ruth J. Hegyeli, Washington, D.C.: U.S. Government Printing Office.

Artificial internal organs: Promise, profits, and problems. MR Management Reports, Boston, 1966. A study prepared by graduate students at the Harvard Business School. By Paul Sullivan et al.

Astor, G. 1970. Heart transplants do work. *Look* 34 (29 December): 43–48.

Austen, W. G. 1978. Heart transplantation after ten years (editorial). *New Eng. J. Med.* 298 (23 March): 682–84.

Bach, F. H. 1969. Histocompatibility genetics and immunosuppression. *Proc. Nat. Acad. Sci. U.S.A.* 63 (August): 1017–38.

————. 1970. Transplantation: Pairing of donor and recipient. *Science* 168 (5 June): 1170–78.

Baram, M. S. 1971. Social control of science and technology. *Science* 172 (7 May): 535–39.

Barber, B. 1970. The structure and process of peer group review. Prepared by the Research Group on Human Experimentation,

Barnard College, for the American Sociological Association sessions, Chicago, December 1970 (mimeographed).

Barber, B.; Lally, J. J.; Makarushka, J.; and Sullivan, D. 1973. *Research on human subjects: Problems of social control in medical experimentation.* New York: Russell Sage Foundation.

Barnard, C. N. 1970. Heart transplants are defined by Dr. Barnard. *Philadelphia Evening Bulletin,* 20 October.

Barnard, C. N., and Pepper, C. B., 1969. *One life.* New York: Macmillan.

Beard, B. H. 1971. The quality of life before and after renal transplantation. *Dis. Nerv. Syst.* 32:24–31.

Beecher, H. K. 1962. Some fallacies and errors in the application of the principle of consent in human experimentation. *Clin. Pharmacol. Ther.* 3:141–46.

———. 1968. Ethical problems created by the hopelessly unconscious patient. *New Eng. J. Med.* 278 (27 June): 1425–30.

———. 1970. Scarce resources and medical advancement. In *Experimentation with human subjects,* ed. Paul A. Freund, pp. 66–104. New York: George Braziller.

Benoit, F. L.; Rulon, D. B.; Theil, G. B.; Doolan, P.D.; and Watten, R. H. 1964. Goodpasture's syndrome: A clinico-pathologic entity. *Amer. J. Med.* 37:424–44.

Bevan W. 1971. On stimulating the gift of blood [editorial]. *Science* 173 (13 August): 583.

Bibliography on human organ transplantation and related aspects. 1969. Transplant Immunology Branch, Collaborative Research Program. National Institute of Allergy and Infectious Diseases, National Institutes of Health, March 1969 (mimeographed).

Bieber, I. 1969. Discussion of a paper by H. H. Sadler, et al. "The human phenomenon of the unrelated kidney donor." American Psychiatric Association Meeting, Miami Beach, Florida, 1969.

Billingham, R. E. 1969. Basic genetical and immunological considerations. In Symposium on organ transplantation in man, *Proc. Nat. Acad. Sci. U.S.A.* 63 (August): 1020–25.

———. 1977. Introduction: Contributions of transplantation to modern biology and medicine. *Transpl. Proc.* 9 (March): xxxix–xlviii.

Blagg, C. R.; Cole, J. J.; Irvine, G.; Marr, T.; and Pollard, T. L. 1972. How much should dialysis cost? *Proceedings of the Workshop on Dialysis and Transplantation,* 16 April, pp. 54–60.

Blagg, C. R.; Hickman, R. O.; Eschbach, J. W.; and Scribner, B. H. 1970. Home dialysis: Six years' experience. *New Eng. J. Med.* 283 (19 November): 1126–31.

Blagg, C. R., and Sawyer, T. K. 1973. Kidney failure (letter to the editor). *New Eng. J. Med.* 289 (6 September).

Blaiberg, P. 1968. *Looking at my heart.* New York: Stein and Day.

Blaiberg's death a signal for surgeons to take stock. 1969. *London Times,* 18 August.

Blakeslee, S. 1969. Heart experts urge caution on implants. *N.Y. Times,* 19 August.

————. 1970. Under the hospital mask are nine ordinary citizens. *N.Y. Times,* 3 December, p. 28.

Blumgart, H. L. 1970. The medical framework for viewing the problem of human experimentation. In *Experimentation with human subjects,* ed. Paul A. Freund, pp. 39–65. New York: George Braziller.

Borel, D. M. 1969. Defining death. *GP* (January), pp. 171–78.

Borgenicht, L.; Younger, S.; and Zinn, S. 1969. Psychological aspects of home dialysis. M.D. thesis, Case Western Reserve University School of Medicine.

Brent, L. 1977. Presidential address. *Transpl. Proc.* 9 (March): 1343–48.

Brettschneider, L., and Starzl, T. E. 1967. Impediments to successful liver transplantation in man, and possible solutions. Proceedings of the nineteenth symposium of the Colston Research Society, Bristol, England, 3–7 April 1967. *Colston Papers* 19: 307–19.

Brewer, L. A., III. 1968. Cardiac transplantation. *JAMA* 205 (2 September): 101–3.

Brown, H. N., and Kelly, M. J. 1976. Stages of bone marrow transplantation: A psychiatric perspective. *Psychosomatic Med.* 38: 439–46.

Brown, N. K.; Bulger, R. J.; Laws, E. H.; and Thompson, D. J. 1970. The preservation of life. *JAMA* 211 (5 January): 76–81.

Burns, F. 1951. Army flies man 1700 miles for rare treatment. *Boston Sunday Globe,* 21 January.

Burton, B. T. 1975. Introduction: Adequacy of dialysis. *Kidney Int.* 7 (suppl. 2): S–1.

Callahan, D. 1969. The sanctity of life. In *The religious situation, 1969,* ed. Donald R. Cutler. Boston: Beacon Press.

Calland, C. 1972. Iatrogenic problems in end-stage renal failure. *New Eng. J. Med.* 287 (17 August): 334–36.

Calne, R. Y. 1977. The present status of liver transplantation. *Transpl. Proc.* 9 (March): 209–16.

Calne, R. Y., and Williams, R. 1970. Survival after orthotopic liver transplantation: A follow-up report of two patients. *Brit. Med. J.* 3 (22 August): 436–38.

Campbell, J. D., and Campbell, A. 1977. End stage renal disease financial dilemmas: A consumer viewpoint. Unpublished manuscript.

Cardiac and other organ transplantation in the setting of transplant science as a national effort. 1968. American College of Cardiology's Fifth Bethesda Conference, 28, 29 September 1968. *Amer. J. Cardiol.* 22:896–912.

Cardiac replacement. 1969. A report by the Ad Hoc Task Force on Cardiac Replacement, National Heart Institute, October 1969. Washington, D.C.: U.S. Government Printing Office.

Cardiac transplantation in man: Statement prepared by the Board on Medicine of the National Academy of Sciences. 1968. *JAMA* 204 (27 May): 147–48.

Cassell, E. J. 1969. Death and the physician. *Commentary* 47 (June): 73–79.

Castelnuovo-Tedesco, P. 1971. Cardiac surgeons look at transplantation: Interviews with Drs. Cleveland, Cooley, DeBakey, Hallman and Rochelle. *Sem. Psychiat.* 3 (February): 5–16.

A change of attitude: From despair to hope. 1969. *Mass. Gen. Hosp. News,* November.

Chedd, G. 1968. Tipping the balance in heart transplant surgery. *New Scientist* (13 July), p. 122.

Childress, J. F. 1970. Who shall live when not all can live? *Soundings* 43 (winter): 339–55.

Christopherson, L. K. 1976. Cardiac transplant: Preparation for dying or for living. *Health and Social Work* 1 (February): 58–72.

Christopherson, L. K.; Griepp, R. B.; and Stinson, E. B. 1976. Rehabilitation after cardiac transplantation. *JAMA* 236 (November 1): 2082–84.

Christopherson, L. K., and Lunde, D. T. 1971*a*. Heart transplant donors and their families. *Sem. Psychiat.* 3 (February): 26–35.

———. 1971*b*. Implications and dilemmas of medical progress: The impact of medical progress on the patient, family, and staff in a transplant unit. Paper read at the American Psychiatric Association Meeting, Washington, D.C., 6 May 1971.

———. 1971c. The selection of cardiac transplant recipients and their subsequent psychological adjustment. *Sem. Psychiat.* 3 (February): 36–45.

Christy, G. 1968. Live better, live longer: Conversations with the world's greatest heart surgeon, Dr. Michael Ellis DeBakey. *Town and Country* 122 (February): 92.

Cleveland, S. E., and Johnson, D. L. 1970. Motivation and readiness of potential human tissue donors and nondonors. *Psychosom. Med.* 32 (May–June): 225–31.

Collins, V. J. 1968. Limits of medical responsibility in prolonging life. *JAMA* 206 (7 October): 389–92.

Comptroller General of the U.S. 24 June 1975. *Report to the Congress. Treatment of chronic kidney failure: Dialysis, transplant, costs, and the need for more vigorous efforts.* Washington, D.C.: General Accounting Office.

Cooley, D. A. 1969. First implantation of cardiac prosthesis for staged total replacement of the heart. *Trans. Amer. Soc. Artif. Intern. Organs* 15:252–63.

Cooley, D.A.; Bloodwell, R. D.; Hallman, G. L.; and Nora, J. J. 1968. Transplantation of the human heart. *JAMA* 205 (12 August): 479–86.

Cooley, D. A.; Liotta, D.; Hallman, G. L.; Bloodwell, R. D.; Leachman, R. D.; and Milam, J. D. 1969. Orthotopic cardiac prosthesis for two-staged cardiac replacement. *Amer. J. Cardiol.* 24 (November): 723–28.

Cooley feared hospital would halt heart project. 1969. *Washington Post,* 25 April.

Cooley sees a permanent "built-in" heart. 1969. *N. Y. Post,* 25 April.

Cooper, T. 1969. Human heart transplantation. *News Report,* June–July, pp. 8–10.

Corbet, B. 1969. Heart transplants in balance. *San Diego (Calif.) Evening Tribune,* 28 January.

Couch, N. P.; Curran, W. J.; Hyg, S. M.; and Moore, F. D. 1964. The use of cadaver tissues in transplantation. *New Eng. J. Med.* 271 (1 October): 691–95.

Cournand, A. 1969. Chairman's introductory remarks. *Proc. Nat. Acad. Sci. U.S.A.* 63:1018.

Crammond, W. A. 1967. Renal homotransplantation: Some observations on recipients and donors. *Brit. J. Psychiat.* 113:1223–30.

_____. 1971. Renal transplantation: Experiences with recipients and donors. *Sem. Psychiat.* 3 (February): 116–32.

Crammond, W. A.; Court, J. H.; Higgins, B. A.; Knight, P. R.; and Lawrence, J. R. 1967. Psychological screening of potential donors in a renal homotransplantation programme. *Brit. J. Psychiat.* 113:1213–21.

Crammond, W. A.; Knight, P. R.; and Lawrence, J. R. 1967. The psychiatric contribution to a renal unit undertaking chronic hemodialysis and renal homotransplantation. *Brit. J. Psychiat.* 113:1201–12.

Crane, D., and Matthews, D. 1969. Heart transplant operations: Diffusion of a medical innovation. Paper presented at the sixtieth annual meeting, American Sociological Association, San Francisco, Calif., September 1969.

Crichton, M. 1968. Heart transplants and the press. *New Republic,* 25 May, pp. 28–30, 34.

Criticism seen halting transplants. 1969. *Washington Post,* 28 February.

Curran, W. J. 1969a. Government regulation of the use of human subjects in medical research: The approach of two federal agencies. *Ethical Aspects of Experimentation with Human Subjects. Daedalus* 98 (spring): 545–46.

_____. 1969b. Public health and the law: New regulations on human experimentation. *Amer. J. Public Health* 59 (September): 1746–47.

Curran, W. J., and Beecher, H. K. 1969. Experimentation in children: A reexamination of legal ethical principles. *JAMA* 10 (6 October): 77–83.

Curtis, F. K.; Cole, J. J.; Fellows, B. J.; Tyler, L. L.; and Scribner, B. H. 1965. Hemodialysis in the home. *Trans. Amer. Soc. Artif. Intern. Organs* 11:7–10.

Cutler, D. R., ed. 1968. *Updating life and death: Essays in ethics and medicine.* Boston: Beacon Press.

Daly, R. J., and Hassall, C. 1970. Reported sleep on maintenance hemodialysis. *Brit. Med. J.* 2 (30 May): 508–9.

David, P. 1955. La recherche est-elle possible dans un hôpital canadien-français? *Un. Med. Canada* 84 (November): 1–6.

DeBakey, M. E. 1968a. Human cardiac transplantation. *J. Thorac. Cardiovasc. Surg.* 55 (March): 447–53.

_____. 1968*b*. Medical research and the golden rule. *JAMA* 203 (February): 574–76.

_____. 1968*c*. Science and humanism. *Mich. Quart. Rev.* 7: 85–91.

DeBakey, M., ed. 1970. *The year book of general surgery.* Chicago: Year Book Medical Publishers.

DeBakey, M.; Diethrich, E. B.; Glick, G.; Noon, G. P.; Butler, W. T.; Rossen, R. D.; Liddicoat, J. E.; and Brooks, D. K. 1969. Human cardiac transplantation: Clinical experience. *J. Thorac. Cardiovasc. Surg.* 58:303–17.

DeBakey, M.; Hall, C. W.; et al. 1969. Orthotopic cardiac prosthesis: Preliminary experiments in animals with biventricular artifical heart. *Cardiovasc. Res. Cent. Bull.* 7 (April-June): 127–42.

A definition of irreversible coma: Report of the Ad Hoc Committee of the Harvard Medical School to Examine the Definition of Brain Death. 1968. *JAMA* 205 (5 August): 85–88.

Delano, B. G. 1977. Home dialysis: A dying entity: *NAPHT News* (May), pp. 5, 19.

Disease by disease toward national health insurance? 1973. Washington, D.C.: National Academy of Sciences.

Doctor in eye transplant ousted by medical group. 1969. *N.Y. Times,* 11 June.

Doctor's wife flown here for care on artificial kidney. 1950. *Boston Herald,* 8 January.

Dole, V. P. 1969. Ethical aspects and sociological implications of organ transplantation as a therapeutic procedure. *Proc. Nat. Acad. Sci. U.S.A.* 63 (August): 1036.

Drake, D. C. 1970. New methods may improve records on heart transplants, *Philadelphia Inquirer,* 25 October.

Drive to transplant vital human organs. 1973. *U.S. News and World Report,* 10 September.

Dukeminier, J., Jr. 1970. Supplying organs for transplantation. *Mich. Law Rev.* 68 (April): 811–66.

Dukeminier, J., and Sanders, D. 1968. Organ transplantation: A proposal for routine salvaging of cadaver organs. *New Eng. J. Med.* 279 (22 August): 413–19.

Eisendrath, R. M. 1969. The role of grief and fear in the death of kidney patients. *Amer. J. Psychiat.* 126:381–87.

Elkinton, J. R. 1970. The literature of ethical problems in medicine: Parts 1–3. *Ann. Intern. Med.* 73 (September–November): 495–98, 662–66, 863–70.

Ellis, R. J.; Lillehei, C. W.; and Zabriskie, J. B. 1970. Detection of circulating heart-reactive antibody in human heart transplants. *JAMA* 211 (2 March): 1505-8.

End-stage diabetic nephropathy. 1974. *Kidney Int.* 6: suppl. 1.

Eschbach, J. W.; Barnett, B. M. S.; Daly, S.; Cole, J. J.; and Scribner, B. H. 1967. Hemodialysis in the home: A new approach to the treatment of chronic uremia. *Ann. Intern. Med.* 67: 1149-62.

Ethical guidelines for organ transplantation. 1968. AMA Judicial Council. *JAMA* 205 (5 August): 89-90.

Eye Man: Three weeks in the dark. 1969. *N. Y. Post,* 23 April.

Fawzy, F.; Wellisch, D.; and Yager, J. 1977. Psychiatric services for the bone marrow transplantation patient, family and staff. *UCLA Cancer Center Bull.* 4 (January/February): 5-7.

Fellner, C. H. 1971. Selection of living kidney donors and the problem of informed consent. *Sem. Psychiat.* 3 (February): 79-85.

Fellner, C. H., and Marshall, J. R. 1968. Twelve kidney donors. *JAMA* 206 (16 December): 2703-7.

_____. 1970. Kidney donors: The myth of informed consent. *Amer. J. Psychiat.* 126 (March): 1245-51.

Fellner, C. H., and Schwartz, S. H. 1971. Altruism in disrepute: Medical vs. public attitudes towards the living organ donor. *New Eng. J. Med.* 284 (March): 582-612.

Fenton, S. S.; Blagg, C. R.; Eschbach, J. W.; and Scribner, B. H. 1968. Treatment of end-stage renal disease by home dialysis. *J. Amer. Med. Wom. Ass.* 23:1096-1103.

Final summary report on six studies basic to consideration of the artifical heart program. 1966. Prepared for the National Institutes of Health. Baltimore, Md.: Hittman Associates.

Fine, R. N.; Brennan, L. P.; Edelbrook, H. H.; Riddell, H.; Stiles, Q.; and Lieberman, E. 1969. Use of pediatric cadaver kidneys for homotransplantation in children. *JAMA* 210 (20 October): 477-84.

First artificial heart planted by cardiowhiz. 1969. *N. Y. Daily News,* 5 April, p. 1.

First annual John F. Kennedy symposium on recent significant developments in medicine and surgery. 1968. Boston, 9 May 1968 (unpublished transcript).

Fletcher, J. 1969. Our shameful waste of human tissues: An ethical problem for the living and the dead. In *The religious situation, 1969,* ed. Donald R. Cutler. Boston: Beacon Press.

Fox, R. C. 1957. Training for uncertainty. In *The student-physician,* ed. R. K. Merton, G. Reader, and P. Kendall, pp. 207–41. Cambridge: Harvard University Press.

———. 1958. The autopsy: Its place in the attitude-learning of second-year medical students. Unpublished paper.

———. 1959. *Experiment perilous.* Glencoe, Ill.: Free Press.

———. 1970. A sociological perspective on organ transplantation and hemodialysis. In *New dimensions in legal and ethical concepts for human research. Ann. N.Y. Acad. Sci.* 169:406–28.

———. 1976. Advanced medical technology: Social and ethical implications. *Ann. Rev. Sociol.* 2:231–68.

———. 1977. The medicalization and demedicalization of American society. *Daedalus* 106 (winter): 9–22.

———. 1976a. Medical evolution. In *Explorations in general theory in social science,* ed. J. C. Loubser, R. C. Baun, A. Effrat, V. Lidz, et al., pp. 773–87. New York: Free Press.

———. 1976b. The sociology of modern medical research. In *Asian medical systems: A comparative study,* ed. C. Leslie, pp. 102–14. Berkeley: University of California Press.

France rejects ban on heart transplants. 1973. *Toronto Globe and Mail,* 12 September.

Francis, V.; Korsch, B. M.; and Morris, M. J. 1969. Gaps in doctor-patient communication. *New Eng. J. Med.* 280 (6 March): 535–40.

Freund, P. A. 1971. Mogoloids and "mercy-killing." Working paper prepared for "Choices on Our Conscience," international symposium, Joseph P. Kennedy, Jr., Foundation, Washington, D.C., 16 October.

———, ed. 1970. *Experimentation with human subjects.* New York: George Braziller.

Friedman, E. A. 1973. Reply to Blagg and Sawyer's letter to the editor. *New Eng. J. Med.* 289 (6 September): 537.

Friedman, E. A.; Delano, B. G.; and Bhutt, K. M. 1978. Pragmatic realities in uremia therapy. *New Eng. J. Med.* 298 (16 February): 368–71.

Friedman, E. A., and Kountz, S. L. 1973. Impact of HR-1 on the therapy of end-stage uremia. *New Eng. J. Med.* 288 (14 June): 1287.

Fulginiti, V. A.; Scribner, R.; Groth, C. G.; Putnam, C. W.; Brettschneider, L.; Gilbert, S.; Porter, K. A.; and Starzl, T. 1968. Infections in recipients of liver homografts. *New Eng. J. Med.* 279 (19 September): 619–26.

Gale, R. P. 1977. Bone marrow transplantation at UCLA. *UCLA Cancer Center Bull.* 4 (January/February): 3–4, 7.

Genest, J. 1969. L'institut de diagnostic et recherches cliniques de Montréal. *Forces* 6 (winter): 25–37.

Glaser, R. J. 1970. Innovations and heroic acts in prolonging life. In *The dying patient,* ed. O. G. Brim, H. E. Freeman, S. Levine, and N. A. Scotch, pp. 102–28. New York: Russell Sage Foundation.

Goldman, L. L. 1970. *The heart merchants.* New York: Paperback Library.

Goldstein, A. M., and Reznikoff, M. 1971. Suicide in chronic hemodialysis patients from an external locus of control framework. *Amer. J. Psychiat.* 127:1204–7.

Goodman, G. E. 1968. Activities of the Kidney Disease Control Program. U.S. Department of Health, Education, and Welfare.

Goodwin, W. E., and Martin, D.C. 1963. Transplantation of the kidney. *Urological Survey* 13 (spring): 229–48.

Gottschalk, C. W. 1971. *Memorandum.* Prepared for the meeting of the Ethics Committee of the American Heart Association, Quail Roost, N.C., 21–22 October 1971.

Graubard, S. R. 1970. Preface. In *Experimentation with human subjects,* ed. Paul A. Freund. New York: George Braziller.

Griepp, R. B.; Stinson, E. B.; et al. 1977. Increasing patient survival following heart transplantation. *Transpl. Proc.* 9 (March): 197–202.

Grimsrud, L.; Cole, J. J.; Eschbach, J. W.; Babb, A. L.; Scribner, B. H. 1967. Safety aspects of hemodialysis. *Trans. Amer. Soc. Artif. Intern. Organs* 17:1–4.

Gross, J. B.; Keane, M. F.; and McDonald, A. 1973. Survival and rehabilitation of patients on home dialysis: Five years experience. *Ann. Int. Med.* 78:341–46.

Gustafson, J. M. 1970. Basic ethical issues in the bio-medical fields. *Soundings* 53 (summer): 151–80.

Hackett, T. P.; Cassem, N. H.; and Wishnie, H. A. 1968. The coronary care unit: An appraisal of its psychologic hazards. *New Eng. J. Med.* 279 (19 December): 1365–70.

Hall, C. W.; Liotta, D.; and DeBakey, M. E. 1967. Artificial heart: Present and future. Conference sponsored by the Subcommittee on Government Research, 27 October 1966, pp. 201–16. Washington, D.C.: U.S. Government Printing Office.

Hall, C. W.; Liotta, D.; Henly, W. S.; Crawford, E. S.; and DeBakey, M. E. 1964. Development of artificial intrathoracic circulatory pumps. *Amer. J. Surg.* 108 (November): 685.

Hamburger, J. 1969. Opening remarks. *Transpl. Proc.* 1 (March), pt. 1, pp. 160–61.

————. 1977. Some implications of transplantation research for biology and medicine. *Transpl. Proc.* 9 (March): 1313–18.

Hardy, J. D.; Alican, F.; Moynihan, P.; Timmis, H. H.; Chavez, C. M.; Davis, J. T.; and Anas, P. 1970. A case of clinical lung allotransplantation. *Thorac. Cardiovasc. Surg.* 60 (September): 411–26.

Harken, D. 1968. Transplantation (editorial). *JAMA* 206 (9 December): 2514.

Harken, D., and Zoll, P. M. 1946. Foreign bodies in, and in relation to, the thoracic blood vessels and heart. III. Indications for the removal of intracardiac foreign bodies and the behavior of the heart during manipulation. *Amer. Heart J.* 32:1–19.

The heart-transplant debate. 1969. *Chicago Daily News,* 22 January.

Heart transplant safeguard falters (editorial). 1969. *JAMA* 205 (5 November): 784.

Heart transplants halted in Montreal. 1969. *N. Y. Times,* 23 January.

Heart transplants tomorrow. 1970. *N. Y. Times,* 19 January.

Heart transplant surgeons find rejection big obstacle. 1969. *Long Island Press,* 2 February.

The heartmakers. 1969. NET science special, produced by David Prowitt, 5 November 1969 (unpublished transcript).

Hegstrom, R. M.; Murray, J. S.; Pendras, J. P.; Burnell, J. M.; and Scribner, B. H. 1961. Hemodialysis in the treatment of chronic uremia. *Trans. Amer. Soc. Artif. Intern. Organs* 7:136.

Higginbotham, L. 1975. Due process in the allocation of scarce lifesaving medical resources. *Yale Law J.* 84:1734–49.

Hilton, A. 1970. *The heart people.* New York: Berkeley Publishing Corp.

Hirsch, P., ed. 1969. *Medical miracles.* New York: Pyramid Books.

Holcomb, J. L., and MacDonald, R. W. 1973. Social functioning of artificial kidney patients. *Soc. Sci. Med.* 7:109–19.

Holton, G. 1970. Lessons of the intellectual biography of science (editorial). *Science* 170 (27 November): 933.

Human rights and scientific and technological developments. II. Protection of the human personality and its physical and intellectual integrity in the list of advances in biology, medicine and biochemistry. 1970. United Nations Economic and Social Council, Commission on Human Rights, 26th session, 19 March 1970.

Hume, D. M. 1968. Kidney transplantaiton. In *Human transplantation,* ed. F. T. Rapaport and J. Dausset, pp. 110–15. New York: Grune and Stratton.

Hume, D. M.; Leo, J.; Rolley, R. T.; and Williams, G. M. 1969 . Some immunological and surgical aspects of kidney transplantation in man. *Transpl. Proc.* 1 (March): 171–77.

Hutchings, R. H.; Hickman, R.; and Scribner, B. H. 1966. Chronic hemodialysis in a pre-adolescent. *Pediatrics* 37 (January): 68–73.

Hyatt, J. 1968. The cost of living: Some kidney patients die for lack of funds for machine treatment. *Wall Street Journal,* 10 March.

Improved methods boost cadaver kidney survival. 1970. *JAMA* 211 (9 March): 1615–17.

Jaffe, L. L. 1969. Law as a system of control. *Ethical aspects of experimentation with human subjects. Daedalus* 98 (spring): 406–26.

Jonas, H. 1970. Philosophical reflections on experimenting with subjects. In *Experimentation with human subjects,* ed. Paul A. Freund. New York: George Braziller.

Kadushin, C. 1968. Power, influence, and social circles: A new methodology for studying opinion makers. *Amer. Sociol. Rev.* 33:685–99.

Kalish, R. A. 1968. Life and death: Dividing the indivisible. *Soc. Sci. Med.* 2:249–59.

Kaplan de Nour, A., and Czackes, J. 1968. Emotional problems and reaction of the medical team in a chronic hemodialysis unit. *Lancet,* 9 November, pp. 986–91.

Kaplan de Nour, A.; Snaltiel, J.; and Czackes, J. 1968. Emotional reactions of patients on chronic hemodialysis. *Psychosom. Med.* 30 (September–October): 521–33.

Kass, Leon R. 1971. The new biology: What price relieving man's estate? *Science* 174 (19 November): 783.

Kass, M. 1969. Moore didn't do animal research at NYU, doctor says, *Houston Post,* 30 April.

Katz, A. H., and Proctor, D. M. 1969. Social-psychological characteristics of patients receiving hemodialysis treatment for chronic renal failure. Public Health Service, Kidney Disease Control Program, July 1969.

Kemph, J. P. 1967. Psychotherapy with patients receiving kidney transplants. *Amer. J. Psychiat.* 124 (November): 623–29.

———. 1971. Psychotherapy with donors and recipients of kidney transplants. *Sem. Psychiat.* 3 (February): 145–58.

Kesten, Y. 1968. *Diary of a heart patient.* New York: McGraw-Hill.

Kidney disease program analysis: A report to the surgeon general. 1967. Washington, D.C.: U.S. Public Health Service, publication no. 1745.

Kidney disease services, facilities and programs in the United States. 1969. Washington, D.C.: U.S. Government Printing Office.

Kimball, C. P. 1969. Psychological responses to the experience of open heart surgery. *Amer. J. Psychiat.* 126:348–58.

Knutson, A. L. 1968. Body transplants and ethical values: Viewpoints of public health professionals. *Soc. Sci. Med.* 2:393–414.

Kraft, I. A. 1971. Psychiatric complications of cardiac transplantation. *Sem. Psychiat.* 3 (February): 58–69.

Kraft, I. A., and Vick, J. 1971. The transplantation milieu, St. Luke's Hospital, 1968–69. *Sem. Psychiat.* 3 (February): 17–25.

Ladimer, I., consulting ed. 1970. *New dimensions in legal and ethical concepts for human research. Ann. N.Y. Acad. Sci.,* vol. 169.

Ladimer, I., and Newman, R. W., eds. 1963. *Clinical investigation in medicine: Legal, ethical and moral aspects.* Boston: Law-Medicine Research Institute, Boston University.

Lally, J. J. 1970. Are medical schools ethical leaders? A comparison of medical schools with other bio-medical research institutions. Prepared by the Research Group on Human Experimentation, Barnard College, for the American Sociological Association sessions, Chicago, 1970 (mimeographed).

Law of 17 March 1970, ch. 378 (1970) Kan. Laws 994, codified at *Kan. Stat. Ann.,* sect. 77–202, supp. 1971.

Lawrence, H. S. 1968. Immunological considerations in transplantation. In *Human transplantation,* ed. F. Rapaport and J. Dausset, pp. 12–20. New York: Grune and Stratton.

Lear, J. 1968. A realistic look at heart transplants. *Saturday Review* 51 (3 February): 53–59.

Lederberg, J. 1971. The dilemma of tainted blood. *Washington Post,* 1 August.

Lee, B. 1969. Behind the surgeon's mask. *Boston Sunday Globe,* 12 January, pp. 24-29.

Lewis, H. P. 1968. Machine medicine and its relation to the fatally ill. *JAMA* 206 (7 October): 387–88.

Lewis, M. O., ed. 1967. *Foundation directory.* 3d ed. New York: Russell Sage Foundation.

Lindeman, B. 1970. Louis Russell, man with a stout heart. *Today's Health,* December 1970, pp. 32–76.

Lindemann, E. 1944. Symptomatology and management of acute grief. *Amer. J. Psychiat.* 101:141–48.

Lives in the balance. 1969. *Wall Street Journal,* 27 January.

Lunde, D. T. 1969. Psychiatric complications of heart transplants. *Amer. J. Psychiat.* 126 (September): 369–73.

Lyons, R. D. 1968. Dr. Cooley sees transplant obstacle in "antiheart antibodies." *N. Y. Times,* 28 November.

————. 1973. Program to aid kidney victims faces millions in excess costs. *N. Y. Times,* 11 January.

McKengney, F. P., and Lange, P. 1971. The decision to no longer live on hemodialysis. *Amer. J. Psychiat.* 128:264–74.

Mackenzie, R. 1971. *Risk.* New York: Viking Press.

McLaughlin, L. 1977. Self-care dialysis center planned in Boston, *Boston Globe,* 18 May, p. 50.

MacNamara, M. 1967. Psychosocial problems in a renal unit. *Brit. J. Psychiat.* 113:1231–36.

Makarushka, J. 1970. Learning to be ethical: Patterns of socialization and their variable consequences for ethical standards. Prepared by the Research Group on Human Experimentation, Barnard College, for the American Sociological Association sessions, Chicago, 1970 (mimeographed).

Malinowski, B. 1948. *Magic, science, and religion and other essays.* Glencoe, Ill.: Free Press.

Man who gave kidney to daughter is dead. 1973. *Int. Herald-Tribune,* 28 August.

Master builder: Willem J. Kolff, M.D. 1973. *NAPHT News* 4 (August): 4.

Mathé, G.; Schwarzenberg, L.; et al. 1977. Of mice and men in bone marrow transplantation. *Transpl. Proc.* 9 (March): 158–68.

Maugh, T. H., II. 1973. Tissue cultures: Transplantation without immune suppression. *Science* 181 (7 September): 929–31.

Mauss, M. 1954. *The gift: Forms and functions of exchange in archaic societies.* Trans. Ian Cunnison. Glencoe, Ill.: Free Press.

Mead, M. 1970. Research with human beings: A model derived from anthropological field practice. In *Experimentation with human subjects,* ed. Paul A. Freund, pp. 152–77. New York: George Braziller.

Means, J. H. 1958. *Ward 4: The Mallinckrodt Research Ward of the Massachusetts General Hospital,* Cambridge: Harvard University Press.

Medawar, P. 1969. The future of transplantation biology and medicine. *Transpl. Proc.* 1, pt. 2 (March): 666–69.

Medical-legal aspects of tissue transplantation. 1968. A report to the Committee on Tissue Transplantation from the Ad Hoc Committee on Medical Legal Problems of the Division of Medical Sciences, National Research Council, 6 June 1968.

Medicarelessness (editorial). 1973. *N. Y. Times,* 14 January 1973.

Mendelsohn, E.; Swazey, J.; and Taviss, I., eds. 1971. *Human aspects of biomedical innovation.* Cambridge: Harvard University Press.

Menzies, I. C., and Stewart, W. K. 1968. Psychiatric observations on patients receiving regular dialysis treatments. *Brit. Med. J.* 1:544–47.

Merrill, J. P. 1959. The transplantation of the kidney. *Sci. Amer.* 201 (October): 57–63.

———. 1961. The artificial kidney. *Sci. Amer.* 205 (July): 56–64.

———. 1968. The clinical transplant unit. In *Human transplantation,* ed. F. Rapaport and J. Dausset, pp. 61–65. New York: Grune and Stratton.

———. 1969*a*. Medical aspects of transplantation. *Transpl. Proc.* 1 (March): 162–70.

———. 1969*b*. Transplantation of a paired organ, the kidney. *Proc. Nat. Acad. Sci. U.S.A.* 63 (August): 1030–31.

Merrill, J. P.; Schupak, E.; Cameron, E.; and Hampers, C. L. 1964. Hemodialysis in the home. *JAMA* 190 (2 November): 468–70.

Merton, R. K. 1957. Priorities in scientific discovery: A chapter in the sociology of science. *Amer. Sociol. Rev.* 22:635–59.

Merton, R. K., and Barber, E. 1963. Sociological ambivalence. In *Sociological theory, values and sociocultural change: Essays in honor of Pitirim A. Sorokin,* ed. E. A. Tiryakian, pp. 91–120. New York: Free Press.

Miller, R. B., and Tassistro, C. R. 1969. Peritoneal dialysis. *New Eng. J. Med.* 281 (23 October): 945–50.

Minetree, H. 1973. *Cooley.* New York: Harper's Magazine Press.

Molish, H. B.; Kraft, I. A.; and Wiggins, P. Y. 1971. Psychodiagnostic evaluation of the heart transplant patient. *Sem. Psychiat.* 3 (February): 46–57.

Moore, F. D. 1950. Report of the surgeon-in-chief. Peter Bent Brigham Hospital, Boston. *Thirty-seventh annual report for the year 1950*, pp. 54–61.

———. 1965. *Give and take: The biology of tissue transplantation.* Garden City, N.Y.: Doubleday Anchor Books.

———. 1968. Medical responsibility for the prolongation of life. *JAMA* 206:384–86.

———. 1970. Therapeutic innovation: Ethical boundaries in the initial clinical trials of new drugs and surgical procedures. In *Experimentation with human subjects,* ed. Paul A. Freund, pp. 358–78. New York: George Braziller.

———. 1972. *Transplant: The give and take of tissue transplantation.* New York: Simon and Schuster.

Moore, G. L. 1971. Who should be dialyzed? *Amer. J. Psychiat.* 127: 1208–9.

Morison, R. S. 1971. Death: Process or event? *Science* 173 (20 August): 694.

Murdered U.S. man's heart transplanted after legal row. 1973. *Toronto Star*, 13 September, p. B 12.

Murray, J. 1966*a*. Organ transplantation: The practical possibilities. In *Ethics in medical progress: With special reference to transplantation,* ed. G. E. W. Wolstenholme and M. O'Connor, pp. 54–65. Boston: Little, Brown.

———. 1966*b*. Transplantation and hemodialysis: The recipients' response to renal transplantation. *JAMA* 198 (17 October): 305–6.

Murray, J.; Barnes, B.A.; and Atkinson, J. C. 1971. Eighth report of the Human Kidney Transplant Registry. *Transplantation* 11:328–37.

Murray, J.; Tu, W. H.; Albers, J. B.; Burnell, J. M.; and Scribner, B. H. 1962. A community hemodialysis center for the treatment of chronic uremia. *Trans. Amer. Sci. Artif. Intern. Organs* 8:315–19.

National Medical Care, Inc. 1976. Forbes special situation survey, 22 October. Forbes Investors Advisory Institute, Inc.

Neoplasms: A complication of organ transplants? *JAMA* 206:246–47.

Ninth report of the Human Renal Transplant Registry, ACS/NIH Organ Transplant Registry. 1971. Preprint copy.

Nora, J., et al. 1969. Rejection of the transplanted human heart. *New Eng. J. Med.* 280 (15 May): 1079–86.

Norton, C. E. 1967. Chronic hemodialysis as a medical and social experiment. *Ann. Intern. Med.* 66 (June): 1267–77.

Oberly, E., and Oberly, T. 1977. Self dialysis today: A spirited conference. *NAPHT News*, May, pp. 4, 27.

O'Reilly, R. J.; Dupont, B.; et al. 1977. Reconstitution in severe combined immunodeficiency by transplantation of marrow from an unrelated donor. *New Eng. J. Med.* 297 (15 December): 1311–18.

Ostrowski, K. 1969. Current problems of tissue banking. *Transpl. Proc.* 1, pt. 1 (March): 126–31.

Page, I. 1969*a*. Ethics and the press (editorial). *Mod. Med.* (13 January).

———. 1969*b*. The ethics of heart transplantation. *JAMA* 207 (6 January): 109–13.

———. 1970. Cardiac replacement. *Mod. Med.* (4 May), p. 84.

Parsons, T. 1952. *The social system.* Glencoe, Ill.: Free Press.

———. 1967. *Sociological theory and modern society.* New York: Free Press.

———. 1970. Research with human subjects and the "professional complex." In *Experimentation with human subjects,* ed. Paul A. Freund, pp. 116–51. New York: George Braziller.

———. 1971. *The system of modern societies.* Englewood Cliffs, N.J.: Prentice-Hall.

Parsons, T.; Fox, R. C.; and Lidz, V. M. 1972. The gift of life and its reciprocation. *Soc. Res.* 39:367–415.

Patel, R.; Glassock, R.; and Terasaki, P. I. 1969. Serotyping for homotransplantation. 19. Experience with an interhospital scheme of cadaver-kidney sharing and tissue typing. *JAMA* 207 (17 February): 1319–24.

Paton, A. 1971. Life and death: Moral and ethical aspects of transplantation. *Sem. Psychiat.* 3 (February): 161–68.

Penn, I.; Bunch, D.; Olenik, D.; and Abouna, G. 1971. Psychiatric experiences with patients receiving renal and hepatic transplants. *Sem. Psychiat.* 3 (February): 133–44.

Plastic heart works. 1969. *Los Angeles Herald Examiner,* 5 April, p. 1.

Porzio, R. 1969. *The transplant age: Reflections on the legal and moral aspects of organ transplants.* New York: Vantage Press.

Première greffe cardiaque réalisée en Belgique. 1973. *Le Soir,* 26–27 August, pp. 1, 4.

Protection of the individual as a research subject. 1969. U.S. Department of Health, Education, and Welfare. Public Health Service.

Quigley, J. 1969. Dr. Cooley sees drug changes in transplants. *Houston Post,* 26 January.

Quinn, J. 1969a. I'm qualified to judge what is right. *N. Y. Daily News,* 10 September, p. 2.

———. 1969b. The surgeons say artificial heart wasn't ready. *N. Y. Daily News,* 9 September, p. 38.

Rabinovitch, N. L. 1968. What is the HALAKHAH for organ transplantation? *Tradition* 9:20–27.

Ramsey, P. 1970. *The patient as a person.* New Haven: Yale University Press.

———. 1971. The ethics of a cottage industry in an age of community and research medicine. *New Eng. J. Med.* (1 April): 704–5.

Randal, J. 1969. Implant raises questions. *Washington (D.C.) Sunday Star,* 17 August, p. A–18.

Rapaport, F. T., and Dausset, J. 1968a. Typing human tissue. *Sci. J.* 4 (July): 51–55.

———, eds. 1968b. *Human transplantation.* New York: Grune and Stratton.

Recommendations for a kidney disease control program. 1968. Proceedings of the Massachusetts Kidney Disease Planning Project. Cosponsored by Tufts University School of Medicine, U.S. Public Health Service, and Massachusetts Department of Public Health, 23 May 1968.

Reed, J. D. 1970. Organ transplant. *New Yorker,* 26 September, p. 126.

Reflections on the new biology (preface). 1968. *UCLA Law Rev.* 15 (February).

Rennie, D. 1978. Home dialysis and the costs of uremia. *New Eng. J. Med.* 298 (16 February): 399–400.

Report of the Committee on Chronic Kidney Disease. 1967. Washington, D.C.: U.S. Government Printing Office.

Research in the service of man: Biomedical knowledge, development and use. 1967. A conference sponsored by the Subcommittee on Government and Research and the Frontiers of Science

Foundation of Oklahoma, 24–27 October 1966. Washington.
D.C.: U.S. Government Printing Office.

Rettig, R. A. 1976*a*. Valuing lives: The policy debate on patient care financing for victims of end-stage renal disease. *Rand Paper Series.*

_____. 1976*b*. Lessons learned from the end-stage renal disease experience. Background paper for conference on Health Care Technology and Quality of Care, Boston University Program on Public Policy for Quality Health Care.

Rider, A. K.; Copeland, J. G.; et al. 1975. The status of cardiac transplantation, 1975. *Circulation* 52:531-39.

Roberts, J. L. 1976. Analysis and outcome of 1063 patients trained for home dialysis. *Kidney Int.* 9:363-74.

Rosenfeld, A. 1968. Heart transplant: The search for an ethic. *Life,* 5 April, pp. 75-81.

_____. 1969. *The second genesis: The coming control of life.* Englewood Cliffs, N.J.: Prentice-Hall.

Rushmer, R. F., and Huntsman, L. L. 1970. Biomedical engineering. *Science* 167 (6 February): 840-44.

Rusk, H. A. 1968. Organ transplantation. *N.Y. Times,* 14 January.

Russell, P. S. 1969*a*. Heart transplantation: Problems and progress (editorial). *New Eng. J. Med.* 280 (15 May): 1123-24.

_____. 1969*b*. Horizons in clinical organ transplantation. *Transpl. Proc.* 1, pt. 2 (March): 659-65.

_____. 1970. Biological problems at the clinical level (review of Thomas E. Starzl, *Experience in hepatic transplantation).* *Science* 16 (23 January): 364.

_____. 1977. Steps toward immediate progress in clinical transplantation. *Transpl. Proc.* 9 (March): 1327-34.

Russell, P. S., and Winn, H. J. 1970. Transplantation. Pts. 1-3. *New Eng. J. Med.* 282 (2, 9, 16 April): 786-93, 848-54, 896-906.

Sadler, A. M., Jr., and Sadler, B. L. 1970. Transplantation and the law: Progress toward uniformity. *New Eng. J. Med.* 282 (26 March): 717-24.

Sadler, A. M., Jr.; Sadler, B. L., eds. 1969. *Organ transplantation—Current medical and medical-legal status: The problems of an opportunity.* Proceedings of a Maryland Academy of Sciences symposium, 24 May 1969. Washington, D.C.: U.S. Government Printing Office.

Sadler, A. M., Jr.; Sadler, B. L.; and Stason, E. B. 1968. The

Uniform Anatomical Gift Act: A model for reform. *JAMA* 206 (9 December): 2501-6.

Sadler, A. M., Jr.; Sadler, B. L.; Stason, E. B.; and Stickel, D. L. 1969. Transplantation: A case for consent. *New Eng. J. Med.* 280 (17 April): 862-67.

Sadler, H.; Davison, L.; Carroll, C.; and Kountz, S. L. 1971. The living, genetically unrelated, kidney donor. *Sem. Psychiat.* 3 (February): 86-101.

Sanders, D., and Dukeminier, J. 1968. Medical advance and legal lag: Hemodialysis and kidney transplantation: *UCLA Law Rev.* 15:357-413.

Sands, P.; Livingston, G.; and Wright, R. G. 1966. Psychological assessment of candidates for a hemodialysis program. *Ann. Intern. Med.* 64:602-10.

Sapperstein, M. 1971. Dialysis: A poem. *NAPH News* 2 (March):8.

Schmeck, H. M. 1969*a*. Dr. Cooley defends his use of artificial heart to save patient. *N. Y. Times,* 11 April.

_____. 1969*b*. Transplantation of organs and attitudes: The public's attitude toward clinical transplantation. *Transpl. Proc.* 1, pt. 2 (March): 670-74.

_____. 1970. Technology gains to facilitate use of artificial kidney. *N. Y. Times,* 10 November.

Schneider, D. M. 1968. *American kinship: A cultural account.* Englewood Cliffs, N.J.: Prentice-Hall.

Schreiner, G. E. 1966. Problems of ethics in relation to hemodialysis and transplantation. In *Ethics in medical progress,* ed. G. E. W. Wolstenholme and M. O'Connor, pp. 126-33. Boston: Little, Brown.

_____. 1967. Achievements and possibilities in artificial organs. In *Research in the service of man,* pp. 173-76. Washington, D.C.: U.S. Government Printing Office.

Schroeder, J. S. 1977. Guidelines for consideration of cardiac transplantation. Stanford University Medical Center (unpublished).

Schwartz, R. S. 1968. Immunosuppressive drug therapy. In *Human transplantation,* ed. F. Rapaport and J. Dausset, pp. 440-71. New York: Grune and Stratton.

Schwartz, S. H. 1970. Elicitation of moral obligation and self-sacrificing behavior: An experimental study of volunteering to be a bone marrow donor. *J. Personality Soc. Psychol.* 15:283-93.

Scribner, B. H. 1964. Ethical problems of using artificial organs to sustain life. *Trans. Amer. Soc. Artif. Intern. Organs* 10: 209–12.

————. 1967. The artificial kidney. In *Research in the service of man,* pp. 182–200. Washington, D.C.: U.S. Government Printing Office.

————. 1972. The problem of patient selection for treatment with an artificial kidney. Unpublished manuscript.

————. 1976. Statement prepared for a hearing of the U.S. Government Council on Wage and Price Stability. San Francisco, 11 August.

Scribner, B. H., and Blagg, C. R. 1968. Maintenance dialysis. In *Human transplantation,* ed. F. Rapaport and J. Dausset, pp. 80–99. New York: Grune and Stratton.

Scribner, B. H.; Buri, R.; Caner, J. E. Z.; Hegstrom, R.; and Burnell, J. M. 1960. The treatment of chronic uremia by means of intermittent hemodialysis: A preliminary report. *Trans. Amer. Soc. Artif. Intern. Organs* 6:144.

Seventh report of the Human Kidney Transplant Registry. 1969. *Transplantation* 8: 721–38.

Shambaugh, P. W. 1969. Spouses under stress: Group meetings with spouses of patients on hemodialysis. *Amer. J. Psychiat.* 125–27 (January): 928–36.

Shambaugh, P. W.; Hampers, C. L.; Bailey, G. L.; Synder, D.; and Merrill, J. 1967. Hemodialysis in the home: Emotional impact on the spouse. *Trans. Amer. Soc. Artif. Intern. Organs* 13:41–45.

Shapiro, F. L. 1970. Comprehensive regional approach to the chronic renal failure problem. *Perspect. Biol. Med.* (summer): 597–617.

Shapiro, F. L.; Leonard, A.; and Comty, C. M. 1974. Mortality, morbidity and rehabilitation results in regularly dialyzed patients with diabetes mellitus. *Kidney Int.* 6 (suppl. 1): S-8–S-14.

Shapiro, H. A., ed. 1969. *Experience with human heart transplantation.* Proceedings of the Cape Town Heart Transplantation Symposium, 1968. New York: Appleton-Century-Crofts.

Sherman, M. n.d. Artificial organs: Kidney, lung, heart. A review of research grants supported by the National Heart Institute, 1949–64. Department of Health, Education, and Welfare, Public Health Service.

Shorr, E. 1955. Emergence of psychological problems in patients requiring prolonged hospitalization. In *Medical and psycho-*

logical teamwork in the care of the chronically ill, ed. Molly Harrower, pp. 32–38. Springfield, Ill.: Charles C. Thomas.

Shumway, N. E. 1969. Transplanta.ion of an unpaired organ, the heart. *Proc. Nat. Acad. Sci. U.S.A.* 63 (August): 1032–33.

Shumway, N. E.; Angell, W. W.; and Wuerflein, R. D. 1968. Heart replacement: The cardiac chimera vs. mechanical man. *Journal-Lancet* 88 (July): 172.

Shumway, N. E.; Dong, E.; and Stinson, E. B. 1969. Surgical aspects of cardiac transplantation in man. *Bull N.Y. Acad. Med.* 45 (May): 387–93.

Shumway, N. E.; Stinson, E. B.; and Dong, E., Jr. 1969. Cardiac homotransplantation in man. *Transpl. Proc.* 1 (March): 739–45.

Simmons, R. G.; Fulton, J.; and Fulton, R. 1970. The prospective organ transplant donor: Problems and prospects of medical innovation. Read at the Second International Conference on Social Science and Medicine, Aberdeen Scotland, 7–11 September 1970.

Simmons, R. G.; Hickey, K.; Kjellstrand, C. M.; and Simmons, R. L. 1971. Donors and non-donors: The role of the family and the physician in kidney transplantation. *Sem. Psychiat.* 3 (February): 102–14.

Simmons, R. G.; Hickey, K.; Kjellstrand, C. M.; and Simmons, R. L. 1971. Family tension in the search for a kidney donor. *JAMA* 215 (8 February): 909–12.

Simmons, R. G.; Klein, S.; and Thornton, T. 1972. Family decision-making and the selection of a kidney transplant donor. Paper read at the American Sociological Association Meetings, New Orleans, La., August 1972.

Simmons, R. G., and Simmons, R. L. 1971. Organ transplantation: A societal problem. *Soc. Prob.* 19:36–57.

Simmons, R. L., and Najarian, J. 1970. Reply to Starzl. *New Eng. J. Med.* 283 (22 October): 934–35.

Simmons, R. L.; Kelly, W. D.; Tallent, M. B.; and Najarian, J. S. 1970. Cure of dysgerminoma with widespread metastases appearing after renal transplantation. *New Eng. J. Med.* 283 (23 July): 190–91.

Smith, H. W. 1953. The kidney. *Sci. Amer.* 188 (January): 40–48.

Smithy, H. G.; Boone, J.; and Stallworth, J. 1950. Surgical treatment of constrictive valvular disease of the heart. *Surg. Gynec. Obstet.* 90:175–92.

Snyder, B. 1968. Where heart transplants were pioneered in Canada. *Montreal,* October, pp. 4–6.

Specialists say eye transplant is doomed. 1969. *Houston Chronicle,* 26 April.

Stanford heart transplant team plans few changes in program. 1969. *JAMA* 209 (22 September): 1825.

Stange, P. V., and Sumner, A. T. 1978. Predicting treatment costs and life expectancy for end-stage renal disease. *New Eng. J. Med.* 298 (16 February): 372–78.

Starzl, T. E. 1964. *Experience in renal transplantation.* Philadelphia, Pa.: W. B. Saunders Co.

————. 1969. *Experience in hepatic transplantation.* Philadelphia, Pa.: W. B. Saunders Co.

Starzl, T. E.; Brettschneider, L.; Martin, A. J.; Groth, C. G.; Blanchard, H.; Smith, G.; Penn, I. 1968. Organ transplantation, past and present, *Surg. Clin. N. Amer.* 48 (August): 817–38.

Starzl, T. E.; Brettschneider, L.; Penn, I.; Bell, P.; Groth, C. G.; Blanchard, H.; Hashiwari, N.; and Putnam, C. W. 1969. Orthotopic liver transplantation in man. *Transpl. Proc.* 1, pt. 1 (March): 216–22.

Starzl, T. E.; Brettschneider, L.; and Putnam, C. W. 1969. Transplantation of the liver. In *Progress in liver diseases,* ed. Hans Popper and Fenton Schaffner, vol. 3, chap. 30. New York: Grune and Stratton.

Starzl, T. E.; Brettschneider, L.; et al. 1969. A trial with heterologous antilymphocyte globulin in man. *Transpl. Proc.* 1, pt. 2 (March): 448–54.

Starzl, T. E., and Marchioro, T. 1965. The past and future of organ transplantation. *Radiology* 85 (August): 369–72.

Starzl, T. E.; Marchioro, T.; and Faris, T. 1966. Liver transplantation (editorial). *Ann. Int. Med.* 64:473–77.

Starzl, T. E.; Penn, I.; and Halgrimson, C. G. 1970. Immunosuppression and malignant neoplasms (letter to the editor). *New Eng. J. Med.* 282 (22 October): 934.

Starzl, T. E.; Putnam, C. W.; et al. 1976. Orthotopic liver transplantation in ninety-three patients. *Surg. Gyn. Obst.* 142 (April): 487–505.

Starzl, T. E.; Weil, R.; and Putnam, C. W. 1977. Modern trends in kidney transplantation. *Transpl. Proc.* 9 (March): 1–8.

Starzl, T. E., et al. 1970. Long term survival after renal transplantation in humans. *Ann. Surg.* 172 (September): 437–72.

Status of transplantation. 1968. A report by the Surgery Training Committee of the National Institute of General Medical Sciences,

National Institutes of Health, U.S. Dept. of Health, Education, and Welfare.

Stinson, E. B.; Dong, E., Jr.; Bieber, C. P.; Schroeder, J. S.; and Shumway, N. E. 1969. Cardiac transplantation in man. 1. Early rejection. *JAMA* 207 (24 March): 2233–42.

Stinson, E. B.; Dong, E., Jr.; Iben, A. B.; and Shumway, N. E. 1969. Cardiac transplantation in man. 3. Surgical aspects. *Amer. J. Surg.* 118 (August): 182–87.

Stinson, E. B.; Dong, E., Jr.; Schroeder, J. S.; Harrison, D. C.; and Shumway, N. E. 1968. Initial clinical experience with heart transplantation. *Amer. J. Cardiol.* 22 (December): 791–803.

Stinson, E. B.; Dong, N., Jr.; Schroeder, J. S.; and Shumway, N. E. 1969. Cardiac transplantation in man. 4. Early results. *Ann. Surg.* 170 (October): 588.

Stinson, E. B.; Dong, E., Jr.; and Shumway, N. E. 1969. Experimental and clinical cardiac transplantation. *Postgrad. Med.* 46 (September): 199–203.

Stinson, E. B.; Griepp, R. B.; Clark, D. A.; Dong, E., Jr.; and Shumway, N. E. 1970. Cardiac transplantation in man. 8. Survival and function. *J. Thorac. Cardiovasc. Surg.* 60 (September): 303–21.

Stinson, E. B.; Schroeder, J. S.; et al. 1969. Experience with cardiac transplantation in fourteen patients. Paper presented at the Second World Symposium on Heart Transplantation, Montreal, Canada, 6–8 June 1969.

Storb, R.; Weiden, P. L.; et al. 1977. Aplastic anemia (AA) treated by allogenic marrow transplantation: The Seattle experience. *Transpl. Proc.* 9 (March): 181–85.

Sullivan, D. 1970. Science versus therapy: The effect of scientific competition on ethical standards and practices. Prepared by the Research Group on Human Experimentation, Barnard College, for the American Sociological Association sessions, Chicago. December 1970 (mimeographed).

Surgeon denies total eye transplant. 1969. *N. Y. Times,* 27 April.

Surgical operation for mitral stenosis. 1902. *Lancet* (15 February), pp. 461–62.

Swazey, J. P., and Fox, R. C. 1970. The clinical moratorium: A case study of mitral valve surgery. In *Experimentation with human subjects,* ed. Paul A. Freund, pp. 315–57. New York: George Braziller.

Symposium on organ transplantation in man. 1969. *Proc. Nat. Acad. Sci. U.S.A.* 63 (August): 1017–38.

Taussig, H. B. 1969. Heart transplantation (letter to the editor). *JAMA* 207 (3 February): 951.

Teacher marks 5 years with a new heart. 1973. *Int. Herald-Tribune,* 27 August.

Technique stops graft rejection without impairing immunity. 1968. *JAMA* 206 (7 October): 245.

Tenckhoff, H., and Boen, S. T. 1965. Long-term peritoneal dialysis in the home: The first one and one half years. Excerpta Medica International Congress series no. 103, pp. 104–8.

Tendler, M. D. 1968. Medical ethics and Torah morality. *Tradition* 9:5–13.

Terasaki, P. I,; Mickey, M. R.; Singal, D. P.; Mittal, K. K.; and Patel, R. 1968. Serotyping for homotransplantation. 20. Selection of recipients for cadaver donor transplants. *New Eng. J. Med.* 279 (14 November): 1101–3.

Tertiary hyperparathyroidism after renal transplantation. 1969. *JAMA* 209 (29 September): 2048.

Texas plea made for heart donor. 1969. *N. Y. Times,* 6 April.

The Texas tornado. 1965. *Time,* 28 May, pp. 46–55.

Thirteenth report of the Human Renal Transplant Registry. 1977. *Transpl. Proc.* 9 (March): 9–26.

Thomas, E. E.; Ranier, M. D.; et al. 1975. Bone-marrow transplantation. Pts. I, II. *New Eng. J. Med. 292:*832–43; 895–901.

Thompson, T. 1970. The Texas tornado vs. Dr. Wonderful. *Life,* 10 April.

———. 1971a. *Hearts.* New York: McCall Publishing Co.

———. 1971b. The year they changed hearts. *Life,* 17 September, pp. 58f.

Thorwald, J. 1971. *The patients.* New York: Harcourt Brace Jovanovich.

Titmuss, R. M. 1971. *The gift relationship: From human blood to social policy.* New York: Pantheon Books.

Total artificial heart is implanted in man. 1969. *Washington D.C. Evening Star,* 5 April, p. 1.

Transplantation immunology. 1968. *Nature* 219 (24 August): 833–35.

Transplantation is only half an answer. 1969. *JAMA* 208 (16 June): 2004.

Transplants: Guarded outlook. 1969. *Newsweek,* 21 July, pp. 109–10.

UCLA bone marrow transplantation group. 1977. Bone marrow transplantation with intensive combination chemotherapy/radiation therapy (SCARI) in acute leukemia. *Ann. Int. Med.* 86: 155–61.

United Nations Economic and Social Council. 1970. *Human rights and scientific and technological developments. II. Protection of the human personality and its physical and intellectual integrity in the light of advances in biology, medicine and biochemistry.* Commission on Human Rights, 26th session, 19 March 1970.

Van Bekkum, D. W. 1977. Bone marrow transplantation. *Transpl. Proc.* 9 (March): 147–56.

Vaux, K. 1969. A year of heart transplants: An ethical valuation. *Postgrad. Med.* 46 (January): 201–5.

_____. ed. 1970. *Who shall live? Medicine, technology, values.* Philadelphia, Pa.: Fortress Press.

Veith, F. J. 1970. Lung transplantation 1970 (editorial). *Ann. Thorac. Surg.* 9 (June): 580–83.

Versieck, J.; Barbier, F.; and Derom, F. 1971. A case of lung transplant: Clinical note. *Sem. Psychiat.* 3 (February): 159–60.

Walsh, A. 1969. Some practical problems in kidney transplantation. *Transpl. Proc.* 1, pt. 1 (March): 178–83.

Wardener, H. E. de. 1966. Some ethical and economic problems associated with intermittent hemodialysis. In *Ethics in medical progress,* ed. G. E. W. Wolstenholme and M. O'Connor, pp. 104–25. Boston: Little, Brown.

Wildevuur, C. R. H., and Benfield, J. R. 1970. A review of 23 human lung transplantations by 20 surgeons. *Ann. Thorac. Surg.* 9 (June): 484–515.

Williams, G. M.; Lee, H. M.; and Hume, D. M. 1970. Renal transplants with children. *Transpl. Proc.* 1, pt. 1 (March): 262–66.

Williams, H. 1971. The first artificial kidney patient. *Seattle Times Magazine,* 11 July, pp. 8–9.

Wolstenholme, G. E. W., and O'Connor, M., eds. 1966. *Ethics in medical progress.* Boston: Little, Brown.

Woodward, K. L. 1971. Death in America. *U.S. Catholic News and Jubilee* (January), pp. 6–18.

Wright, R. G.; Sand, P., and Livingston, G. 1966. Psychological stress during hemodialysis for chronic renal failure. *Ann. Intern. Med.* 64 (March): 611–21.

Young, C. 1969. *The Todd dossier: A disquieting novel about a change of heart.* New York: Delacorte Press.

Index